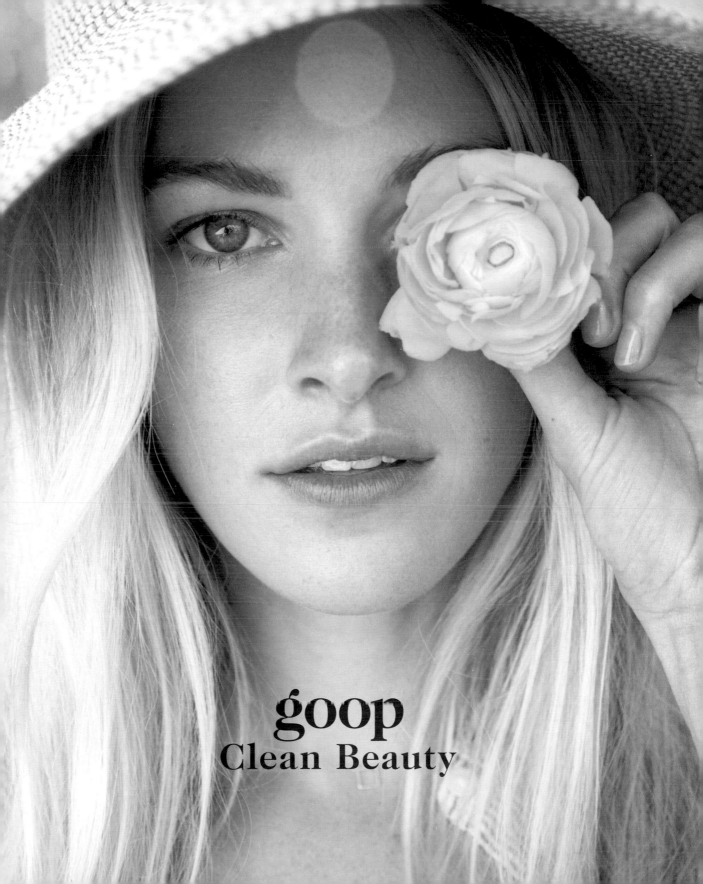

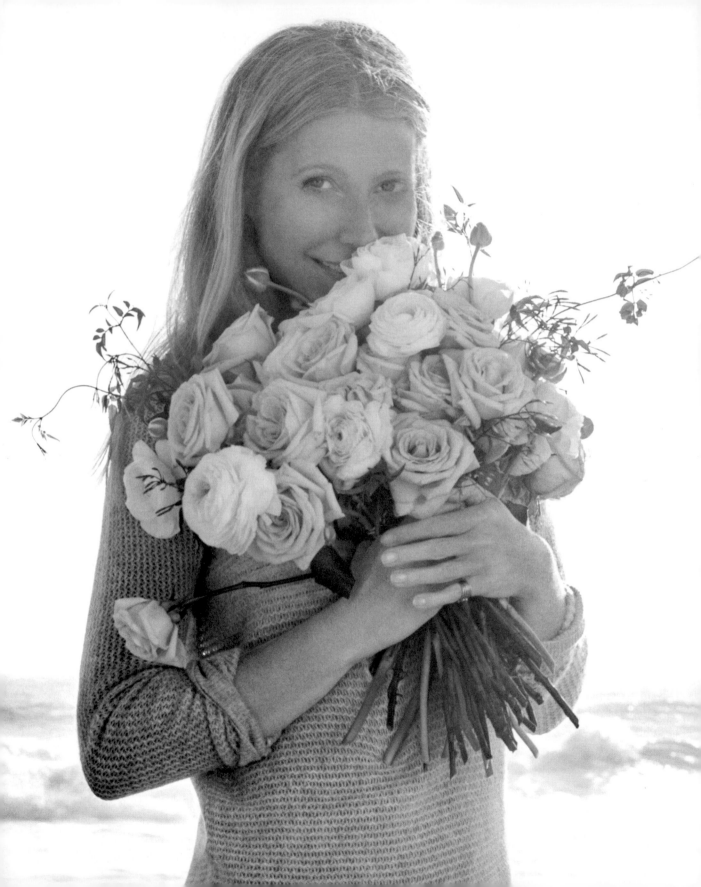

goop
Clean Beauty

THE EDITORS OF **goop**

FOREWORD BY

Gwyneth Paltrow

**goop
press**

GRAND CENTRAL
Life&Style
NEW YORK · BOSTON

Copyright © 2016 by Goop, Inc.
Photographs by Brigitte Sire
Photograph on page xiv by Cydney Puro
Book and jacket design by Shubhani Sarkar, sarkardesignstudio.com
Cover copyright © 2016 by Hachette Book Group, Inc.

Grand Central Life & Style
Hachette Book Group
1290 Avenue of the Americas, New York, NY 10104

www.GrandCentralLifeandStyle.com

First Edition: December 2016

Grand Central Life & Style is an imprint of Grand Central Publishing. The Grand Central Life & Style name and logo are trademarks of Hachette Book Group, Inc.

The publisher is not responsible for websites (or their content) that are not owned by the publisher.

The Hachette Speakers Bureau provides a wide range of authors for speaking events. To find out more, go to www.hachettespeakersbureau.com or call (866) 376-6591.

Library of Congress Cataloging-in-Publication Data

Names: Goop, Inc.
Title: Goop clean beauty / The editors of Goop ; foreword by Gwyneth Paltrow.
Description: First edition. | New York : Grand Central Life & Style, 2016.
Identifiers: LCCN 2016024113| ISBN 9781455541553 (hardback) | ISBN 9781455541560 (ebook)
Subjects: LCSH: Beauty, Personal—Popular works. | Women—Health and hygiene—Popular works. | Detoxification (Health)—Popular works. | BISAC: HEALTH & FITNESS / Beauty & Grooming. | HEALTH & FITNESS / Women's Health.
Classification: LCC RA776.98 .G66 2016 | DDC 646.7/2—dc23 LC record available at https://lccn.loc.gov/2016024113

Printed in the United States of America

Q-MA

10 9 8 7 6 5 4 3 2 1

To the GOOP readers, who have allowed us to
keep the lighthouse going all these years,
and whose insatiable curiosity and desire to make
every choice count have helped us build a brand.

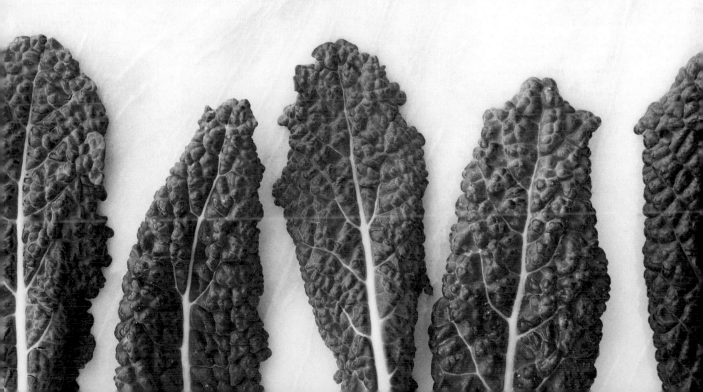

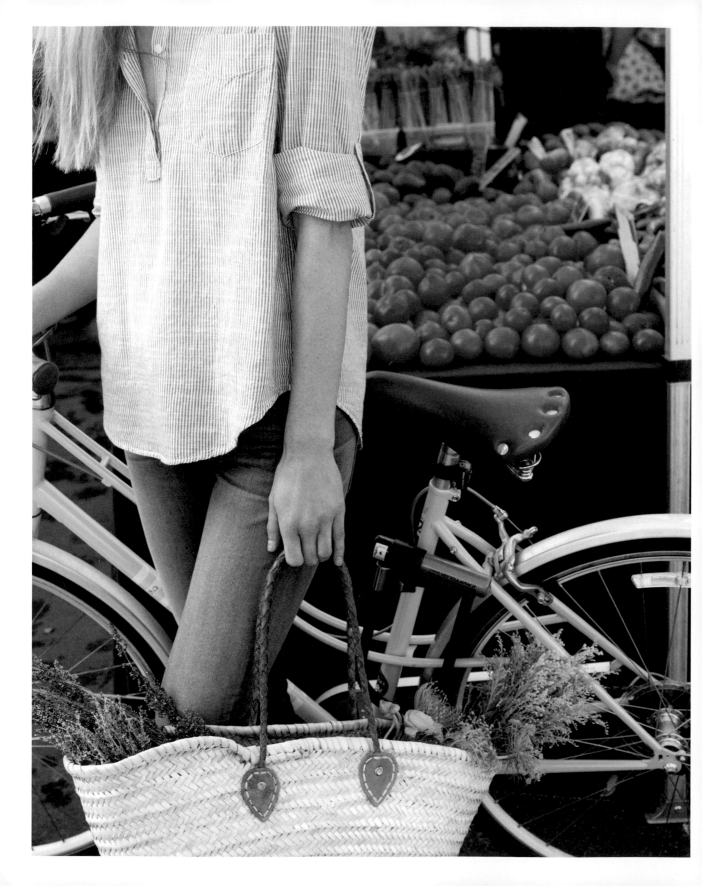

Contents

Foreword by Gwyneth Paltrow   ix

PART 1
Beauty from the Inside Out

1. A Detox Life   3
2. Next-Level Detoxing   65
3. Beauty Superfoods vs. Sapping Foods   89
4. The Impact of the Environment   117
5. Sleeping Soundly   133

PART 2
Your Clean Beauty Routine

6. What's in a Product   153
7. Ultimate Hair Health   171
8. Your Skin As You Age   183
9. Breakout-Prone Skin   201
10. Dry and Sensitive Skin   219
11. Easy Makeup—Made Easier   233
12. Effortless Hair   243

Last Gloss   259
Acknowledgments   261
Index   263

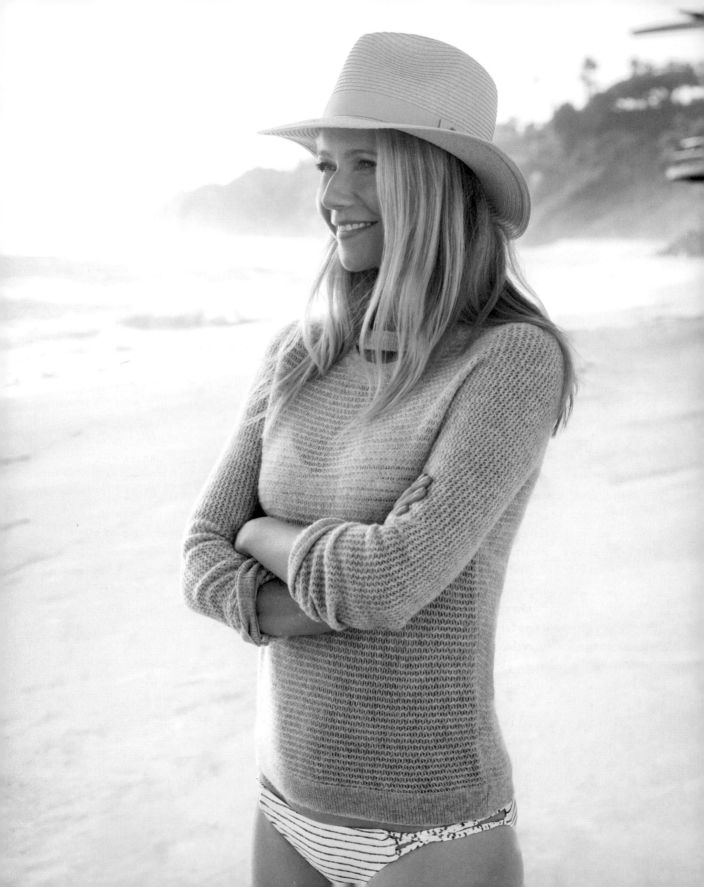

Foreword

BY Gwyneth Paltrow

The whole concept of beauty is complicated. It's kind of like love—you know it when you see it—but that only really holds when it's in the flesh, unbiased by Photoshop, Instagram filters, Glam Squads, and really great lighting and photography.

As someone who has been in the public eye for many decades, having even been heralded by *People* magazine as the world's most beautiful person (I mean, *what?*), I can tell you firsthand that the concept of beauty in popular culture is all fantasy. It can be a fun one, but the reality is a bit like pulling back the curtain in Oz, under-eye circles, freckles, and all. And I find myself preferring the reality: There's me, Gwyneth, in my everyday life—and then there's Gwyneth Paltrow with the super-slick blow-out and fake lashes. I generally feel much more comfortable as the former and can be found wiping off my makeup in the car on the way home after parties and awards shows have wrapped.

This is not to say that I'm not interested in beauty: While I may not have had a Kaboodle kitted out with every shade of Bonne Bell as a child, or been a masterful nail artist in high school, or be

capable of making myself look even halfway done before a dinner out with friends (people are always surprised that after decades of sitting in the hair and makeup chair, I still don't know how to use bronzer), I am devoted to the concept, particularly under the lens of self-preservation and aging. Call it vanity, call it health, but I know that there's a huge correlation between how I feel internally and what I look like when I roll out of bed in the morning (preferably after 8 hours of sleep). And my goal, in general, is to look and feel as good as possible.

That's really the thesis of this book. Those of you who have spent time on GOOP, the lifestyle site I founded in 2008, or dabbled in any of my three cookbooks, particularly *It's All Good*, will recognize the underlying philosophy in the following pages: There's a little bit about foundation and concealer in the final section, along with a tutorial for a basic smoky eye (which I, evidently, need to study), but a majority of the pages explores the lifestyle we try to abide by at GOOP, which is predicated on eating clean, getting good sleep, and making sure that everything else—adrenals,

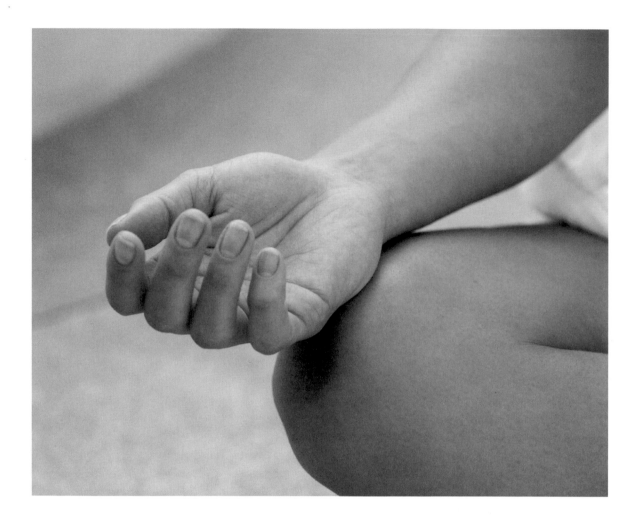

hormones, micronutrients, hydration, mood—is in balance. It's an entire system: beauty from the inside out.

I saw this for myself the first time I launched into a whole-foods, organic, sugar-free diet (and then some). My father had recently been diagnosed with throat cancer, and I became obsessed with the idea that diet could heal the body, particularly by eliminating the things that could make us unwell (pesticides, processed foods, growth hormones). What I learned during this time always

stuck with me, and when I became a mom, the idea of eliminating as many toxins as possible from my kid's world became all the more important.

Still, while I've long-aimed to be healthy, there have been periods of time when I have decidedly not been (I'm a fan of french fries and martinis, for starters, and like all moms, I don't always get enough sleep). Those periods of time always seem to have a way of catching up with me, physically and mentally. The day I swear off red wine and gluten for life isn't coming (ever), but I've settled into a way of mostly clean living that lets me indulge and stay balanced while feeling really good. And when I inevitably get too far off track, I'm diligent about going back to this way of eating and living until I feel pretty brand-new again. Sometimes it takes only a week.

This way of eating, exercising, detoxing, sleeping, dealing with stress, and interacting with the environment is outlined in the rest of this book, and is informed by all the experts featured within it. We are eternally curious about health and wellness, but by no means experts ourselves, which is why we've built a roster of incredible mentors to ask. You'll meet many of those people here. You'll also find a pretty comprehensive survey of all things GOOP, from detox hacks to our chosen workout sessions, staff favorite recipes, vitamins and minerals that make hair shine, sauna practices, nighttime skin routines, and some simple hairstyles and makeup looks modeled by some of GOOP's finest. Because what's the point in doing all the research and trying things out if you're not going to share what you've learned with your friends?

There's another important message about beauty in this book, which I'd love you to share as well. It revolves around the standards of the completely unregulated personal care industry. Throughout the world, you'll find rigorous testing and regulation—for example, the European Union bans about 1,300 ingredients from personal care products, while in the United States, there are only eleven ingredients on the list (the last federal regulation passed in 1938). It is completely legal to use known carcinogens and endocrine disruptors in the products we use every day—the latter are most potent in teeny tiny doses because they mimic the way our hormones naturally behave. So many of us eat well, exercise, and then unknowingly slather ourselves with hundreds of toxins before we even leave the house in the morning. At GOOP, we find it ironic that many of the U.S.'s biggest beauty companies use ingredients that are known to be harmful and then set up foundations and charities to support breast, cervical, and ovarian cancer research.

To do our part, we fill the shelves in the GOOP Clean Beauty Shop only with products from companies that are doing better by all of us. And last year we launched our very first product line GOOP by Juice Beauty, a collection of nontoxic skincare that delivers clinically proven, age-defying results that mirror exactly what you would find from the big guys with huge research and development budgets and no ingredient restrictions. Instead of plastics, which you would be surprised to learn are found in so many expensive face creams, our collection is loaded with organic, naturally occurring ingredients that are actually good for you. It's a skincare line that's safe enough for our daughters and powerful enough for those of us who have maybe spent too much time in the sun. (Speaking of sun, there's a lot about both vitamin D and clean sunblock in this book, too.) We will walk you through the steps of ensuring that your own home is free of as many of these toxins as possible.

I hope this book serves as an ongoing resource for you—the goal was to create something that you could return to again and again, whether for a detox-friendly recipe or for some tips on combatting jet lag and looking pretty great on the other end of a long-haul flight. It really is a guide to looking and feeling beautiful. I would like it to be a book you can come back to on any day when, for whatever reason, you don't feel that way.

Love,

gp

goop
Clean Beauty

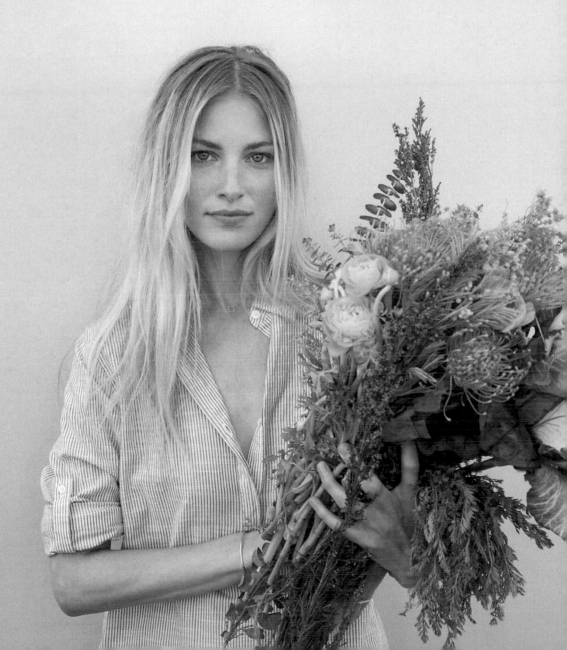

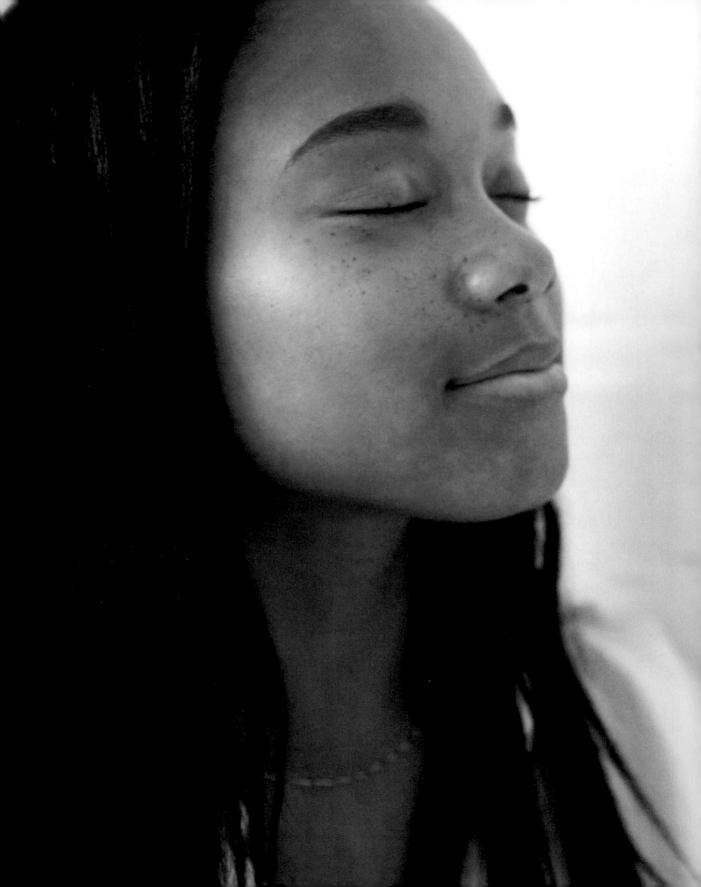

PART 1

Beauty from the Inside Out

Our moms were right: Beauty really does begin on the inside—and perhaps more specifically, in the gut—after all, haven't you met those people who glow from within? And so it goes without saying that feeling and looking beautiful don't begin with perfectly turned-out hair or makeup—it ends there, as does this book.

At GOOP, we subscribe to a more foundational approach to beauty that's deeply tethered to diet and health. Layered on top of that is really our relationship to the world, and how we all navigate stress, environmental factors, rest, and repair. Then comes the fun stuff, like the right shade of lip sheer and the most flattering haircut. But before we can get to that, let's begin with the gut, and the quality of the food that we're putting into it.

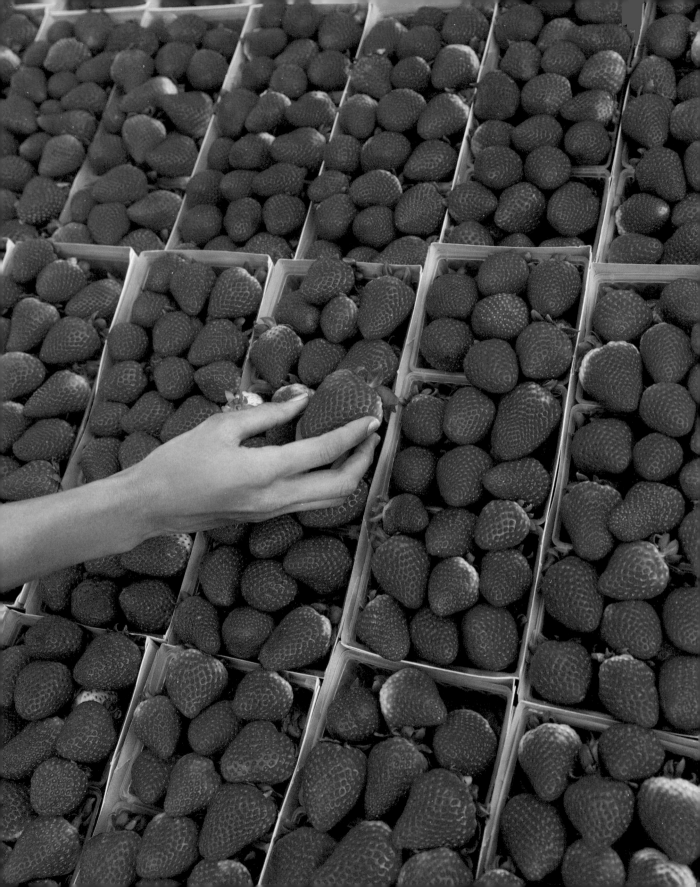

1.
A Detox Life

This Is Not a Fad

Let's get real for a moment. Whether you're contemplating a physical, emotional, or spiritual change in your life, there is no such thing as a quick fix. In the health and wellness world, those words are repeated *again and again,* yet we all find ourselves chasing fad diets, exercise trends, and miracle products in the hopes of cutting out the work and jettisoning ourselves to an overnight fix. Lasting transformations take work. That doesn't mean that everything we'll outline is hard; it just requires commitment—a little time, energy, careful thought, and practice. While there is more than one way to achieve health, happiness, and beauty, there is no getting around the fact that no magical shortcuts exist—but the effort, in our experience, is well worth it for lasting wellness that you can both see and feel. In the following pages, we'll be highlighting the methods that have borne the most fruit for us, in part because they're grounded in real food and real science. Besides general feelings of wellness, your hair, your skin, and your immune system will likely flourish, too.

Beauty Detox

Beauty may start on the inside, but the picture is more complicated than "you are what you eat." While there are ways in which our bodies function very much like machines, what goes in is not always what comes out, and our health can become quite dependent on how efficiently we can support and supplement the body's natural detox process. Sounds exhausting, but your body is detoxing all the time—that said, it's possible to significantly ease the load by eating the right foods and limiting exposure to toxins where possible.

The body has an extraordinary and innate capacity to detox. It's what a number of our organs, such as the liver and kidneys, do naturally—they get rid of the impurities in our system. And in a perfect world—or, one that more accurately represents the conditions in which humans evolved—we would just let these organs do their thing. Today, however, as you are likely already well aware, we are faced with an unprecedented number and volume of harmful chemicals that make it impossible for our bodies to keep up without

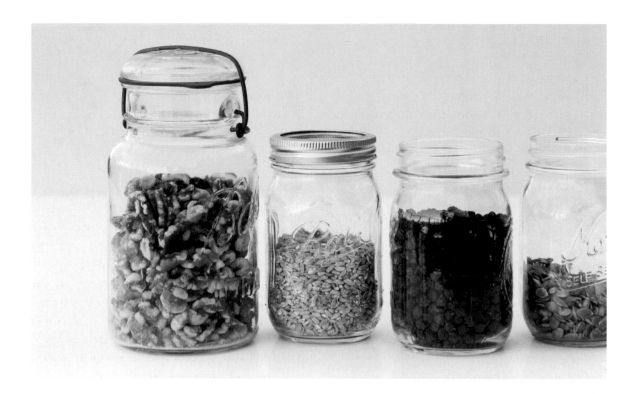

some help. Our detox organs suffer from overload, leaving the toxins circulating in our system (and, thanks to an obesity problem in this country, clinging to our fat). This nonstop work also means our organs have no downtime to repair themselves. There are chemicals in food, makeup, plastic water bottles, hand soaps, laundry detergent, nonstick pans—even the mattresses we sleep on. These toxins have been linked to nearly every health issue imaginable, and they steal our glow one way or another—whether through inflamed skin or indigestion. Often without knowing it, we are ingesting, breathing, and absorbing these toxins through our skin (our largest organ) every day—at home, in the office, sitting in our cars, eating out.

As much as we are all for reducing our exposure to the big ones when we can (more on that throughout this book), toxins are too omnipresent to avoid completely. (In fact, babies are born with more than 200 toxic chemicals in their umbilical cords—see more on page 153—so in a sense, one of the purest things around is born pre-polluted.) While there are plenty of people who believe that "detoxing" is a silly fad, there's no doubt that giving your body a little bit of a helping hand can make a real difference. And the best way, of course, is to try to minimize the amount of detoxing it needs to do in the first place. Think of it as the ultimate efficiency play: The less energy we have to spend on getting rid of toxins that are bad for our insides (i.e., fatal to our organs) and our outsides (i.e., causing allergic skin reactions, drying out the scalp, and so on)—the better. It's really the secret to a palpable glow.

Clean Eating

As painful as it may be to put aside the french fries, anyone who has ventured into clean eating—even if for only a week—would probably agree that mental clarity and an uptick in energy are really nice side effects. When your body has to spend less time breaking down processed foods, it can spend more time on stuff that advances the eight ball, so to speak. And those are generally the upsides that reveal themselves every time you look in the mirror. There are no makeup tricks or hairstyle hacks that can truly give the same results as eating the right things.

We're going to explore some of the creative ways that you can reduce your toxic load, and boost your body's own ability to detox. And we're also going to break down gut health, which goes hand in hand with your detox lifestyle. Eating within a detox lifestyle is eating "healthy" and avoiding foods that contain known toxins, but the true picture is more nuanced than that. There are foods that tend to cause inflammation in the body, food allergies, and sensitivities, ranging from dairy and gluten to shellfish and nightshades (a family of plants that includes tomato, eggplant, and potato). While many detoxes revolve around week-long juice cleanses (which, incidentally, have a ton of sugar), we're bigger fans of eating mostly clean (emphasis on eating, not "eating" liquids) or in a "detox" way all the time—or at least for as many meals as you can throughout the week. We do end up making plenty of exceptions, but in our books, it's kind of a tradition to kick off the New Year with a 10-day detox (or occasionally longer) of completely clean eating—no exceptions—that really gives the gut a chance to take a break and repair itself. (If you want a detox in kit form,

Dr. Alejandro Junger's 21-Day Clean Program—cleanprogram.com—is pretty incredible.)

The rules of clean eating are relatively simple (if not a little painful, particularly for those who rely on a latte to kick-start the day, and a glass of rosé to wind it down), but if you can follow them for your own 10-day detox, we promise that not only will you feel amazing by the end, but you'll look pretty amazing, too. And keep in mind that if you have concerns that you might have food allergies, there's really no better way to test the thesis than to clean out your system and then reintroduce the potentially problematic foods (generally gluten and dairy) to see if they actually affect you. As our good friend and go-to expert on many matters of health, Dr. Junger explains: "After a cleanse, you're working with a white wall and it's easy to see the paint—when your system is chronically inflamed, it's hard to tell what's making the marks."

But if you're ready to look and feel better, here are the rules:

1. No alcohol.
2. No caffeine.
3. No dairy.
4. No eggs.
5. No beef, no pork.
6. No shellfish, no raw fish.
7. No gluten.
8. No soy.
9. No nightshades (potatoes, tomatoes, eggplant, peppers).
10. No strawberries, oranges, grapefruits, grapes, bananas.
11. No corn.
12. No white rice.
13. No added sugar.
14. No peanuts, though other nuts are fine.

15. No processed oils and butters (margarine, spreads, and the like), and no vegetable seed oils like canola and corn. Stick to cold-pressed olive oil and coconut, sesame, almond/walnut, and pumpkin seed oils.

Don't panic! This actually leaves a lot of delicious foods! Think brown rice, most animal proteins, most vegetables, most fruits, beans and legumes. And if you've done a full detox before and you know that foods like strawberries and eggs are not problematic for you, they can stay in your personalized rotation.

Don't think we're leaving you alone to fend for yourself, either. We wouldn't take away your wine and cheese without offering some help! Thea Baumann, our food editor, has put together a menu of twenty-four simple, ridiculously delicious recipes, which you can easily stretch into a thirty-day GOOP Clean Beauty detox. (You can improvise, too: Basic salads, rice bowls, and simply prepared chicken and fish always make the cut.)

If a 30-day detox sounds overwhelming, use the recipes that follow to start with a 10-day burst. We've found this is a manageable amount of time to stick strictly to the rules preceding, planning around celebratory events on the calendar (be it a big birthday or dinner out with friends). We've also found this to be a satisfactory amount of time to reset our systems after we've been hitting the bottle for too long and we're feeling run-down, with puffier skin and darker circles to match. You'll want to amplify your better eating habits by drinking lots of water and getting some exercise, which points to another huge benefit of detoxing with food: You'll have the energy to actually move.

Regardless of how long you stretch your detox, though, and whether you make it a seasonal or annual ritual, the hope is that you'll add these recipes to your arsenal and turn to them even when you're not eating full-on clean. While the results won't be as marked, pivoting your weekly routine to be even a bit less processed can net some good results. Everyone has to start somewhere!

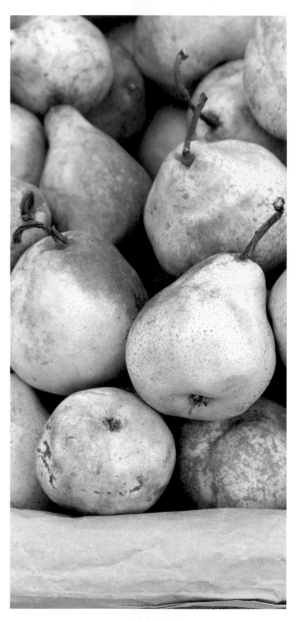

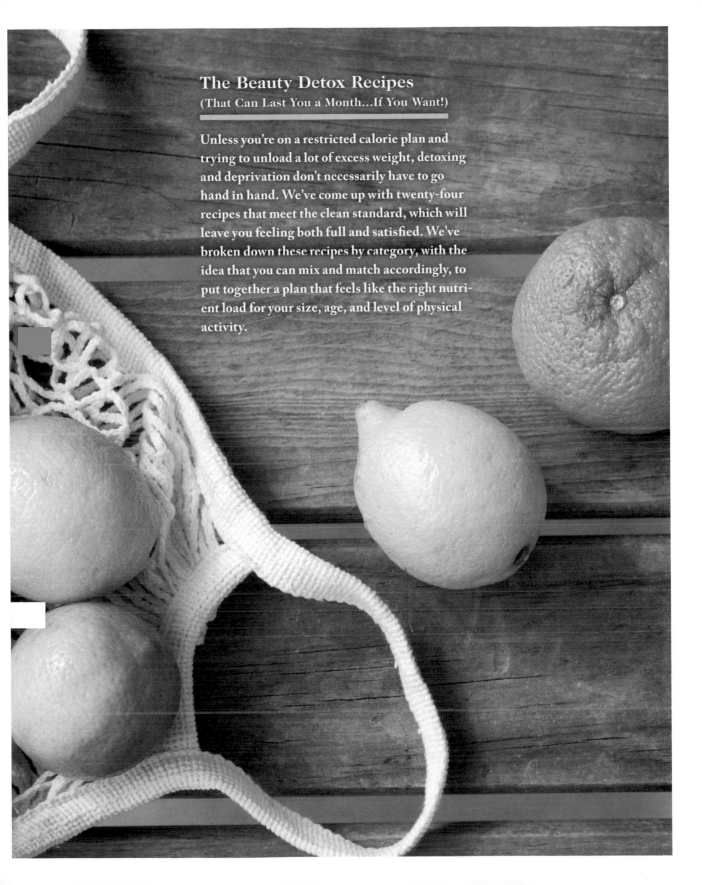

The Beauty Detox Recipes
(That Can Last You a Month...If You Want!)

Unless you're on a restricted calorie plan and trying to unload a lot of excess weight, detoxing and deprivation don't necessarily have to go hand in hand. We've come up with twenty-four recipes that meet the clean standard, which will leave you feeling both full and satisfied. We've broken down these recipes by category, with the idea that you can mix and match accordingly, to put together a plan that feels like the right nutrient load for your size, age, and level of physical activity.

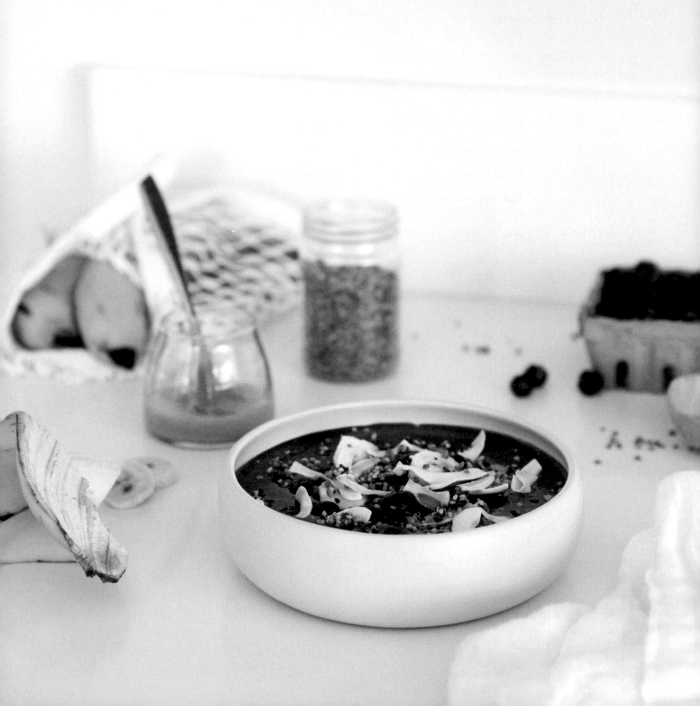

GOOD MORNINGS

Chocolate Milkshake Smoothie

This tastes like a chocolate milkshake but is detox-friendly and actually good for you. It's perfect to drink in the morning after a workout or as a sweet treat after a light dinner. Include the ice if you like your smoothie cold.

SERVES 1

1 cup almond milk

⅛ large avocado, about ¼ cup

2 pitted dates

1 tablespoon almond butter

2 teaspoons cacao powder

Pinch sea salt

2 to 4 ice cubes, optional

Combine all ingredients in a powerful blender and blitz until smooth.

Breakfast Porridge with Cinnamon and Blueberries

This warming porridge, made creamy with almond and coconut milks, is packed with calcium, protein, and fiber thanks to oats and teff flour (a traditional Ethiopian grain that can be found at most health food stores). We love the combo of antioxidant-rich blueberries and ground cinnamon, but feel free to play around with other clean toppings.

SERVES 2

½ cup almond milk

½ cup coconut milk

Pinch kosher salt

⅔ cup gluten-free oats

¼ cup whole-grain teff

2 tablespoons coconut oil

Fresh blueberries

Ground cinnamon

1. Combine 1 cup water, the almond milk, coconut milk, and salt in a small saucepan and bring to a gentle boil.
2. Add the oats and teff, stir to combine, and turn the heat down to maintain a low simmer. Simmer, partially covered and stirring occasionally, for 15 minutes, until the oats are cooked and most of the liquid has been absorbed.
3. Stir in the coconut oil and top with fresh blueberries and a generous pinch of cinnamon.

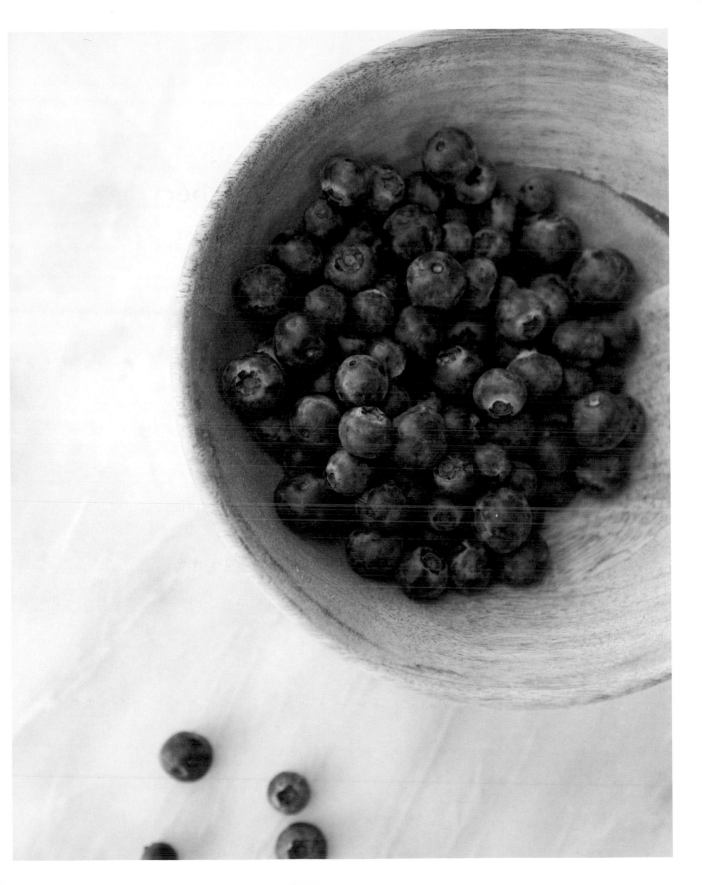

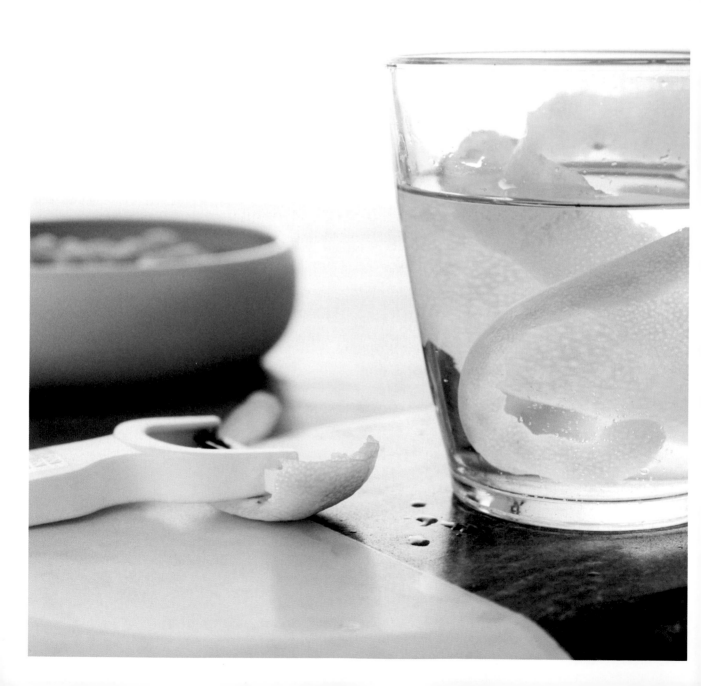

Canarino

It's always a good idea to start your day with canarino while detoxing, as the alkalizing lemon helps balance pH in the body, and the vitamin C helps neutralize harmful free radicals in the skin. While a room-temperature glass of lemon water works just fine, we're particularly into this soothing, warm Italian tea. The goal is to remove the colored part of the peel of the whole lemon in one continuous piece, but don't worry if your peeler skills aren't that good—you'll still get all the benefits.

SERVES 2

1 unwaxed organic lemon   Boiling water

1. Wash the lemon and carefully peel it, trying to leave as much white pith as possible on the lemon.
2. Place the lemon peel in a small teapot and fill with boiling water.
3. Let sit for 5 minutes to steep before drinking.

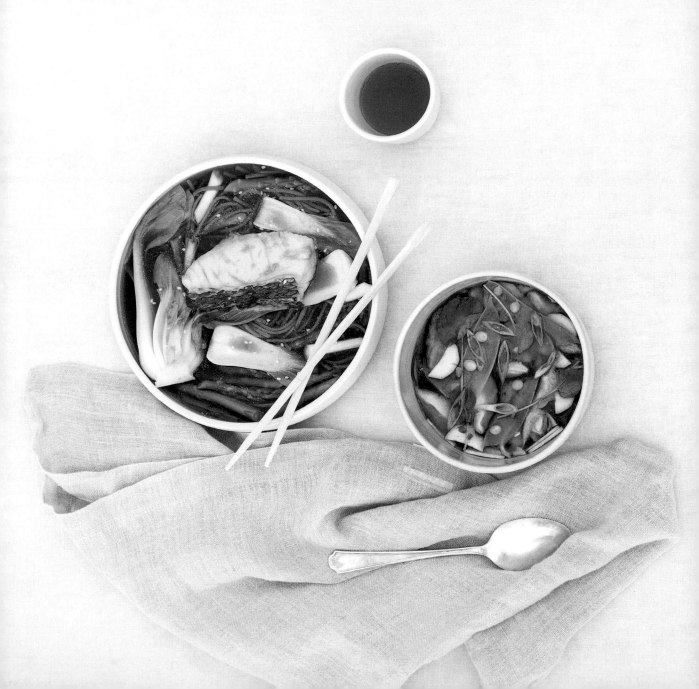

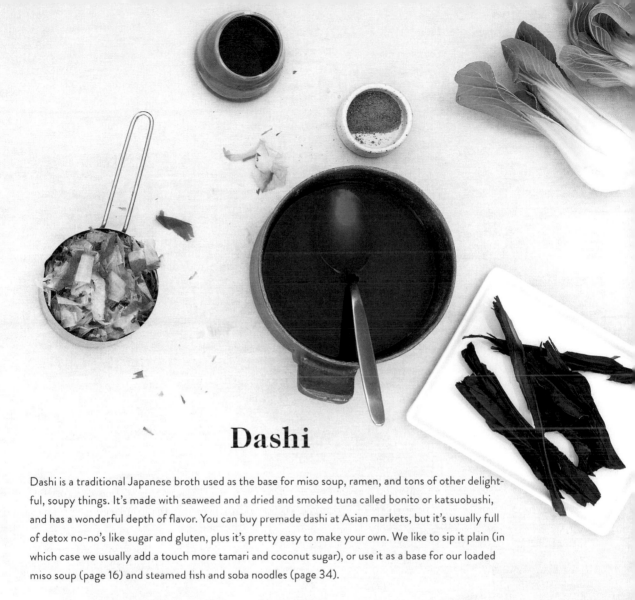

Dashi

Dashi is a traditional Japanese broth used as the base for miso soup, ramen, and tons of other delightful, soupy things. It's made with seaweed and a dried and smoked tuna called bonito or katsuobushi, and has a wonderful depth of flavor. You can buy premade dashi at Asian markets, but it's usually full of detox no-no's like sugar and gluten, plus it's pretty easy to make your own. We like to sip it plain (in which case we usually add a touch more tamari and coconut sugar), or use it as a base for our loaded miso soup (page 16) and steamed fish and soba noodles (page 34).

MAKES 8 CUPS; SERVES 1 TO 6

¼ cup wakame	2 tablespoons tamari
1 cup bonito flakes	1 tablespoon coconut sugar

1. Bring 8 cups water to a gentle simmer. Add the wakame and simmer very gently for 10 minutes. Add the bonito flakes and simmer another 5 minutes. Turn off the heat, cover, and let the mixture steep for 2 minutes.
2. Strain through a fine-mesh sieve and season with the tamari and coconut sugar.

Loaded Miso Soup

Miso soup makes a great breakfast, lunch, or dinner while detoxing, and this one, packed with green veggies, is particularly satisfying.

SERVES 2

4 cups Dashi (page 15)

3 tablespoons white miso paste

1 cup watercress leaves

1 small zucchini, cut in half and thinly sliced into half moons

4 shiitake mushrooms, stemmed and thinly sliced

16 snow peas

2 tablespoons thinly sliced scallions, optional

1. Heat the dashi in a small saucepan over medium heat, being careful not to let it boil.
2. Place the miso paste in a small bowl and add about 1 tablespoon of the hot dashi from the saucepan, stirring to dissolve the miso in the hot broth.
3. Add the miso and dashi mix back to the saucepan along with the watercress, zucchini, mushrooms, and snow peas. Simmer gently for 1 minute, or until the veggies are just tender.
4. Serve hot, topped with sliced scallions if desired.

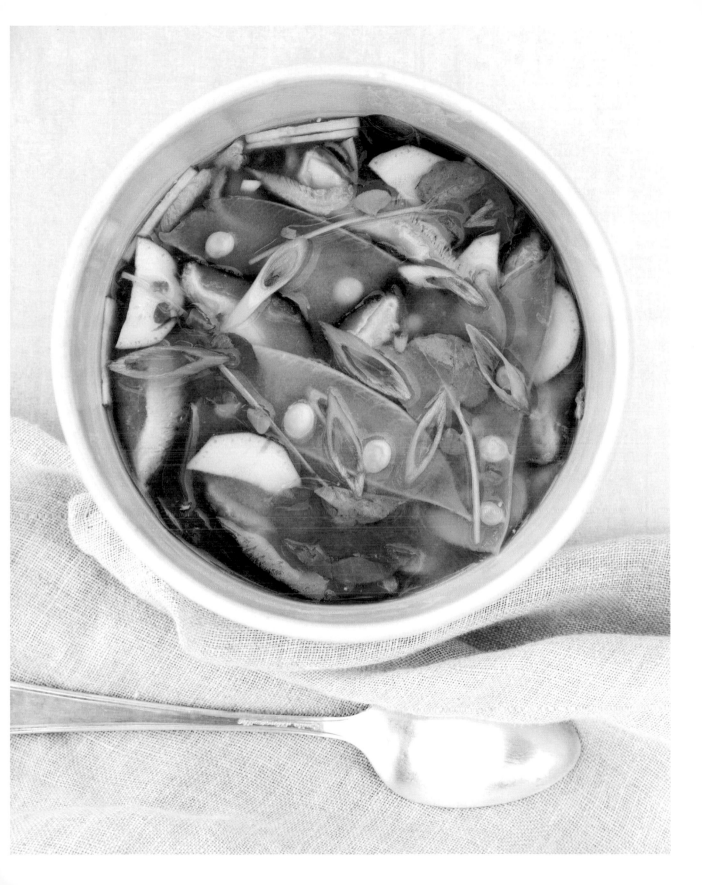

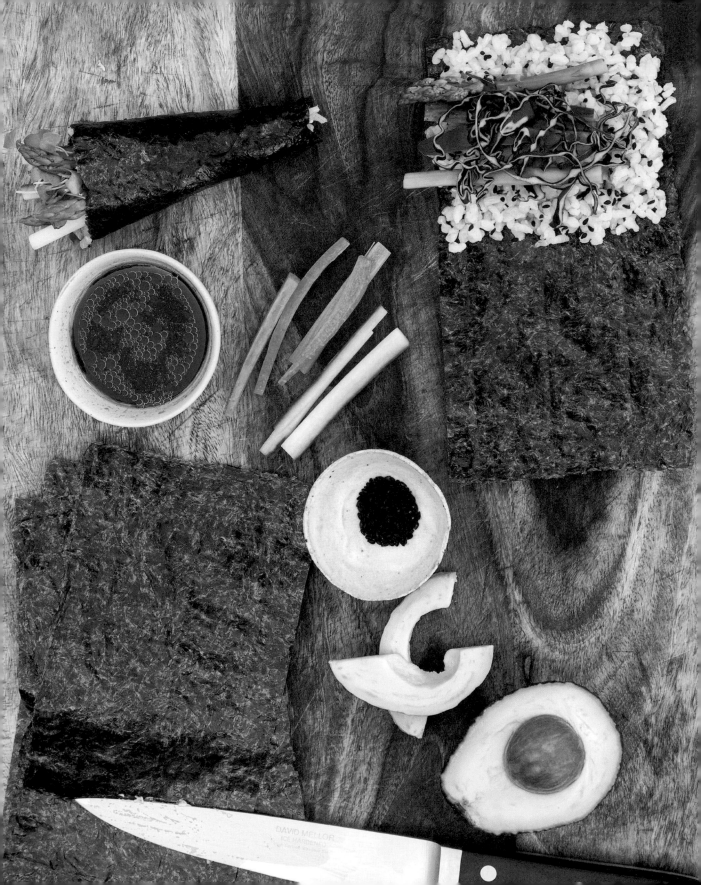

Hand Rolls

Hand rolls are an awesome detox lunch or snack—they're crunchy, satisfying, and actually fun to make. Plus they're extremely versatile, as you can fill them with any raw or cooked vegetables you like. Just be sure your veggies are all roughly 2 inches long and ¼ to ½ inch wide so they fit nicely in the hand roll.

SERVES 1 TO 2

2 nori sheets, cut in half to make 4 (7½ × 8-inch) rectangular pieces

1 cup cooked brown sushi rice

1 scallion, thinly sliced

Sesame seeds

Veggies of choice, such as thinly sliced avocado, julienned cucumber, grated carrot, lightly steamed asparagus, shaved radishes, julienned bell pepper, sprouts, shredded cabbage, etc.

2 tablespoons tamari

1 tablespoon rice wine vinegar or fresh lemon juice

½ teaspoon toasted sesame oil

1. Place the 4 nori sheets on a flat surface and spoon ¼ cup of rice on the right side of each one. Wet your fingers with water, and spread the rice into an even square over the right half of each nori sheet. Sprinkle with the scallion and some sesame seeds, then arrange your vegetables of choice along the center of the square of rice.
2. Starting at a bottom right hand corner, carefully roll up the nori and rice toward the upper left hand corner, wetting the nori with water so it sticks as you roll. Repeat to make 4 rolls.
3. Combine the tamari, vinegar, and sesame oil in a small bowl and serve on the side for dipping.

Little Gem Salad
with Vegan Green Goddess Dressing

Cashews are a magical ingredient. They are full of healthy fat, and when soaked and blended they lend an incredibly creamy texture to sauces and dressings while still keeping them detox-friendly. This green goddess dressing is so good we'd eat it with a spoon, but it's also perfect drizzled over any mixed greens or as a dip for crudités. If you want to make this salad a bit more filling, grilled salmon makes a particularly nice addition.

SERVES 2

FOR THE GREEN GODDESS DRESSING

¼ cup cashews, soaked in water for at least 2 hours and drained

¼ cup packed spinach

¼ cup packed fresh mint

¼ cup packed fresh basil

1 tablespoon minced shallot

¼ cup extra-virgin olive oil

2 tablespoons red wine vinegar

½ teaspoon coconut sugar, or to taste

Kosher salt and freshly ground black pepper

FOR THE SALAD

2 Little Gem lettuces, leaves separated, cleaned and dried

1 cup baby arugula leaves

1 small fennel bulb, cored and very finely sliced

1 Armenian cucumber, thinly sliced

½ avocado, diced

2 radishes, thinly sliced

1. To make the dressing, combine all the ingredients (except the salt and pepper) with ¼ cup water in a powerful blender and blend until smooth. Season to taste with salt and pepper.
2. To make the salad, combine all ingredients in a medium bowl and toss with half the dressing. Taste for seasoning, and serve with extra dressing on the side.

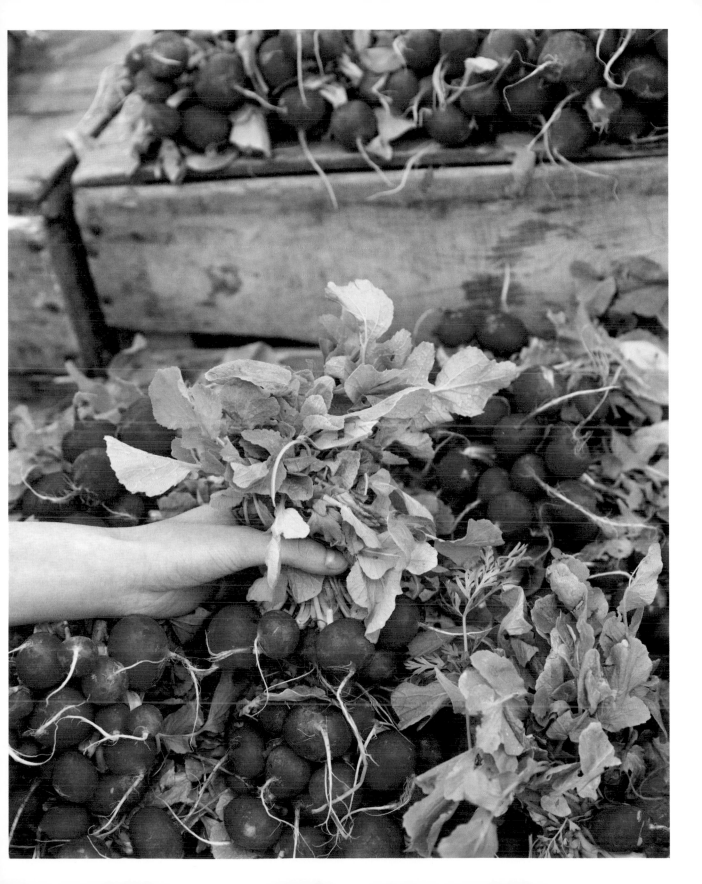

Kimchi Turkey Burgers

Kimchi-spiked burgers have quickly become a favorite in the GOOP office. Easy to make, and satisfying enough for non-detoxing friends and spouses, our slightly spicy turkey burgers are definitely a winner.

SERVES 1 TO 2

¼ cup packed kimchi, liquid squeezed out

2 large scallions, thinly sliced

1 tablespoon tamari

1 large carrot, grated

1 clove garlic, finely minced (or grated with a Microplane)

½ pound ground dark turkey meat

Olive oil, for brushing

4 butter lettuce leaves

Thinly sliced red onion, to taste

½ large or 1 small avocado, sliced

1. Place the kimchi and scallions in the bowl of a food processor and pulse until finely chopped (alternatively, finely chop the kimchi and scallions with a knife).
2. Transfer to a medium bowl and add the tamari, carrot, garlic, and turkey. Use your hands to mix well, then divide into 4 equal patties. You can make these up to 1 day in advance and refrigerate, covered, until ready to use.
3. To cook, heat a grill pan over medium-high heat. Brush the pan with oil and grill the burgers for about 3 minutes per side, or until very firm to the touch.
4. Serve the burgers on butter lettuce leaves with red onion and avocado.

Root Vegetable Soup

This recipe makes a lot of soup, but it lasts in the fridge for almost a week and freezes really well, too. We like a mix of celery root, sweet potato, and turnips, but you can use any root vegetables you like (except potatoes, which are in the nightshade family).

SERVES 4 TO 6

2 pounds mixed root vegetables such as turnips, celery root, and sweet potato

4 tablespoons olive oil

Kosher salt and freshly ground black pepper

1 small yellow onion, thinly sliced

1 medium leek, very well rinsed and cut into ½-inch slices

1 small carrot, diced

1 celery stalk, diced

2 large cloves garlic, minced

1 large sprig fresh rosemary

2 sprigs fresh thyme

Pinch red chili flakes

1. Preheat the oven to 400°F.
2. Peel all of the root vegetables and cut into roughly 1-inch pieces. Place on a large baking sheet and toss with 2 tablespoons of olive oil, a large pinch of salt, and a generous grind of black pepper. Roast for 30 minutes, or until the vegetables are browned and tender.
3. Meanwhile, heat the remaining 2 tablespoons olive oil in a large heavy-bottomed stockpot or Dutch oven over medium heat. Add the onion and leek plus a generous pinch of salt, partially cover with the lid, and cook, stirring occasionally, until translucent and just starting to brown, about 10 minutes. Add the carrot, celery, garlic, rosemary, thyme, and chili flakes, and cook for 5 more minutes.
4. When the root vegetables are roasted, scrape them directly into the soup pot and add 4 cups water, a very generous pinch of salt, and a few grinds of black pepper. Bring to a boil, then reduce to a simmer, and cook for 15 to 20 minutes.
5. Use an immersion blender or Vitamix to blend the soup, then season with salt and pepper to taste.

Clean Fish Tacos

We all love Baja-style fish tacos, but just because the classic breaded and deep-fried version is out of the question when detoxing, it doesn't mean you have to give up tacos completely. These clean fish tacos taste amazing and are completely gluten, dairy, and corn free. The cashew crema takes a bit of advance prep (the cashews need to be soaked in water for at least 2 hours before blending), but is really worth making.

SERVES 2

FOR THE FISH

⅔ pound halibut fillet, skin removed, cut into 2 large rectangular pieces

2 tablespoons olive oil

Juice of 2 small or 1 large lime

3 tablespoons roughly chopped fresh cilantro

1 teaspoon ground cumin

Kosher salt

FOR THE CASHEW CREMA

1 cup raw cashews, soaked in water for at least 2 hours or up to overnight

Juice of 1 lime

1 teaspoon ground chipotle powder

½ teaspoon ground cumin

Kosher salt

FOR THE TACOS

4 taco-size brown-rice tortillas (or burrito-size tortillas cut into taco size)

1 avocado, thinly sliced

¼ cup finely chopped fresh cilantro

¼ cup finely diced white onion

2 tablespoons finely diced jalapeño pepper

1 cup shredded white cabbage

Lime wedges, for serving

1. To marinate the fish, in a medium bowl, toss the halibut with the olive oil, lime juice, cilantro, cumin, and a generous pinch of salt. Cover the bowl and marinate in the fridge for at least 10 minutes and up to 1 hour.
2. To make the cashew crema, drain the soaked cashews and combine with ½ cup water, the lime juice, chipotle powder, and cumin in a powerful blender. Blitz until smooth and creamy. Season to taste with salt and set aside.
3. To cook the fish: Heat a grill pan over medium-high heat. When very hot, add the halibut and cook until it has nice grill marks on both sides and is firm to the touch, about 2 minutes per side.
4. To assemble the tacos, heat the tortillas in a small sauté pan over medium heat until soft, then fill each with a piece of halibut and top with avocado, cilantro, onion, jalapeño, cabbage, and a drizzle of cashew crema. Serve with lime wedges.

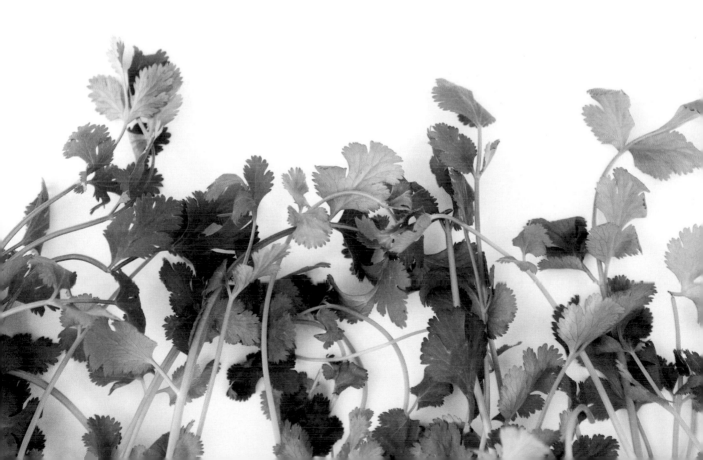

Grain Bowls, Two Ways

Grain bowls are perfect when you're detoxing. Since they're densely packed with healthy nutrients, they're satisfying enough to keep you full all afternoon. Here are two of our favorites, though it's easy to customize your own: Start with cooked brown rice or quinoa and top with any veggies, proteins, and sauces you like.

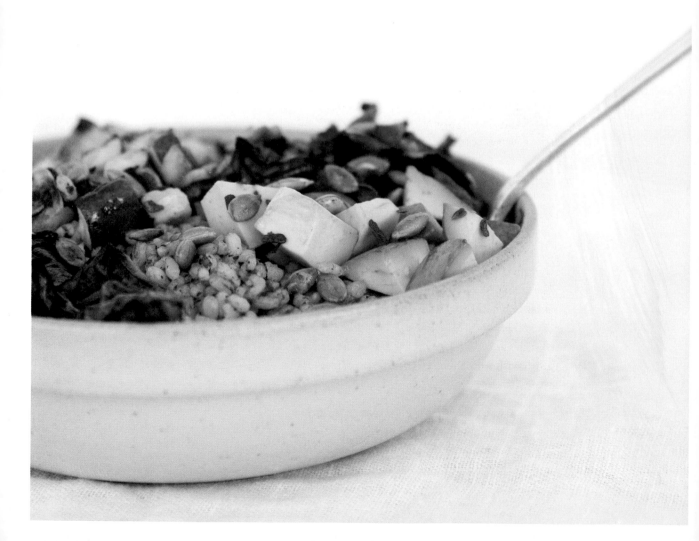

Green Grain Bowls

SERVES 2

FOR THE PESTO

$\frac{1}{3}$ cup lightly packed fresh basil leaves, roughly chopped

$\frac{1}{3}$ cup lightly packed fresh mint leaves, roughly chopped

$\frac{1}{3}$ cup walnut halves, roughly chopped

$\frac{1}{3}$ cup extra-virgin olive oil

Kosher salt

FOR THE BOWLS

1 medium zucchini, cut into 3 long strips

1 teaspoon extra-virgin olive oil

Kosher salt and freshly ground black pepper

1½ cups cooked brown rice or quinoa

Zest and juice of ½ lemon, plus more juice to taste

¾ cup Sautéed Cavolo Nero (page 38), or any simply sautéed greens such as chard or rapini

½ large ripe yet firm avocado, diced

3 tablespoons toasted pumpkin seeds

Red chili flakes to taste, optional

1. To make the pesto, combine the herbs, walnuts, olive oil, and 2 tablespoons water in a food processor and blend until almost smooth. Season to taste with salt.
2. To cook the zucchini, heat a grill pan over medium-high heat. Toss the zucchini with the olive oil and season with salt and pepper to taste. When the grill pan is hot, add the zucchini strips and cook for about 2 minutes per side, until the zucchini is tender and has nice grill marks. Remove to a cutting board and dice when cooled.
3. To assemble the bowls, toss the brown rice with ¼ cup of pesto and the lemon zest and juice; divide between two bowls. Top each bowl with half the zucchini, half the sautéed greens, half the avocado, and half the toasted pumpkin seeds. Finish with a pinch of red chili flakes and some fresh lemon juice, if desired, and serve with the remaining pesto on the side.

Sweet Potato and Avocado Grain Bowls

SERVES 2

FOR THE SAUCE

1 teaspoon white miso

½ teaspoon hot water

1 tablespoon extra-virgin olive oil

Juice of ½ small lime

½ teaspoon tamari

¼ teaspoon toasted sesame oil

FOR THE BOWLS

1½ cups cooked brown rice or quinoa

¾ cup diced Roasted Sweet Potatoes (page 39)

½ to 1 avocado (depending on size), diced or sliced

¼ cup chopped fresh cilantro leaves

½ cup Sautéed Cavolo Nero (page 38), or any simply sautéed greens such as chard or rapini

2 radishes, thinly sliced with a mandoline

½ sheet nori, cut into thin strips

1. To make the sauce, combine the miso and hot water in a small bowl and whisk to dissolve the miso. Add the remaining ingredients and whisk to combine and emulsify.

2. To assemble the bowls, divide the cooked grains between two bowls. Top each bowl with half the sweet potato, half the avocado, half the cilantro, half the cavolo nero, half the sliced radishes, and sprinkle the nori strips over the top. Pour over the sauce or serve on the side.

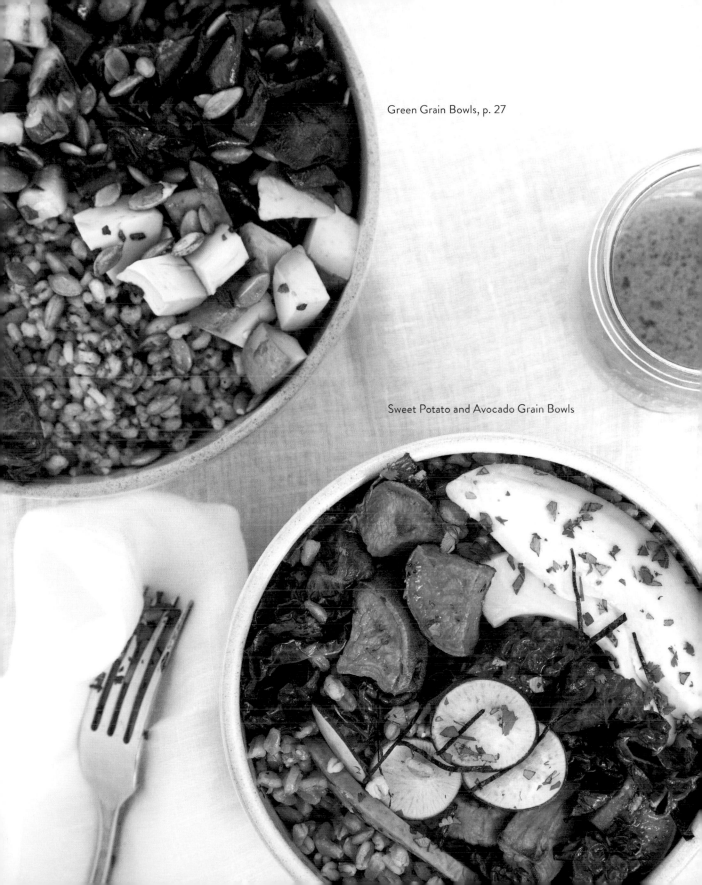

Green Grain Bowls, p. 27

Sweet Potato and Avocado Grain Bowls

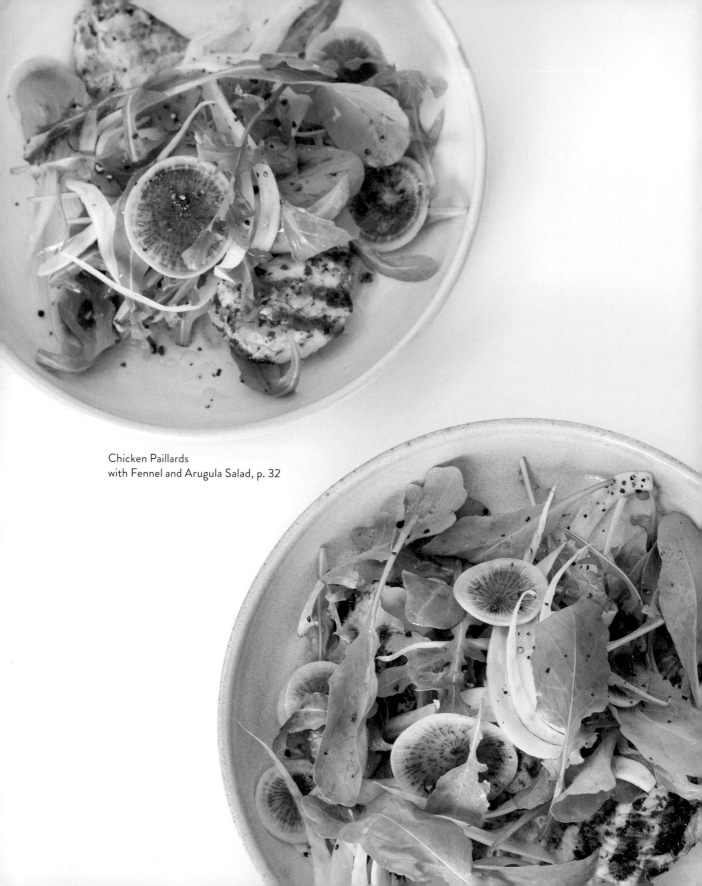

Chicken Paillards
with Fennel and Arugula Salad, p. 32

Chicken Paillards, Two Ways

A grilled chicken paillard is the perfect detox lunch or dinner. It's quick and easy to cook, a great source of lean protein, and can be topped with pretty much any salad you like. Here are two versions, but feel free to play around with whatever ingredients you have in the fridge or find at the farmers' market.

Chicken Paillards with Radicchio Salad

SERVES 2

FOR THE CHICKEN AND MARINADE

1 boneless skinless chicken breast, cut into 2 cutlets

1 teaspoon finely grated lemon zest

Juice of ½ small or ¼ large lemon

1 teaspoon finely chopped fresh thyme

1 teaspoon finely chopped fresh rosemary

1 teaspoon finely chopped fresh basil

1½ tablespoons olive oil

Kosher salt

FOR THE CAPER DRESSING

1 tablespoon red wine vinegar

2 teaspoons capers, roughly chopped

2 teaspoons finely minced shallot

1 teaspoon Dijon mustard

½ teaspoon anchovy paste

3 tablespoons extra-virgin olive oil, plus more for brushing the pan

Kosher salt and freshly ground black pepper

FOR THE RADICCHIO SALAD

½ cup thinly sliced radicchio

½ cup thinly sliced endive

½ cup baby arugula

3 large cauliflower florets, thinly shaved using a mandoline

1. To prepare the chicken, place it between two large pieces of wax or parchment paper and, using a heavy mallet, frying pan, or the side of a cleaver, pound until each cutlet is about ⅓ inch thin. This may take some time and some elbow grease, but it's worth it.
2. In a medium bowl, combine the lemon zest, lemon juice, herbs, olive oil, and a large pinch of salt and stir to mix well. Add the chicken and turn to coat. Cover and marinate at room temperature for at least 15 minutes and up to 1 hour.
3. To make the caper dressing, whisk together the vinegar, capers, shallot, mustard, and anchovy paste. Slowly whisk in the olive oil and season to taste with salt and pepper.
4. Heat a grill pan over medium-high heat and brush it lightly with olive oil. When the pan is hot, grill the chicken breasts until charred and cooked through, about 3 minutes per side.
5. To assemble the salad, toss the radicchio, endive, arugula, and cauliflower with the dressing in a medium bowl. Arrange the salad on top of the grilled paillards and serve.

Chicken Paillards with Fennel and Arugula Salad

We use a mandoline to shave the fennel and watermelon radish for the salad, but you can also use a sharp knife to very thinly slice them.

SERVES 2

FORE THE CHICKEN AND MARINADE

1 boneless skinless chicken breast, cut into 2 cutlets	1 teaspoon finely chopped fresh rosemary
1 teaspoon finely grated lemon zest	1 teaspoon finely chopped fresh basil
Juice of ½ small or ¼ large lemon	1½ tablespoons olive oil, plus more for brushing the pan
1 teaspoon finely chopped fresh thyme	Kosher salt

FOR THE FENNEL AND ARUGULA SALAD

2 handfuls baby arugula	Juice of 1 small lemon
1 small fennel bulb, cored and very finely shaved	2 tablespoons extra-virgin olive oil
1 small watermelon radish, very finely shaved	Kosher salt and freshly ground black pepper

1. To prepare the chicken, place it between two large pieces of wax or parchment paper and, using a heavy mallet, frying pan, or the side of a cleaver, pound until each cutlet is about ⅓ inch thin. This may take some time and some elbow grease, but it's worth it.
2. In a medium bowl, combine the lemon zest, lemon juice, herbs, olive oil, and a large pinch of salt and stir to mix well. Add the chicken and turn to coat. Cover and marinate at room temperature for at least 15 minutes and up to 1 hour.
3. Heat a grill pan over medium-high heat and brush it lightly with olive oil. When the pan is hot, grill the chicken until charred and cooked through, about 3 minutes per side.
4. To assemble the salad, toss the arugula, fennel, and radish with the lemon juice, olive oil, and salt to taste, and arrange on top of the grilled paillards. Finish with cracked black pepper to taste.

Steamed Fish with Dashi and Soba Noodles

This is a perfect dish to serve for company if you double or triple the recipe—it's easy, elegant, and super-healthy.

SERVES 2

2 cups Dashi (page 15)

2 tablespoons tamari

2 teaspoons coconut sugar

½ teaspoon finely grated fresh ginger

½ teaspoon finely grated garlic

2 (6-ounce) portions firm white fish such as sole, black cod, or sea bass

1 large or 2 small baby bok choy, broken into individual leaves if large or cut into halves if small

6 to 10 asparagus spears, cut into 2-inch pieces

6 scallions, cut into 2-inch pieces

3 ounces 100 percent buckwheat soba noodles, cooked according to package instructions

1. Combine the dashi, tamari, sugar, ginger, and garlic in a large, shallow, straight-sided sauté pan just large enough to fit all of the fish and veggies in a single layer and bring to a simmer.
2. Add the fish, cover, and simmer for 3 to 5 minutes (depending how thick your fish is), then add the bok choy, asparagus, and scallions. Cover again, and simmer for another 2 minutes, until the fish is firm to the touch and the veggies are just tender.
3. Divide the cooked soba noodles between two shallow bowls and top each pile with one piece of fish and half of the steamed veggies. Ladle over the dashi and serve immediately.

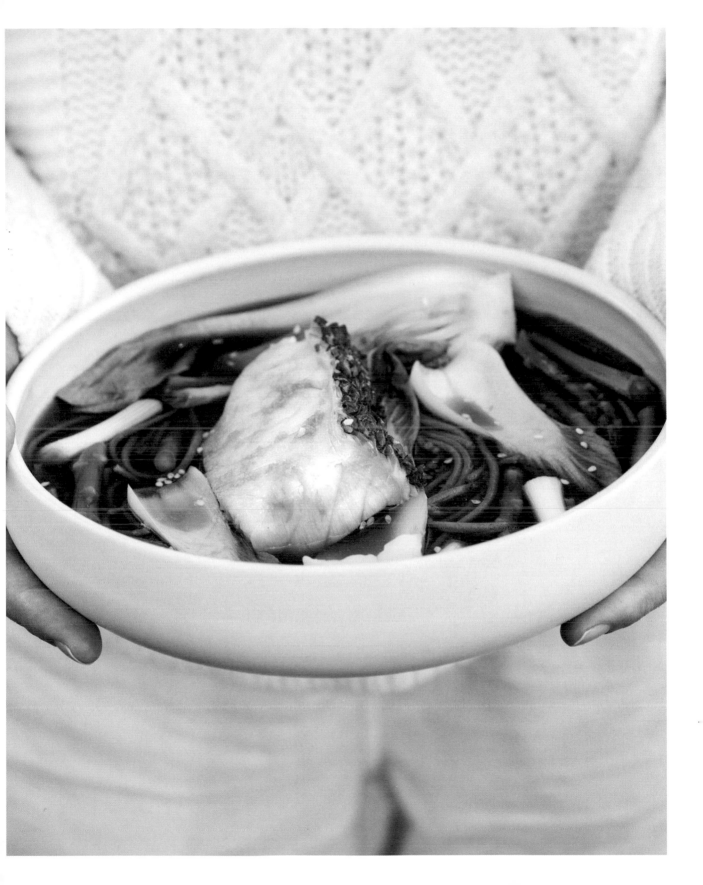

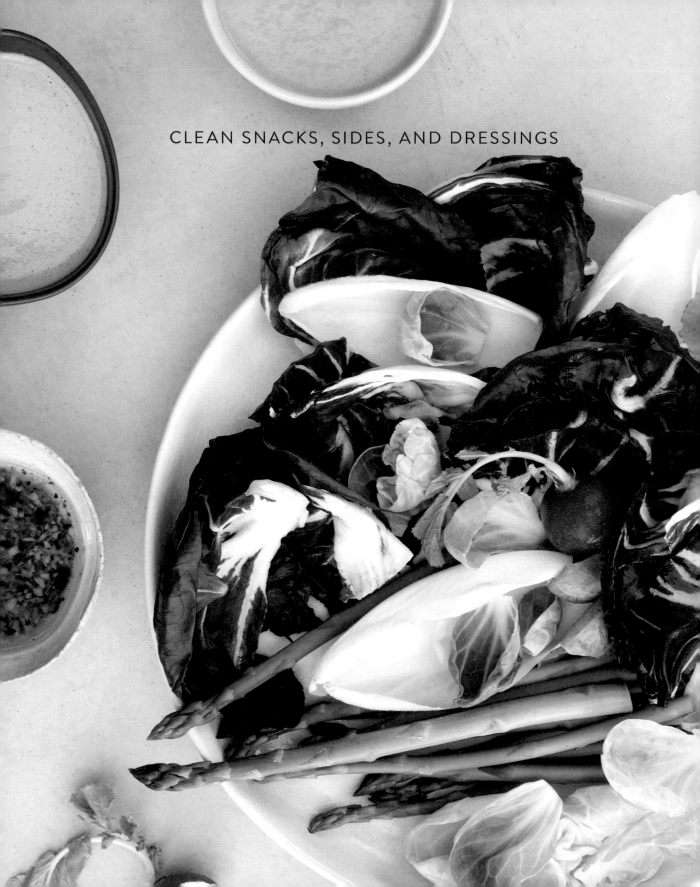

Bagna Cauda

This classic warm Italian dip is salty, spicy, and super-satisfying—great as an afternoon snack with veggies or even as a light lunch.

SERVES 2 TO 4

FOR THE BAGNA CAUDA

¼ cup olive oil

Large pinch red chili flakes

4 oil-packed anchovy fillets, finely chopped

10 grinds freshly ground black pepper

1 clove garlic, finely minced or grated

Zest and juice of ½ lemon

CRUDITÉS OF CHOICE, SUCH AS...

1 head endive, separated into leaves

8 asparagus spears, quickly blanched and cut in half

½ small head radicchio, cut into large pieces

6 Brussels sprouts, separated into individual leaves

1 small head fennel, cored and cut into large pieces

1. To make the bagna cauda, combine the olive oil, anchovies, garlic, red chili flakes, and black pepper in a small saucepan. Cook over medium-low heat, stirring constantly with a wooden spoon, until the anchovies have melted and the garlic is fragrant but not burned, about 3 minutes. Add the lemon zest and juice, and taste for seasoning.
2. Transfer the warm dip to a bowl and serve with assorted crudités.

Sautéed Cavolo Nero

This easy kale dish is a total detox staple. It's great as a side dish with a simply cooked protein, but we particularly love making a big batch and adding it to dishes throughout the week like our grain bowls (page 26) or a quinoa and veggie stir-fry.

SERVES 4

2 tablespoons olive oil

2 cloves garlic, thinly sliced

Pinch red chili flakes

1 bunch cavolo nero (also called dinosaur kale), washed, dried, and chopped into 1-inch pieces

Kosher salt

1. Heat the olive oil in a large sauté pan over medium heat. Add the garlic and red chili flakes and cook for 30 seconds, until the garlic is fragrant but not browned.
2. Add the kale and a large pinch of salt. Use a wooden spoon to stir, mixing everything well so that the garlic doesn't stick to the pan and burn. Sauté for 3 to 5 minutes, until the kale is starting to wilt and the garlic is lightly toasted.
3. Cover with a lid, turn the heat down to low, and cook for 5 minutes, until the kale is tender.

Roasted Sweet Potatoes

This one doesn't really need a recipe, but it's such a great snack when you're detoxing that we wanted to include it. We roast two sweet potatoes at a time, enjoying one as a snack straight out of the oven with coconut oil and flaxseed, and storing the other in the fridge to use in our Sweet Potato and Avocado Grain Bowls (page 28) or to bulk up a breakfast porridge.

SERVES 2 TO 4

2 medium sweet potatoes

1. Preheat the oven to 450°F.
2. Scrub the sweet potatoes to remove any dirt, prick them all over with a paring knife or fork, and place directly on the oven rack. Place a foil-lined baking sheet underneath to catch any drippings.
3. Roast for 1 hour, until very tender when pricked with a knife. Eat immediately or allow to cool to room temperature, then peel and store in the fridge until ready to use.

Roasted Fennel

Roasting fennel yields the sweetest, most tender vegetable side dish you can imagine. We love it as a side with any fish or chicken dish, but it also makes a great snack. It's so sweet it could almost stand in for candy.

SERVES 4

2 large fennel bulbs

About 3 tablespoons olive oil

Kosher salt and freshly ground black pepper

Red chili flakes

1. Preheat the oven to 375°F.
2. Peel the tough outer layer off the fennel bulbs, wash to remove any dirt, then cut vertically into 1-inch slices. Cut out the tough core from any center slices and pat dry.
3. Place on a baking sheet and toss with the olive oil, a couple good pinches of salt and black pepper, and red chili flakes to taste. Roast for 1 hour, flipping halfway through so the slices brown evenly on both sides, until tender and caramelized.

Ginger-Carrot Miso Dressing

We're addicted to this. It's perfect as a dressing for salad or a dip for crudités. We like to make a big batch on the weekend to have on hand all week. If you're using it as a salad dressing, you might want to add a splash more water or rice vinegar to thin it a bit.

MAKES ABOUT 1 CUP

1 large carrot, peeled and roughly chopped

1 medium shallot, roughly chopped (about ⅓ cup)

1 (3-inch) piece fresh ginger, peeled and roughly chopped (about ¼ cup)

¼ cup neutral oil, such as grapeseed or safflower

2 tablespoons white miso

2 tablespoons tamari

2 tablespoons rice wine vinegar

1 teaspoon coconut sugar

Kosher salt and freshly ground black pepper

Combine 2 tablespoons water with all the ingredients except salt and pepper in a powerful blender and blitz until smooth. Season to taste with salt and pepper.

Kohlrabi Slaw

Refreshing and light, this slaw is the perfect light lunch or accompaniment to simply grilled chicken or fish. If you have a mandoline, use it to julienne all your fruits and veggies—it's a real time-saver.

SERVES 4

1 small fennel bulb, tough outsides peeled, julienned

1 medium kohlrabi, peeled, julienned

1 small Granny Smith apple, core removed, julienned

Zest and juice of 1 lemon

1 small shallot, thinly sliced

2 tablespoons extra-virgin olive oil

Kosher salt

⅓ cup roughly chopped fresh mint leaves

Combine the fennel, kohlrabi, and apple in a large bowl. Toss with the lemon zest and juice, shallot, and olive oil and season to taste with salt. Mix in the mint just before serving.

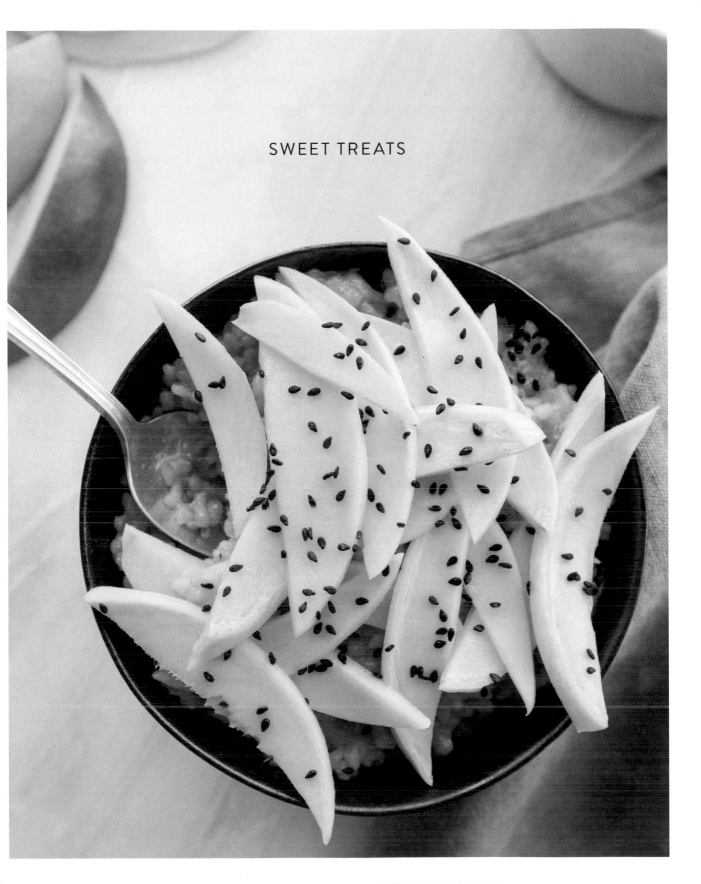

SWEET TREATS

Coconut Rice with Mango

Coconut sticky rice might be the best treat ever, and this version, made with nutrient-dense brown rice and sweetened with coconut sugar, is totally addictive. We like a ratio of mostly mango and a little rice, but if you're looking to fill up, increase the amount of rice.

SERVES 2

$^2/_3$ cup cooked brown rice

½ cup light coconut milk

2 teaspoons coconut sugar

Pinch sea salt (depending on how salty your rice is)

1 ripe mango, peeled and thinly sliced

Sesame seeds, for garnish, optional

Combine the rice, coconut milk, sugar, and salt in a small saucepan and bring to a simmer. Simmer over low heat, stirring often, for 2 minutes, until the mixture has thickened and most of the liquid has evaporated. Top with the mango and sesame seeds, if using.

Almond Butter and Sea Salt Cookies

Yum. These are salty, sweet, and dangerously poppable. They're also totally detox-friendly so go ahead and pop with abandon. Since almond butter textures vary dramatically from brand to brand, add another tablespoon if your dough is looking too dry.

MAKES 24 SMALL COOKIES

1½ cups gluten-free oats, divided

⅔ cup almond butter (be sure to get one with no added sugar), plus more as needed

½ cup coconut sugar

2 tablespoons coconut oil

1 teaspoon coarse sea salt, such as Maldon

1. Preheat the oven to 350°F.
2. Place 1 cup of oats in the bowl of a food processor and blend until smooth, about 10 seconds. Transfer to a medium bowl and add the remaining ½ cup oats, the almond butter, sugar, oil, and salt. Use your fingers to combine the ingredients, making sure they are very well incorporated. Add additional almond butter if necessary.
3. Roll the mixture into 24 small balls and arrange evenly, 1 inch apart, on a large baking sheet. Bake for 12 minutes, until lightly browned. Allow to cool completely before serving. Store in an airtight container at room temperature for up to 5 days.

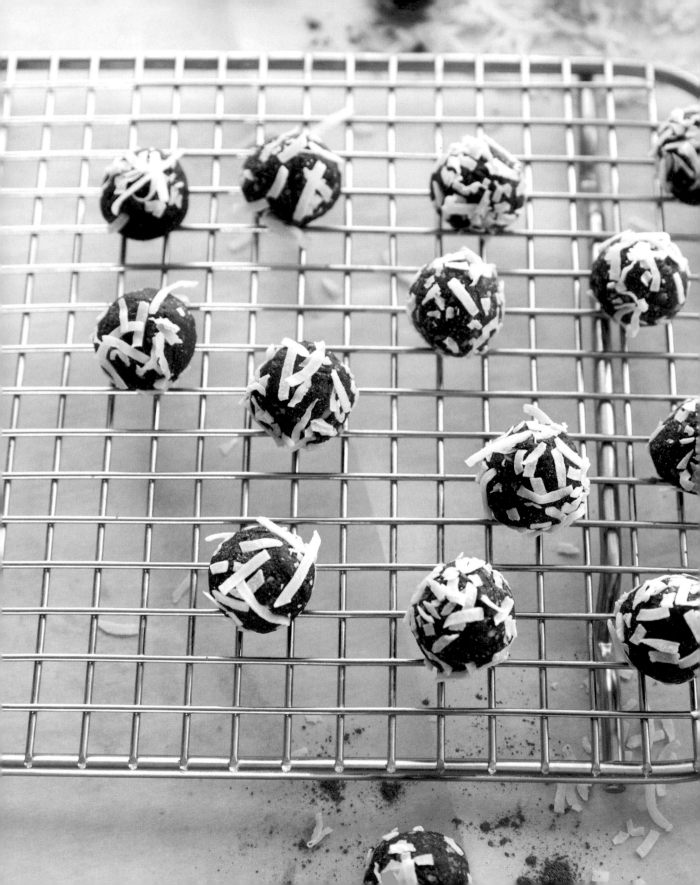

Detox Truffles

These raw, three-ingredient truffles are the perfect bite to satisfy your detoxing sweet tooth. We recommend making a double batch and keeping them in the fridge so you're always ready to combat those cookie cravings.

MAKES 24 SMALL TRUFFLES

12 pitted dates

¼ cup raw cacao powder

¼ cup unsweetened shredded coconut, plus extra for rolling

1. Blend the dates, cacao, and coconut in a food processor until smooth.
2. Wet your hands with water and roll the mixture into 24 small balls (about 1 teaspoon each), then roll each one in additional shredded coconut to coat. Store in the refrigerator for up to a week.

Beauty Detox Food Hacks

If the preceding recipes feel insurmountable, we hear you. Or, at least the less culinary inclined of us at GOOP hear you. It's true that we all love food. But for some of us, there are significant hurdles between our intentions and actually getting into the kitchen. Coming home and turning on the stove after a long day of meetings, traffic, and errands can sound downright overwhelming— and then facing a sink full of dishes later sounds crazy. So that's why we're happy to have Shira Lenchewski on speed dial—another good GOOP friend who happens to spend most of her time as a nutritionist coaching busy women who don't have time to do much beyond opening up Seamless and ordering in some Chinese. (Her best friend? The salad bar at Whole Foods.) Below, she shares some shortcuts for eating a bit better through the day.

Shira Lenchewski
TELLS US WHAT TO EAT WHEN WE DON'T HAVE THE TIME TO THINK

We know you've coached your fair share of busy women. Can you give us five tips for making the day a little healthier?

1. Gauge hunger with crudités: "Eat when you're hungry, stop when you're full." It's not bad advice, but what if you're not really sure? Keep fresh crudités (cut and washed) at eye level in your fridge at all times. If it's between meals or at snack time and you're feeling like a snack, go for the crudités. If you don't want crudités, you're probably not really hungry.

2. Put it on a plate: Many of us go out of our way to present food beautifully when we're serving it to others, but wind up eating from paper containers (or hurriedly over the sink) when it's just us. When food is plated, it prevents overeating because it gives the meal dignity, and because we're able to visualize what and how much we're actually eating. I'm not saying go full-on French Laundry, but do yourself a favor and put your food on a plate.

3. Banish all-or-nothing thinking: I'll fill you in on what I share with every one of my clients: No matter who you are, or how far you've come in maintaining your wellness goals, at some point you'll inevitably take a small step backward. It can be so frustrating and heartbreaking, but it's normal and part of life. The key isn't making sure you never veer off the path, it's forgiving yourself for taking a step back, so that you regroup and take another two steps forward.

4. Wait 15 minutes: We all have internal cues that help us figure out what we actually want and need, but those lines of communication travel at AOL dial-up speed, while our cravings run on broadband. If you're jonesing for something, say a doughnut, try waiting 15 minutes before acting on the impulse. If you still want the doughnut after the 15 minutes are up, put it on a plate, and slowly enjoy every bite. Then move on. But you may find that acting on the craving is not as important to you as you initially thought.

5. Check online before you dine: Just like you want to avoid going into meals starving, you also ideally want to enter a restaurant with a plan, so you're not forced to make a hasty game-time decision that's not in line with what you *really* want. So check out the restaurant menu online and decide what you want to eat before heading out. This will also help you from being corrupted by your more decadent dining pals.

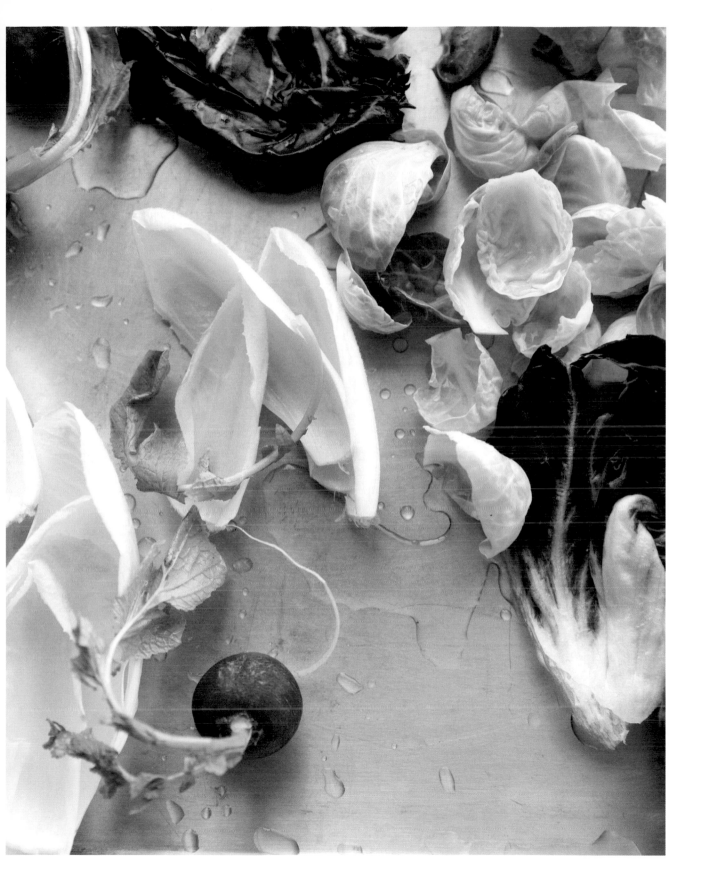

For those of us who are continually on the go, how do we avoid resorting to granola bars, baked goods from a coffee shop, and the same repeat takeout order from the place across the street from the office?

I'm a big believer in the idea that the more structure and planning you incorporate into your nutritional life, the less self-discipline you actually need. If you know you're always ready for a snack in the mid-afternoon, think about flavorful, healthy options you'll enjoy, and make a point of having them on hand. One of my all-time favorite snacks is half an avocado with sea salt. If you're tired of dinner just happening *to* you, get ahead of it. Think about the things you'll need to have standing by in order to throw together no-brainer meals, like a simple stir-fry, or a breakfast-for-dinner veggie omelet. I recommend always having enough stuff in your fridge or pantry to make a non-*meh* meal that isn't primarily carbs. I'm also not against takeout, as long as you have some good options bookmarked, so

it's a conscious choice rather than a heat-of-the-moment decision made when you're tired and starving.

What are the small changes that we can make—on the phone with the delivery guy / in the kitchen / at the grocery store—that can make a big difference?
On the phone with the delivery guy: Save sweeteners for dessert. Get in the habit of asking how things are prepared, and nixing anything that includes added sugar: We're talking salad dressings, sauces, marinades—all those places where sugar doesn't need to be. Another thing that seems so simple but makes a huge difference: Order before you leave the office, so your food is there when you get home. A lot of times we're so famished when we get home that we end up polishing off half a box of cereal before we can even deal with sorting out dinner. Take that factor out of the equation.

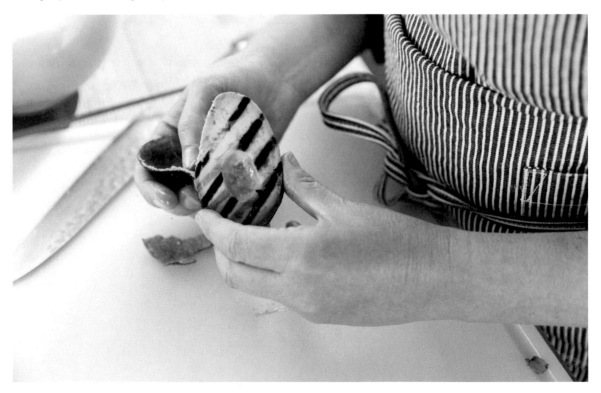

In the kitchen: "Out of sight out of mind" is a real thing. Keep healthy food at eye level in your fridge and store sweets and treats in opaque containers.

At the grocery store: Don't forget about the salad bar! Sliced veggies can be a lifesaver when you're pinched for time! I'm also a huge fan of pre-portioned nuts, because they're easier to regulate.

It's dinnertime on a weeknight and we didn't prepare ahead with a big batch of anything on the previous Sunday. What to do?
Forget about the idea that dinner needs to be an event—it can be a one-plate meal and you don't even have to do any heavy lifting if you don't have time.

I heard versions of this question so often in my practice (because let's be real, batch cooking isn't always realistic), that I came up with a sort of proactive, realistic, and somewhat scrappy approach to doctoring up meals. My advice: When you're pinched for time, try sprucing up high-quality, pre-prepared stuff, like organic rotisserie chicken and cooked brown rice from the salad bar, by making them feel mildly fussed-over with herbs, spices, and easy aromatics like onions, shallots, chives, and garlic. Then all you have to do is throw some vinaigrette on greens, or sauté your ingredients in olive oil and top them off with sea salt, and you're done. Zero heavy lifting required!

Planes, Trains, and Automobiles

Things are looking a bit better at the food courts of major airports these days, but it can still be hard to find a basic apple, or a simple salad that hasn't been hanging out a few days too long. More often than not, the only options are fast and greasy: burgers and fries, quesadillas, and (gulp) Cinnabons. You can either embrace the idea that what

happens at 20,000 feet stays at 20,000 feet, or you can pack yourself a lunch and get through your flight with a minimal amount of gas and bloating—and save those calories for something worth it, like wine. Next, a few hearty go-to salads that pack well.

goop TIP

As you likely already know, plastic containers, while convenient, are potentially hazardous to our health. BPA (bisphenol A), a toxic component of polycarbonate plastics, can leach out of food containers (and water bottles) into the food (or water) inside. It's often recommended that you avoid plastic containers marked with a PC (for polycarbonate) or the recycling numbers 3, 6, 7. We try to pack our to-go lunches and leftovers in glass containers as much as possible—which can also be safely heated up. We have regular rectangular glass containers on hand at home, and are also fans of packing in jars—classic Mason jars are great, as are jars from the brand Weck. Stainless steel is also a safe bet. But when you're traveling you probably don't want to make your luggage load any heavier. So, consider buying biodegradable takeout containers (like what you'd find at the Whole Foods salad bar) online for ease.

Asian Chopped Salad

Full of fresh herbs and a salty, sweet, tangy dressing, this Vietnamese-style chopped salad is a GOOP team favorite. If you don't like shrimp (or if you're not packing an ice pack to keep things cold), substitute grilled chicken or tofu, or keep it simple with just the veggies. To save time, consider buying some ingredients from the salad bar, such as chopped lettuce, grated carrots, cabbage, and cooked protein.

SERVES 1

FOR THE SHRIMP

⅓ pound medium shrimp, peeled and deveined

Olive oil

Kosher salt and freshly ground black pepper

FOR THE DRESSING

1 tablespoon minced shallot

1 tablespoon fish sauce

1 tablespoon maple syrup

1 tablespoon fresh lime juice

Pinch red chili flakes

FOR THE SALAD

1 baby bok choy, leaves thinly sliced (about ½ cup)

½ cup shredded romaine

½ cup shredded napa cabbage

⅓ cup snap peas, sliced into ⅓-inch pieces

½ small zucchini, thinly sliced into half moons (about ⅓ cup)

⅓ cup grated carrot

2 tablespoons packed, roughly chopped fresh mint leaves

2 tablespoons packed, roughly chopped fresh cilantro leaves

1. To cook the shrimp, heat a grill pan over medium-high heat. Toss the shrimp with a little olive oil and salt and pepper, and cook until each piece has nice grill marks and is firm to the touch, about 2 minutes per side. Set aside to cool.
2. To make the dressing, whisk together all the ingredients in a small travel container and taste for seasoning.
3. To assemble, arrange the shrimp and all the salad ingredients in a travel container, keeping them separate so the lettuce doesn't get soggy.
4. When ready to eat, drizzle on the dressing and replace the lid. Shake to combine all ingredients and enjoy.

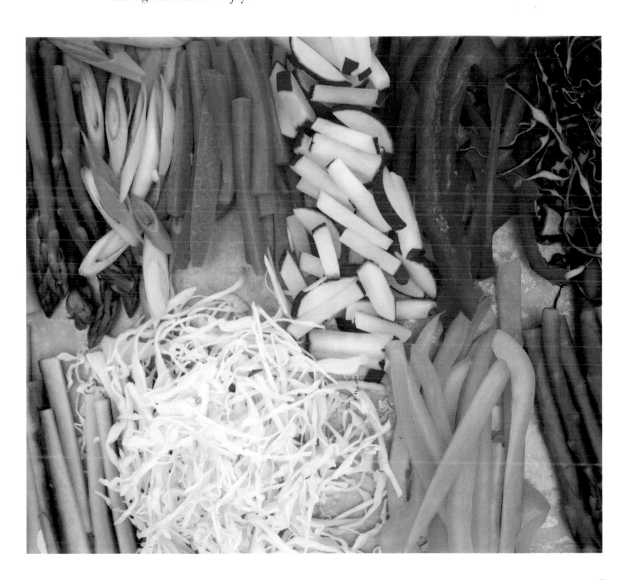

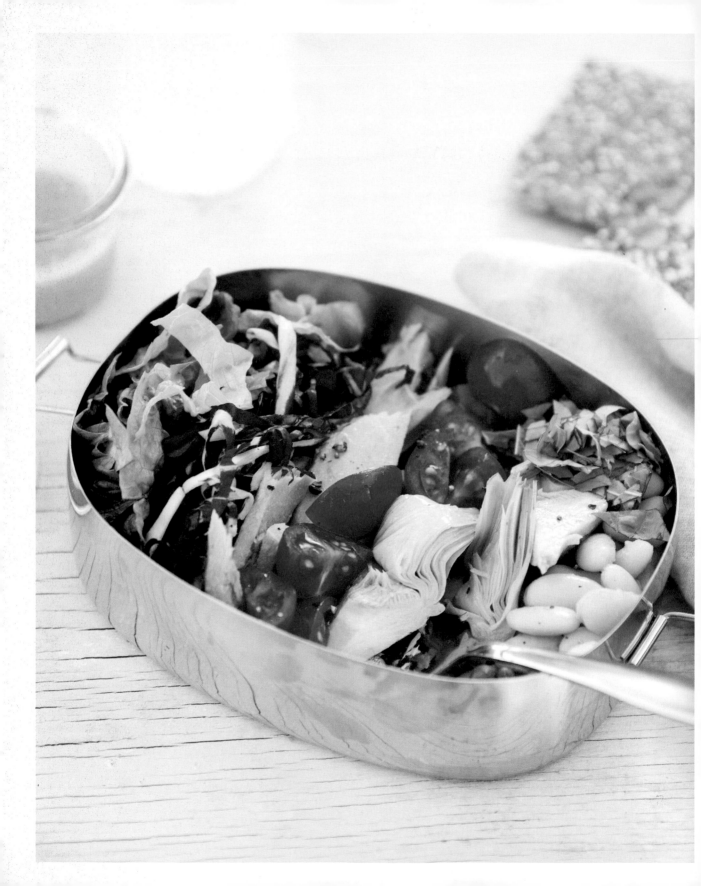

Italian Chopped Salad

We love the salty, briny flavors of anchovy and capers in this colorful, Italian-inspired chopped salad. Since you need only 3 ounces of tuna, use a good jarred brand that can easily be stored in the fridge.

SERVES 1

FOR THE SALAD

½ cup finely chopped romaine

½ cup finely chopped radicchio

⅓ cup canned cannellini beans, drained and rinsed

8 cherry tomatoes, cut in half

1 whole marinated artichoke, quartered or diced depending on preference

3 ounces oil-packed tuna, broken into small pieces

2 oil-packed anchovy fillets, finely chopped, optional

1 tablespoon capers

1 tablespoon chopped fresh basil

FOR THE DRESSING

3 tablespoons extra-virgin olive oil

1 tablespoon red wine vinegar

1 teaspoon Dijon mustard

1 very small clove garlic, grated

Kosher salt and freshly ground black pepper

1. For the salad, carefully arrange all the ingredients in a travel container, trying to keep each one separate.
2. To make the dressing, combine all the ingredients except the salt and pepper in a jar or small Tupperware container and shake to combine; season with salt and pepper to taste.
3. When ready to eat, pour on the dressing and replace the lid. Shake to combine all the ingredients and enjoy.

Mediterranean Chopped Salad

This refreshing, protein-packed salad is killer. To make life easier, consider buying some ingredients, such as the romaine, cucumber, chickpeas, and cooked chicken, from the salad bar.

SERVES 1

FOR THE SALAD

1 cup finely chopped romaine

½ cup finely diced cucumber

⅓ cup canned chickpeas, drained and rinsed

6 thin slices watermelon radish, cut into halves or quarters depending on size

1 grilled chicken cutlet (about ⅓ pound), cooled and diced

1 scallion, thinly sliced

2 tablespoons roughly chopped fresh mint

2 tablespoons roughly chopped fresh cilantro

2 tablespoons roughly chopped fresh flat-leaf parsley

FOR THE DRESSING

2 tablespoons extra-virgin olive oil

1 tablespoon fresh lemon juice

2 teaspoons vegan mayonnaise, such as Vegenaise

1 teaspoon tahini

½ small clove garlic, very finely minced or grated

Kosher salt and freshly ground black pepper

1. To make the salad, carefully arrange all salad ingredients in a travel container, trying to keep each one separate.
2. To make the dressing, combine all the ingredients except the salt and pepper in a jar or small Tupperware container and shake to combine; season with salt and pepper to taste.
3. When ready to eat, pour on the dressing and replace the lid. Shake to combine all the ingredients and enjoy.

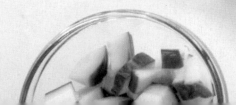

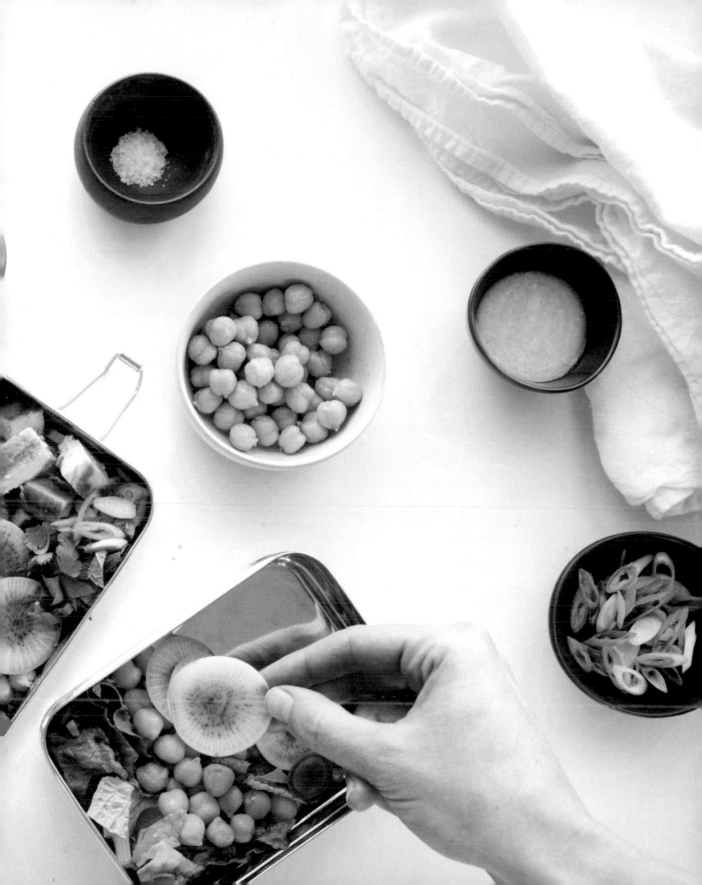

Gut Matters

The cleaner we eat, the better we feel and look. A detox life means less bloating, more energy, and clearer skin, which is usually motivation enough. But we find it helps, too, to understand why this is. So, we're going to go deeper for a minute into the science and biology that support the benefits of a detox life. In other words, if you're not convinced, or if you're wondering why detoxing could be the answer to a beauty concern like inflamed skin, keep reading.

At GOOP, we believe that everything—not just beauty but basic health—begins and ends with the gut: Whether it's in learning to trust our intuition, or pushing toxins out of our system, there's

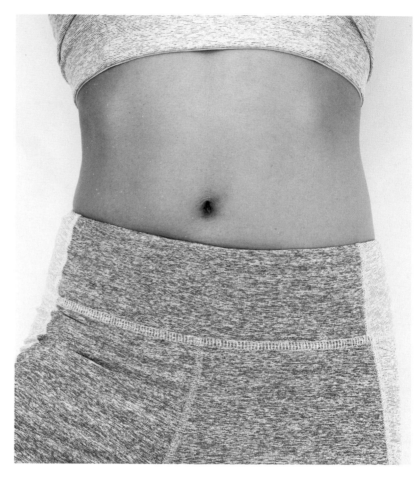

good reason that this nebulous inner system is often called the second brain. As Dr. Alejandro Junger has taught us, the gut is home to a nervous system that is actually physically larger than the one inside our skulls—and holds three-quarters of our immune system tissues. More and more doctors believe that chronic disease is rooted in chronic inflammation—which often begins with our digestive system. And if the gut is off and the body is inflamed, no amount of surface-level beauty tricks are going to make you look or feel good enough.

Although the word *gut* is commonly used as a synonym for the intestines, it's more than our digestive tube. The four major parts of the gut system that affect our health are: the intestinal wall (the lining of the digestive tube); the intestinal flora (the good bacteria that live along the intestinal wall, also called the microbiome); the gut's immune system, or gut-associated lymphatic tissue (GALT); and its nervous system, the small nerve filaments that are spread throughout the gut.

When the gut is healthy, the intestinal wall keeps harmful pathogens and toxins from passing through to the bloodstream while allowing the nutrients we need to get in. Picture the lining as a net with very small holes. There are many elements that can cause this net to break, and several of the more alarming threats (some of which we've already touched on) have been multiplying. For instance, exposure to toxins (mercury, pesticides, BPA, and so on), antibiotic overuse, and sugar consumption can all irritate the gut lining, along with stress, infections, alcohol (sigh), and gluten (but of course you already knew that). This irritation can cause actual holes in the wall, which is known (simply but unpleasantly) as *leaky gut*, which makes it possible for undigested food particles and other foreign organisms to pass through the intestinal lining. This impairs the functioning of the gut's immune system and nervous system, leading to a host of unwanted side effects, ranging from food allergies and sensitivities, to un-fun symptoms like indigestion, bloating, and inflammatory skin conditions, as well as more serious health concerns.

The leaky gut process, as we at GOOP have come to understand via Dr. Junger, is too complex for us to examine every mechanism and possible outcome, but it's also entirely logical when you begin to break it down. For one, when the gut lining (and intestinal flora) is compromised, the GALT becomes vulnerable to an increased number of organisms, undigested food, and toxins—all foreign particles as far as the body is concerned. And the GALT springs to action to attack the foreign particles. (Which, again, could be food, like milk, pasta, soy.) If the gut's immune system is incessantly under siege, we experience the responses of our hyperactive GALT as "mistakes," as Dr. Junger puts it. And we think his analogy for explaining why is perfect: "If you were able to isolate all the cells of the GALT and bulk them together, they would produce a mass larger than one of your quadriceps,

the biggest muscles in your body. Imagine how exhausted you would feel if you had a disease that forced your quads to constantly contract."

In the case of the hyperactive GALT, the "mistakes" often manifest as vague symptoms whose causes can be tricky to pinpoint: fatigue, allergies, sneezing, mucus secretion, itchiness, coughing. (For instance, over time, your body may have decided that cheese, sadly, is a foreign invader, tagged it with antibodies, and now, whenever you overdo it on the cheese platter, your immune system responds with inflammation.)

Autoimmune disorders are also associated with leaky gut. It's another complex relationship, but on a basic level here's how it works: With an autoimmune disease, the immune system becomes confused and is unable to identify what is part of the body and what is not, so it attacks not just foreign cells, but also its own cells. And as Dr. Junger has found with his patients, this confusion often occurs in the gut—when the gut is leaky and the GALT is at risk. If you feel off or look unwell and don't understand why, cleaning up the gut will paint a much clearer picture of what's going on (and it might solve the problem in and of itself).

The gut's nervous system performs different functions from its immune system—mainly sending and receiving information to and from the neurons in the gut; taking care of peristalsis (contractions of the muscles within the intestinal tube) and digestion; as well as coordinating hormonal responses and signals to and from the GALT and the rest of the body's immune system. But like the GALT, the gut's nervous system is similarly bombarded by leaky gut—instead of being able to do all its many important jobs, the gut's nervous system must concentrate on the urgent tasks of coordinating the responses of the immune system.

Again, the effects on our bodies vary, but none are desirable. Often, constipation occurs because the gut's nervous system isn't able to send out the typical signals to move the bowels (peristalsis). Another problem: The neurons in the gut's nervous system are not able to function properly when the gut is unwell, because they lack the nutrients (e.g., B vitamins, magnesium, calcium, potassium) needed for neurotransmitter production (essential to neuron communication). As a result, as outlined by Dr. Junger, we can experience mood swings, anxiety, brain fog, and so on.

We've all been plagued by a case of brain fog and we're not fans of any of the other symptoms of leaky gut. So we've culled some of the best and easiest ways to repair the gut lining and promote gut health, which has a far-reaching impact on every component of our body and health, as well as, in turn, the way we look in the mirror. These are all Dr. Junger–approved and tested:

- Reduce the amount of gluten you consume— whether or not you are celiac or intolerant. Gluten causes the body to produce increased amounts of the molecule zonulin, which controls the open- ing and closing of junctions in the intestinal wall. Although we need zonulin, if there is too much of the molecule in our system, the intestinal wall will be open too wide or too often—leaky gut.

- Get more of the nutrients that the cells of the intestinal wall need to rebuild and repair. Dr. Junger has identified two of the most important ones: L-glutamine and butyrate. L-glutamine, which supports cellular production, is found in its highest concentrations in grass-fed beef, bison, chicken, and free-range eggs. As for vegetables, you can find it in red cabbage and parsley—and in oats. And you'll find it in high concentrations in dairy prod-

ucts (e.g., milk, yogurt, cottage cheese)—obviously less useful if you're one of many for whom dairy is problematic. Butyrate, a fatty acid, is actually produced by our intestinal flora—using indigestible fiber (e.g., cellulose and pectin) that we consume in fruits, vegetables, sweet potatoes, grains, beans, and nuts.

- If/when possible (it isn't always), avoid potential threats to the intestinal flora—the health of the intestinal flora is key to the strength of the gut lining, and these beneficial bacteria help protect our immune system against invaders, and help with food digestion and B vitamin absorption, as well as with detoxification as it gets rid of 40 percent of the toxins in food. The list of threats to the intestinal flora, as outlined by Dr. Junger, includes: C-sections (baby is not exposed to bacteria in the birth canal, which serves as a natural vaccine), antibiotics (more on page 62), chlorinated water (get shower and water filters), chemicals and food preservatives, and organisms like yeast fungus and parasites.

- To support the intestinal flora, consider taking a multi-strain probiotic and incorporate fermented foods (like kimchi and sauerkraut) into your diet. Many of the beneficial bacteria we're referring to in the gut are lactic acid–producing bacteria (like lactobacillus and bifidobacteria), which fermented foods are rich in.

- Find out what your personal trigger foods are— maybe you do well with dairy and nightshades, but gluten is tough on your body—and consume less of them. Dr. Junger has deemed foods that cause indigestion, inflammation, bloating, fatigue, and other ailments *toxic triggers*. The best way to dis- cover what is most troubling to your gut and health is to test them through diet—again, this is where a set, clean-slate detox is very handy.

Below, Dr. Junger answers some more of our questions.

Dr. Alejandro Junger
ON THE GUT

What does gut health boil down to?
It is very hard to boil down gut health since it is the most complex system in the body. It processes food, absorbs it, eliminates toxins, regulates mood, hosts around 70 percent of our immune system, and holds a nervous system that is larger than the one inside our skulls. If you consider what most often and most commonly goes wrong for the majority of people, it becomes a little simpler. The integrity of the gut lining and the health of the intestinal flora are the two Achilles' heels of the gut. Their breakdown is at the root of so many of the chronic health issues that we are dealing with today and only just now beginning to understand.

How can you tell if you might have an unhealthy gut or perforated lining?
An unhealthy, perforated gut lining (more commonly known as a leaky gut) can lead to so many different symptoms, from really subtle to devastating. Also, more and more chronic diseases that until now were thought to be independent are being linked to a leaky gut, such as asthma, eczema, arthritis, and many other inflammatory diseases. Clinically, it is not that easy to diagnose a leaky gut. The best way would be to eliminate most foods that are known to be toxic triggers and then reintroduce them, closely observing if any symptoms flare up with specific foods. But even then, these flare-ups may be related to other problems than a perforated gut.

There is a test for leaky gut that involves consuming different sugars that would normally *not* be absorbed through the gut, and then later measuring their presence in the blood or the urine. These tests are getting more popular by the day.

In your experience, do a lot of people have at least one food sensitivity that aggravates the gut, or is it not as common as popular culture would have us believe?
The subject of food sensitivities and food allergies is somewhat confusing. Lots of people get tested for food allergies these days. I have found that these tests mostly add to the confusion because they exclusively measure "allergic reaction components in the blood," such as immunoglobulins—but not all food sensitivities are caused by problems of "allergic reactions." It is my experience that most people have one or more foods that affect them negatively when consumed, and it is evident when they stop eating them. (I call them *toxic triggers* since they initiate some kind of negative cause and effect.) This is one of the tools that I use the most: an elimination diet for 2 or more weeks, and then one-by-one reintroduction of the potential trigger foods. I have yet to find one person who does not benefit in some way or another from eliminating one or more of these foods, but it is a very individual matter. And it needs the process of investigation.

We're aware that inflammatory foods and poor digestion have a wide range of effects on our bodies—including our skin. Why does this happen, and how does it manifest?
Within and around our intestines is the majority of our immune system and a massive nervous system (our second brain). When the different components of the gut get disrupted—such as the intestinal flora, the intestinal wall, the immune system, and the nervous system—the survival and adaptation mechanisms that are triggered in an attempt to compensate can have an impact on every cell of our body. The skin particularly reflects gut health. The lining of the intestine is similar to the skin covering our body, and there are immune system cells below our skin as well. Problems in the gut tend to show up in the skin because in

a way they are an extension of each other. In our mouth, our nose, and anus, the outside skin just turns inward into intestinal lining. They are continuous.

When our body is busy adapting and surviving, a lot of energy and resources are directed toward these functions, taking away from basic functions that are not considered immediately essential by the body. The body's wisdom continuously sacrifices certain things for others. When this becomes chronic, different organs and systems are negatively affected and can fail, potentially leading to almost any possible disease that we know of.

The Truth About Antibiotics

The antibiotics issue is pretty much out in the open now. While antibiotics are sometimes absolutely necessary, a lot of doctors are bringing awareness to the personal health and societal dangers that are associated with their overuse. (As one of our doctors told us on a recent sick visit: "When it comes to antibiotics, less is more.") Many, like Dr. Junger, argue that antibiotics are still prescribed and taken excessively. What's the big deal? In a nutshell:

One, antibiotics attack our intestinal flora—the good bacteria that line the wall of the intestines.

And, two—bigger picture—the overuse of antibiotics has contributed to a dangerous and pervasive level of antibiotic resistance, when bacteria change so that the antibiotics that once effectively treated an infection no longer work. According to the Centers for Disease Control and Prevention, every year at least two million people in the U.S. become infected with antibiotic-resistant bacteria. And at least 23,000 people die because of these infections. A more specific, but global, example: The World Health Organization (WHO) has reported that resistance to antibiotics used to treat life-threatening hospital-acquired infections (pneumonia, bloodstream infections, infections in newborns and ICU patients) has spread to all regions of the world. And (also reported via WHO) resistance to one of the most commonly used antibiotics for urinary tract infections is "very widespread." We've largely demolished what was once a powerful weapon—and as a result, as WHO alarmingly puts it, we are all at serious risk.

To address this, it's crucial that antibiotics be used only when necessary—and, again, sometimes they certainly are—and that they be taken properly. Antibiotics are meant to treat infections; they should not be used when no infection is present—so, not for when you have the flu (caused by a virus). And if you are taking an antibiotic, you should finish the full prescription; don't stop as soon as you feel better.

To further address the effect antibiotics have on our gut, here's Dr. Junger again:

Dr. Alejandro Junger
ON INTESTINAL FLORA

How do antibiotics compromise our intestinal flora and, ultimately, our health?
Antibiotics kill bacteria—and the intestinal flora is bacteria. Antibiotics can decimate our flora and lead to all kinds of health issues. Antibiotics can be lifesaving and they are incredibly useful in many situations. The problem is that we are prescribing them too often and without much thought, leading to two main problems: In the short term, we negatively affect the intestinal flora. In the long term, we create antibiotic-resistant bacteria, which one day may become an insurmountable problem.

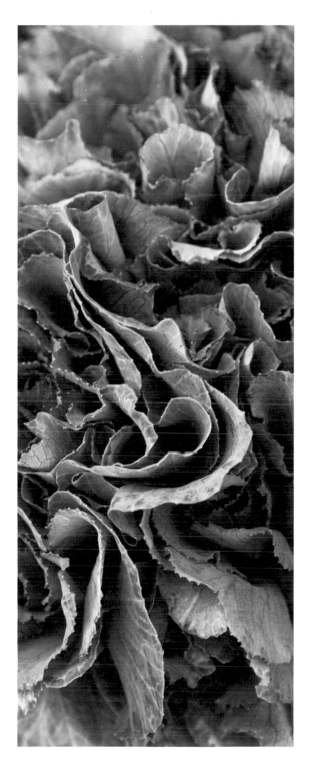

After taking antibiotics, is it possible to mitigate their effect on the intestinal flora?

Depending on the person, age, diet, constitution, and the antibiotic used, the damage can be permanent. For most people, though, it is possible to restore a good flora with probiotics during and after antibiotic use.

If You Remember Anything from This Chapter, Remember These Points

Gut matters. A lot of what ails us on the inside and out is related to problems in our gut. So be good to it. Eat less of what bugs it (e.g., gluten) and more of what's best for it (e.g., fermented foods).

The detox diet rules aren't necessarily easy to follow (almond latte withdrawal, anyone?), but clean eating can be simple and satisfying—and make you feel and look pretty brand-new. And though it's not realistic for most of us to follow the detox rules compulsively outside of a set cleanse, our bodies can still reap some serious rewards even if we're not religious about it—the "cleaner" our everyday diet, the better. So while it feels good to eat well, don't bang yourself up over the slip-ups—that never feels good.

The pursuit of beauty—in all its many forms—begins with detox lifestyle changes that work their magic internally first. Clean eating is number one on the list. When we're eating well, we're better prepared to tackle some of the environmental factors that can set us back, as well as the stress from everyday life. And it all reflects in the mirror, by way of more lustrous hair and foundational, glowing skin that needs little in the way of makeup.

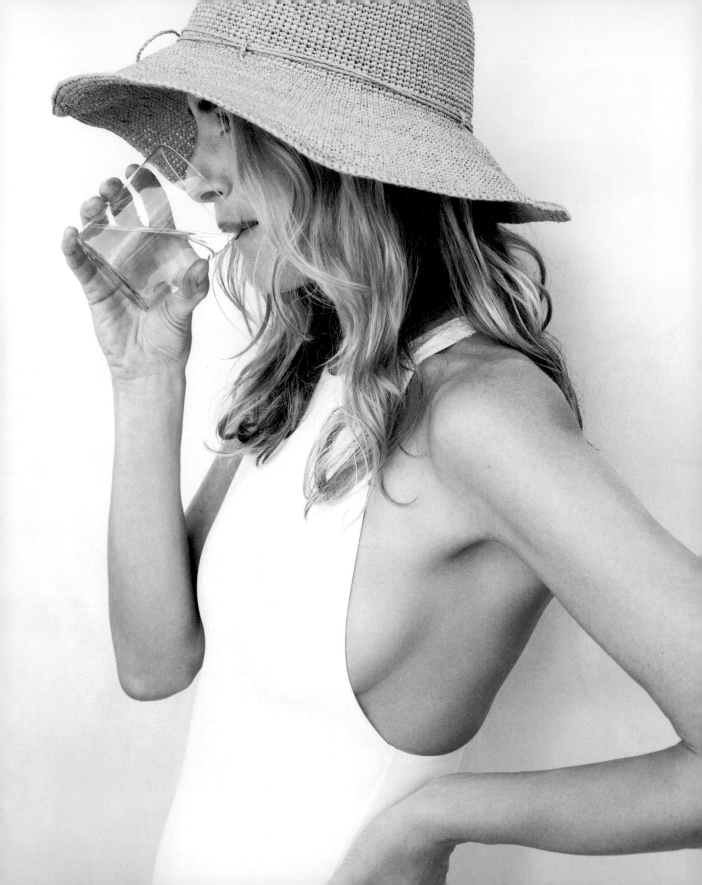

2.
Next-Level Detoxing

What Actually Works

While clean eating is the main pillar of detox, there are other ways to speed the process along. One great resource on what works—and what absolutely doesn't—is environmental thought leader Bruce Lourie, who has not only studied and researched every detox method under the sun, but also personally tried them. He details his detox experiences with great humor with his environmentalist co-author, Rick Smith, in *Toxin Toxout: Getting Harmful Chemicals Out of Our Bodies and Our World*. The ionic footbath, FYI, didn't work, but the good news is that other things did. Although the duo had never detoxed before, and approached the whole concept with skepticism, they scientifically prove throughout the book that it is possible to speed up detoxification—that it's not just mumbo jumbo and marketing money—and that the benefits of doing things that actually work are worth it.

What is most meaningful when it comes to detoxing? Beyond avoiding toxins (which, again, we'll talk more about later) and eating well (with an emphasis on whole, unprocessed foods, and

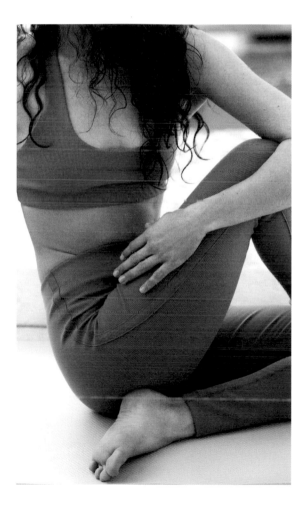

vegetables in particular, which we've already begun to cover), the duo boiled it down to this:

- Drink a lot of water: This is essential for flushing the liver and kidneys, our primary detox organs.
- Sweat as much as possible: Turns out that we sweat out toxic plastics, for one, and that some chemicals are actually easiest to sweat out (as opposed to eliminating through urine). Exercise is a great place to start, as are infrared saunas.
- Burn and avoid fat: Most of the synthetic chemicals and toxins that Lourie has shown to be the most worrisome are *lipophilic,* which means they are attracted to fat. This is problematic for two reasons. First, the more animal fat we consume, the more toxins we're consuming that they were, themselves, storing. And the more fat we hold and store in our own bodies, the more places there are for fat-seeking chemicals to live. These toxins hang out in our fat until we burn it off.

HELLO, SAUNA

The idea of sweating inside a heated space has been around since ancient times, popular across cultures from the Greeks to the Native Americans. It's a cleansing ritual that's been scientifically proven to be effective: As Lourie found, we sweat out plastic toxins in the sauna, and it's also been proven to help with heavy metal detoxification. To name a few more bonuses, sauna sessions have been shown to have positive effects on endorphin levels, musculoskeletal ailments, blood flow, and the immune system's cell activity. And, by the way, we swear that it makes our skin clearer, fresher looking, and dewier. Dr. Junger likes to get in an infrared sauna every day until he breaks a sweat—sometimes for less than 15 minutes, with a few

longer sessions (30 minutes, three to four times a week) thrown in for good measure. The golden rule: Do it as often as you can.

What is an infrared sauna? In the spectrum of light, the infrared band is the one we feel as heat. That may sound otherworldly, but our bodies naturally give off and receive infrared heat. Whereas traditional saunas warm us by heating the air, infrared saunas heat the body more directly and they do it using light. Not entirely unlike the sun, but minus the unwanted side effects of solar radiation. Compared to regular saunas, an infrared sauna penetrates the skin up to three inches, which is big for burning fat—this is nice when it comes to weight loss, particularly because we know that toxins are linked to fat. Another plus of infrared saunas over regular saunas is that you sweat at a lower temperature in an infrared sauna, so if you are typically bothered by the heat in a sauna, infrared is a good choice. If you don't have access, a traditional sauna will do the trick, too.

WORKING IT OUT

There's no mystery as to why exercise is on this list—as they say, sitting is the new smoking. Beyond the rush of endorphins exercise releases—which can make any day infinitely better—it tends to be the root of all good habits and a litmus test for how we intend to treat our bodies. While all exercise is good—even just taking 10 minutes during the day for a walk—anything that involves sweating and a little bit of jumping speeds detox.

Besides the sauna-like situation you can create on any treadmill, exercise burns fat, which in turn releases all those lipophilic (i.e., fat-loving) toxins. Meanwhile, you also want to get the lymphatic system going—which you can do via exercise.

The lymphatic system moves lymph back into the bloodstream, and also supports the immune system by filtering out toxins and other foreign elements. To stay healthy, and look our best, we need to keep this system moving.

Below, our primary exercise guru, Tracy Anderson, explains how to maximize the detox-boosting benefits of exercise, along with all the other bonuses, like younger-looking skin.

Tracy Anderson
ON GETTING PHYSICAL

What's the best kind of exercise for us, and how much should we be doing?
There isn't an absolute one-size-fits-all answer to this. Every body has different imbalances, and you want the exercise you're doing to help bring the body into balance. Cardio, for a multitude of reasons, is extremely important. High-performance cardio—like my dance aerobics program, which doesn't just fire the same muscles over and over again but promotes balance—incorporates calorie burn, coordination, focus, and mental connection. Your brain is actively participating, and your healthy muscle mass is being strengthened as your body burns fat. For the best payoff, combine cardio with muscular structure work (e.g., lifting weights).

I know it isn't always possible to exercise for a full hour, but if you can, I recommend 30 minutes of cardio and 30 minutes of muscular structure work. If you only have half an hour, focus on just one. As for how many times a week... my general rule is usually not a super-welcome one. But if you want to get great results, you have to put in the time—working out isn't magic. Although it can be fun, it *is* work. So, I suggest working out four to seven days a week—with six days seeming to be a sweet spot.

goop TIP

If you happen to be in a position where you can install a personal sauna, keep in mind that infra-red saunas tend to be smaller than regular ones, easier to install, and less expensive. Just be sure to take a look at the materials the sauna is made from—some have hidden toxins and allergens in their wood and/or glue. We like Clearlight's Essential Nordic Spruce models.

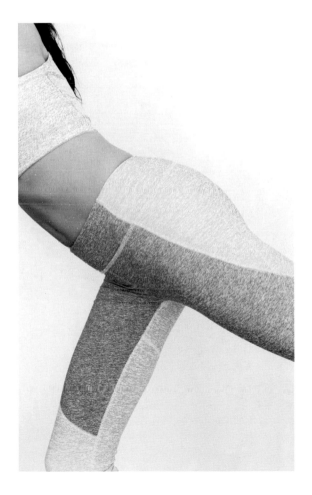

How does exercise (and rebounding, i.e., exercising on a mini trampoline, which we know you're a fan of) stimulate the lymphatic system?

The lymphatic system is complex, and it sits between two incredibly vital parts of our bodies: our blood circulation and our immune system. On a basic level, this is what the lymphatic system is responsible for: For every passage that blood makes through the body (heart to arteries to capillaries to veins and back to the heart), 1 percent of the fluid's volume essentially escapes—it leaves through the capillaries and cannot get back to the vein again. And it's the lymphatic system that picks up the fluid and brings it back to the heart while also filtering out what the body considers foreign (i.e., toxins).

Our lymphatic system works through movement: Gravity, breath, daily activity, even sometimes the touch of someone else can stimulate it. Exercise, though, keeps the system functioning optimally to fight disease, as well as maintain a healthy weight. (Someone who doesn't exercise much but doesn't seem to have pounds to lose may still be carrying too much "toxic weight.") So, the simple solution is to keep moving—all exercise benefits the lymphatic system.

One particularly great form of exercise for supporting healthy circulation is rebounding: jumping on a mini trampoline. And this goes double for anyone who struggles with back/knee/ankle/feet/fatigue issues, as rebounding has a much lower impact on the joints. Rebounding increases blood and oxygen flow as well as bone mass, improves muscle and skin tone, and the coordination involved promotes a strong brain/body connection.

Why do you recommend working out in heat?

The basics of exercise and lymphatic stimulation are simple, but optimization comes from adding X factors like heat and humidity. When your body is put in heat, our built-in thermoregulating system is challenged, and more systems are called into action, including the brain. At the same

time, we're sweating and our muscles become warm, which means we have an enhanced ability to sculpt them, and in a gentler way. So the heat and humidity isn't for weight loss or detoxification specifically—it's about creating a habitat that allows you to best work your body and brain.

goop PICKS

It's no secret that the GOOP staffers are huge fans of the Tracy Anderson Method. (Anderson is GP's business partner and a big part of the reason she's in such good shape.) If you haven't been to one of her dance cardio classes yet—go. She has studios in New York (City and State), LA, London, and a live streaming service—for details, check out tracyanderson.com.

TA classes—both cardio and "muscular structure"—are really our tried-and-true, but a few of us like to experiment with other workouts, too. For one, see the Q&A with Taryn Toomey of The Class on page 75. Our beauty buyer, Ivy Benavente, likes intenSati (developed by Patricia Moreno), which combines empowering affirmations with exercise (interval training, martial arts, dance, yoga). It's sort of like choreography to spoken poems with lots of team energy. Our beauty director, Jean Godfrey-June, swears by Jivamukti yoga, which combines a vigorous practice with mind-focusing meditation and mood-elevating chanting.

As we age, why is exercise increasingly important?

Exercising is the key to delaying the effects of aging and increasing our beauty span. Women are often surprised to hear that our muscle decreases by about 1 percent each year beginning at around the ripe old age of...thirty! Dynamic workouts that engage a variety of muscle groups in different ways, as well as the mind, keep us strong without wearing down our joints. Exercise also supports our bone structure as we lose density. It helps us process hormonal shifts and changes; and it supports our immune system so we can recover faster from injuries and illness. And exercise is so important for our mental health—for feeling in control and connected, comfortable, happy, and confident in our bodies.

When you think you are too old to exercise is the time when it's most important that you do. Whether you are forty, fifty, or older, it is imperative that you continue to move your entire body, creating healthy challenges for your muscles and brain.

More specifically, what can exercise do for our skin, and what impact does it have on skin elasticity?

To keep the skin tight, we need to exercise, which allows us to maintain a strong, healthy muscle design. Without exercise, as we age our skin can become disconnected from our muscles because our connective tissue doesn't have anything to pull the skin tight to, which results in skin that looks thinner and weaker. Another reason it's beyond vital to exercise as you get older: Our production of collagen—the main protein in connective tissue—decreases with age and as a result of poor circulation. We're going to get older whether we like it or not, but by exercising and increasing circulation, we can look fresher and healthier for much longer.

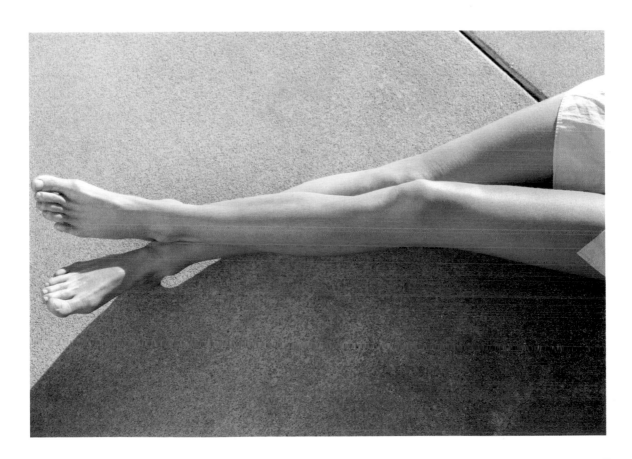

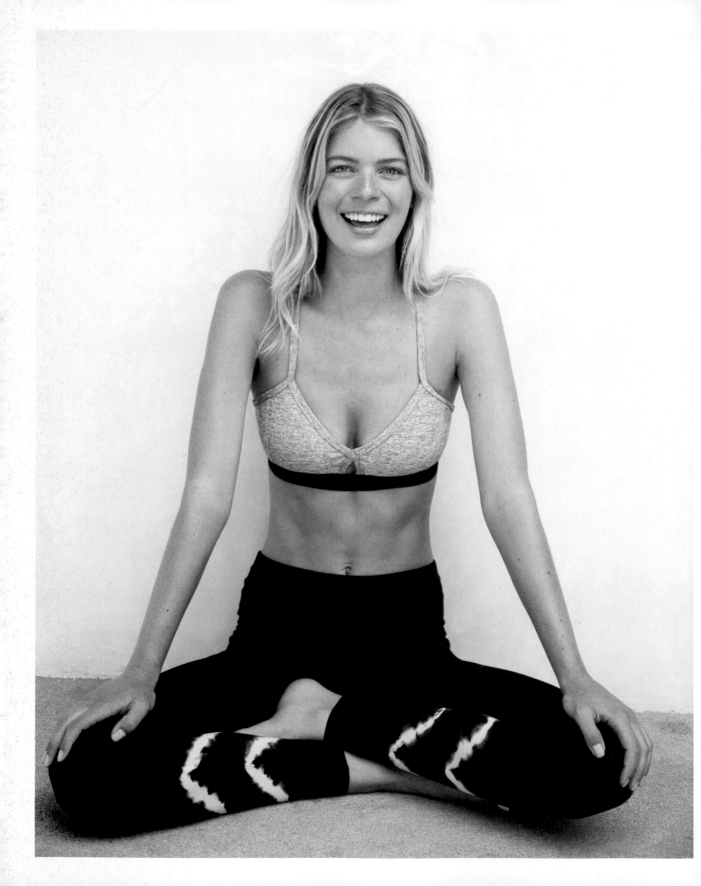

A great complement to more traditionally "active" exercise, yoga also has amazing detox side effects. We asked favorite yoga authority, Eddie Stern, director and co-founder with his wife of Ashtanga Yoga New York, how to get the best results.

Eddie Stern
ON YOGA'S FORCE

What kind of effects can yoga have on the body?
The effects of yoga on our bodies are amazingly varied. Recent studies have shown that a regular practice of yoga—even in modest amounts—may help to lower blood pressure; reduce back pain; reduce symptoms of PTSD; reduce occurrences of asthma attacks; improve posture, strength, and coordination; improve breathing and cardio-vascular health; support self-regulation in children, and so on. It's remarkable that one simple practice can have such a wide range of effects—yet, it does.

The premise of yoga is quite straightforward: By moving, breathing, and concentrating the mind in a particular way, we will bring our body, nervous system, and mind all into a unified state. One of the meanings of *yoga*, after all, is "union"—that special time when all things come together. Another meaning is "concentration." Concentration indicates that yoga is a practice—the practice, in fact, of learning how to pay attention. Whether it is in meditation, being in the zone with a physical or work activity, or listening to our partner or children, there is a linkage, a sameness, and most importantly, a full and complete presence to that which is in front of us.

So, what does this have to do with our bodies? Well, our bodies are the homes that we live in. The philosophical systems of both yoga and Western philosophers like Aristotle held that our body is the home of our soul, and that one cannot exist without the other. The words *psyche* and *spirit* both come from the root words in Greek and Latin that mean "breath," and it is through our breath that our lives are maintained. When the breath leaves our body, life is finished. So the first hint to how we can nourish our bodies is through proper breathing and paying attention to our breath, whether through breathing practices or observing the breath in meditation. Fully breathing periodically throughout the day will refresh our energy levels, refocus the mind, and reduce stress.

The ancient yogis presented the idea that we have not just one body, but three. The first is our physical body, made up of the food we eat and water we drink. The physical body can be strengthened, stretched, molded, and changed through diet and exercise. The second body is called the subtle body, and it is made up of breath, the mind, and our intellect. Our mind, according to the yogis, is the seat of thought, emotions, desire, and memory, which differs from our intellect, which is the faculty of discrimination. While in our mind we might desire, say, a doughnut, our intellect will be the one who says, maybe have some raspberries instead. Our intellect lies closer to our sense of self. Our third body is the body of bliss, the bliss of contact with knowing who we really are—our potential, our infinite creativity, our source of being as pure consciousness. Bliss here is not the bliss of a fleeting indulgence, but the unlimited joy of being; something we have all felt when we experience an uncaused joy—when for no reason, we feel inexplicable happiness, contentment, and everything feels okay.

Yoga is a practice that was designed explicitly to address, strengthen, and purify all three bodies: Through postures and clean eating we purify the physical body; through breathing, meditation, and chanting we purify the subtle body; and through service and thinking of others first we purify the body of bliss.

Can yoga (or other lifestyle choices) affect the way we age?
Research over the past thirty years has shown that the practice of yoga and meditation, and clean diet and

lifestyle, can greatly reduce the fraying of telomeres, the part of our DNA that is related to aging.

The telomere is like the plastic cap on the end of a shoelace that prevents the shoelace from fraying, and hence becoming unusable (or hard to get through a lace hole). In actuality, the telomere is a cap at the end of our DNA that protects our chromosomes. The telomere is related to our biological age, and as it frays, or gets shortened, our longevity decreases. Telomeres naturally shorten with age as our cells replicate themselves; however, stress, smoking, poor diet, and lack of exercise have been shown to lead to a quicker shortening of the telomeres. Research by Nobel Prize–winning scientist Elizabeth Blackburn has shown that after four to six months of regular mindfulness practices, the activity of the enzyme that impacts the length of the telomeres, called telomerase, goes up 30 percent, and reduces their rate of decay. (Her book, *The Telomere Effect*, is a great read.)

Our ability to influence our DNA is part of a science called epigenetics. Epigenetics holds that our genetic activity is not completely fixed—our genes do not entirely rule our destiny—and that our genes, which are like on and off switches, turn on or off depending on the environment that we either are exposed to, or expose ourselves to. Epigenetics is primarily related to diet, and adding a healthy dose of methyl-rich food (beets, onions, garlic, and dark, leafy greens such as kale—but not kale chips!) has been shown to have a beneficial effect on gene expression.

Activities that will help strengthen our healthy genetic activity are:

- Exercise
- Meditation
- Loving kindness practices
- Building and engaging in community
- Self-expression

By consciously placing ourselves in a healthy environment, and by doing practices like breathing, yoga, and meditation with regularity, we can increase our baseline response to challenging situations. Our genes will begin to respond to stressful situations in a constructive manner, rather than going into a hyper-stress response. We can't remove excess stress completely from our lives, but we can change our baseline response to it, which will lead to greater physiological and emotional health.

Another important function of our physiology is called *neuroplasticity,* which is a process that happens within our brain whenever we learn something new, whether it's while reading a book or attempting a new pose on the yoga mat. There is a saying in neuroscience that "nerves that fire together, wire together"—each time we learn something, or are introduced to a new idea, our neural axons fire electrical messages seeking dendrites to connect with in order for the brain to understand the new information.

We have more than a hundred billion neural cells in our brain, which have a potential for making more connections than there are stars in the universe. When we speak of having unlimited potential and infinite creativity within us, we can see that within our own physiology this is an actual fact. As babies, when we experience the world around us, our neurons begin to wire together in response to situational needs. As we begin to lift our heads, roll over, crawl, walk, and eventually speak, neurons make the connections that allow us to perform all of those basic functions without having to continually think or remember how to perform them. We make neural connections when we are held, fed, loved, or abandoned. Every human and environmental interaction leaves its mark upon our nervous system.

As we get older, we can maintain our brain health by learning new languages, doing crossword puzzles, reading a variety of books, studying new subjects, learning to cook or play an instrument, exercising, and generally staying active. Sleep, as well, is a very important part of brain health.

When we sleep, the glymphatic system of the brain, which is connected with the glial cells, drains the plaque debris that collects in the brain due to all the thinking and brain activity we have during the day. This is why consistent good nights of sleep truly are refreshing. When we do not sleep enough, our body releases neurotransmitters such as cortisol and adrenaline that under balanced circumstances are flushed from the body without causing excess conditions of inflammation.

If we want to create lasting habits of health, wellness, happiness, and longevity, all we have to do is support the synaptic connections that will fix those habits as part of who we are. How do we do that? Not only by making choices and setting intentions and goals, but also by identifying what is truly important in our lives and making those things our priority, and consciously remembering those priorities when it comes to decision making.

What role does yoga play in detoxification?
Yoga has been traditionally called a practice of inner purification. Through connecting breath and movement in a particular way, we create an inner heat that warms the blood. The warmed blood flows through all of the internal organs and draws out toxins, which are removed via lymph glands and sweat. The breathing along with yoga poses is similar to when we wring out a sponge that is soaked with dirty water from washing dishes; we wring it in one direction, then another, and then all the dirty water and gunk is cleaned out from the sponge, and it's ready to use again. This is the purpose of the technique of *vinyasa*, which means to breathe and move together in a special way, leading to internal purification.

Detoxification in particular refers to the cleansing of the blood by the liver. The liver is a very complicated organ that takes part in an estimated 500 bodily functions, including the breakdown of toxins and metabolism of both proteins and carbohydrates. Yogic breathing, in particular, is a very good detoxification practice, because the

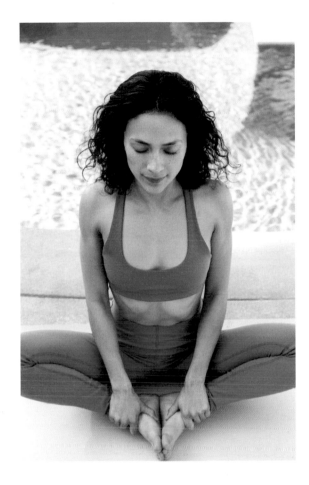

liver literally sits on top of the diaphragm. Every time we inhale and exhale, the liver is getting massaged. For many people who are under stress, whether mild or extreme, the diaphragm begins to tighten, constricting the organs above and below it, like how you feel your chest sometimes gets tight when you are under pressure, yet there are no problems with your heart. When the diaphragm releases, and the breath becomes long, free, and deep, the pressure goes away. The same is true with the liver stress and poor lifestyle choices will impact the liver's ability to perform its natural role as the body's detoxifier. When you combine yoga poses with deep breathing, the purification of the liver is increased, and the benefits are more pronounced.

How often and for how long does someone need to practice yoga in order to really feel and see meaningful change?
The effects of yoga can be felt usually after just one class, but it doesn't last until you make it a regular practice. For meditation, it's recommended to do a little every day; even 5 minutes can be enough to get you started in developing a meditation practice. For yoga, it is the same. You don't need to do a 90-minute class every day, or even three times a week. If you can do 15 to 30 minutes every day, you will begin to build it into a habit—which is, of course, what neuroplasticity is. Practicing yoga or meditation (or both) will eventually become hardwired into our system, and not only does it become easier and easier for us to do, but, when we don't do it, we can tell that we need to address those unseen parts of us: our breath, our spirit, our inner sense of self. As well, that little bit of yoga practice will help you stabilize your metabolism, keep your blood circulation healthy, improve your breathing, focus your mind, and keep your body flexible. Real change will be felt after 3 months of doing just a little every day, and you will come to depend on it, which is a good thing. Those few minutes will be a time for you to reconnect to yourself, to feel calm, centered, and feel that your body, breath, nervous system, and mind are all pulled back together into a state of cooperation and coherence. This indeed is a state of union within us—in our body, breath, and mind; the home within which we live and navigate through the world.

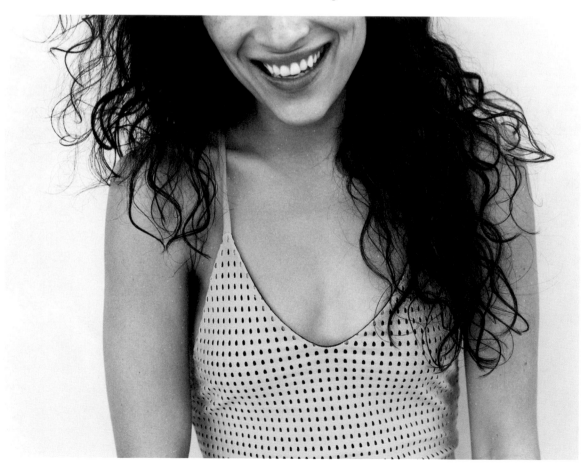

Feeling Stuck?

Admittedly, sometimes, even after a good exercise session or mid-day yoga break, we still feel a bit pent up. For that, there's Taryn Toomey's The Class—an intense, cardio, mind/body experience that has an interesting way of relieving the most stubborn tension. Toomey explains why people come to her find catharsis—and why it's important.

Taryn Toomey
ON KICKING AND SCREAMING

What was the impetus for creating The Class?
After years of "running to yoga," I left my corporate fashion job to pursue yoga teacher training. I taught for many years, but always needed a practice that had more *fire* in it; I needed to move all of the energy, emotion, and residue that had accumulated through my youth. The Class slowly and organically developed from there.

Making noise is a huge part of the practice—yelling, screaming, even crying—why is this so important?
Energy that has been trapped in the body—whether from heartbreak, grief, disappointment, or other negative emotions—needs a vehicle for release. Sound is like a surfboard for that energy; it carries that tension up and out of the body, leaving you with a feeling of relief. Women, especially, are conditioned to be polite, quiet, and nonconfrontational. Think about all the times that you've held in tears or words and lost your voice because you were afraid of upsetting someone else. We like to give people permission to feel. What we offer is a place for people to break some of those societal norms. We give them a place to find raw emotion and let it move.

You talk about undoing layers of emotional trauma and unease through movement and sound—can you explain how this works, and why it is so effective?
What happens to us out there in the world is not just a matter of the brain. You cannot *think* your way out of trauma or heartbreak. It affects us on a cellular level. We hold on to these memories, to feelings, to certain thought patterns—through movement, sound, sweat, tears, all of it, we begin to unwind those holdings. We use the body to access the "storage units" or crevices that the brain doesn't have access to because, again, these layers aren't about *thinking*, they are about *feeling*.

What tends to come up for people who do The Class?
Conversations that people wish they had or *did not* have; memories from childhood; grief; ways of speaking to one's self; thoughts that got stuck on repeat; love lost and gained—it really runs the gamut.

goop TIP

You can take The Class in LA or NYC—visit taryntoomey.com to sign up.

Lessons from
the Body Whisperer

In addition to exercise, you can also stimulate the lymphatic system with a foam roller. If you've ever used a foam roller, you might know that feeling of physically rolling out the day—the way it can release the tension that builds up in our back, neck, and other places after hours of typing, texting, driving, slouching. But the foam roller is a lot more powerful than that—and it happens to be one of the most affordable ways to make a major and noticeable physical difference (whether you're purchasing one to use at home, or using the ones available at your local gym). The benefits of foam rolling are numerous. It can help your lymphatic system get rid of toxins; reduce inflammation, puffiness, *and* cellulite; tighten skin; elongate muscles; and bring the body into alignment.

Structural integrative specialist, fascia expert, and author of *Taller, Slimmer, Younger* Lauren Roxburgh is a master of the foam roller. (At GOOP, she's known as the office body whisperer.) Following, she explains how foam rolling can help detox and improve skin. Plus, she shares a foam roller sequence designed specifically to make you glow.

Lauren Roxburgh
ON FOAM ROLLING TO BRAND-NEW

What exactly is fascia and why is it so important? What does it hold on to, and how does it shape the body?
Fascia is the thin layer of connective tissue that encases your body under your skin like a wetsuit and actually wraps itself around every muscle, joint, and organ. If you've ever cut into a piece of raw chicken or steak and seen that thin, white, filmy layer, then you've seen fascia. Your ligaments are also part of your fascia, so it plays a key role in our structural integrity—in a way it is like the scaffolding of the body. The fascia lies between the skin and the muscles like a web, and it is also where the nerves and the lymph nodes sit—so it has also been called a sensory organ because this is where pain originates and is communicated to the brain.

While fascia is incredibly thin, it plays an important role in the shape, health, and vitality of our bodies. Fascia can store toxins (my orthopedic surgeon friends tell me that when they cut through thickened or "blocked" fascia during surgery, it sometimes actually spurts pus—nasty, right?). Most importantly, it can thicken and harden when it is not used correctly: When you have a stiff shoulder, for example, often it is not damage to the muscle that's causing it, but a hardening or thickening of the fascia around the shoulder muscles and joint.

Poor posture, stress, emotional trauma, poor flexibility, and repetitive movements pull the fascia into ingrained patterns. Adhesions form within the stuck, hard, and blocked fascial tissue like snags in a sweater, and make our bodies feel heavy, thick, uncomfortable, and run down.

The amazing thing about fascia is that it is only now being medically recognized for its importance in maintaining a healthy, fit, toned, calm, and aligned body. In fact, it wasn't until 2007 that the First International Fascia Research Congress was held at Harvard Medical School, bringing a new awareness to the importance of the fascial webbing system.

These days, "myofascial release" has become a bit of a buzzword in the fitness and wellness communities. Medical science is finally catching on that fascia is a major player in every movement you make and every trauma you've experienced, making it largely responsible for "shaping" the body. And the good news is that your fascia is incredibly malleable and has almost ridiculous self-healing abilities—which is where the foam roller comes in! Use a foam roller regularly, even just for 10 minutes a day, and you'll feel better, reduce pain, improve posture and confidence,

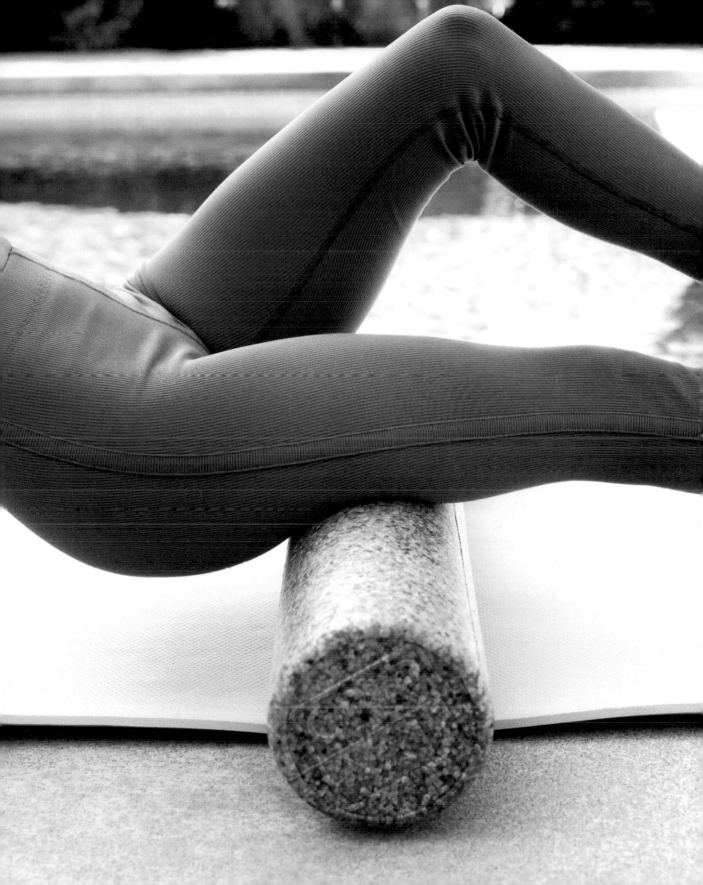

banish cellulite, and reduce stress—all of which will help you both feel and look your best. Once your body is aligned, and you have a full range of motion, you will look, feel, and *be* longer and leaner.

How does foam rolling help the body detox?

Many people turn to radical measures in an effort to detox. Personally I think that torturing yourself with things like extreme juice cleanses is neither fun nor sustainable—and research shows most people put almost all the weight they lose on a cleanse back on within two weeks. The key to detoxing and having a gorgeous glow is maintaining a healthy lymphatic system, reducing inflammation, and boosting circulation. This is where the roller comes in because, like a massage, it helps increase blood flow to your connective tissue and breaks up the areas where toxins become stored within the fascia. The result is your body is able to "flush" those toxins out more efficiently. It facilitates physical and emotional cleansing.

Obviously, ridding your body of toxins is good for health, but how does rolling help you actually *look* better? I called my foam rolling book *Taller, Slimmer, Younger* for a reason. First, aside from its benefits in boosting your lymphatic system, the roller can also help you decompress your joints, align your spine, and activate your core and intrinsic muscles—all of which helps you stand taller and healthier in your own body. In fact many of my clients have gained an inch and a half in height as a result of doing this work.

One of the results of standing taller is that your body effectively narrows out—you may be holding the same weight, but because your posture is more upright, you become longer and leaner—hence you lose a pant size or two.

As far as becoming more youthful, well it's not rocket science to know that the result of holding toxins and blockages within your body as well as living with pain and poor posture are all things that prematurely age us. Because rolling stimulates blood flow, flushes toxins, and

replenishes the body's white blood cells, it actually helps promote a more youthful appearance.

And why is it beneficial for our skin?

As I've outlined, one of the most beneficial things about foam rolling is that it helps detoxify and regenerate the body—and detoxing is one of the best things you can do for your skin. And, because rolling also boosts circulation, it will give your skin a natural glow that no makeup can.

Plus, rolling banishes those pesky dimples that haunt us as we age—the dreaded cellulite. Cellulite occurs when underlying fat pushes through weakened, dry, or brittle fascia. This weakened or imbalanced fascia is caused by gravity, aging, dehydration, lack of movement, and poor muscle tone and/or circulation. But foam rolling rejuvenates the fascia, and strengthens it, meaning that cellulite isn't able to push through to the skin. So foam rolling can not only help your skin get that healthy, glowing look, it can also help get rid of cellulite.

When you add this up, plus the other benefits of foam rolling, such as increasing flexibility and improving muscle tone, you can see why I'm such a fan.

ROXBURGH'S GO-TO BEAUTIFYING FOAM ROLLER SEQUENCE
Benefits of this sequence:

- Helps boost collagen and circulation to the face and improve digestion and elimination.
- Reduces stress levels and decreases inflammation in the body while promoting detoxification.
- Gives you a facelift by incorporating inverted moves, which allows fresh oxygenated blood and nutrient flow to your face.
- Helps fight free radicals, encourages skin cell renewal, and gives a healthy, youthful glow.

Relax and breathe deeply through this practice and you'll see a difference in your complexion when you're done.

Criss-Cross Back Bend

Benefits

- Promotes better blood flow through the neck and face.
- Opens your chest and heart, reduces stress, and rejuvenates skin.
- Increases lung capacity and allows you to breathe more efficiently.
- Increases oxygenated blood circulation to the brain and face.

Sit up tall on your knees with your ankles crossed, knees wide. Place the roller about six inches behind you and press your palms into the roller, thumbs out to the side and chest open. Inhale as you press your palms into the roller to lift up and press your pubic bone forward, gazing up as you lift and open your heart, hips, and neck. Exhale as you release back down to the starting position.

Repeat this movement, alternating which leg is crossed on top, for eight to ten total sets.

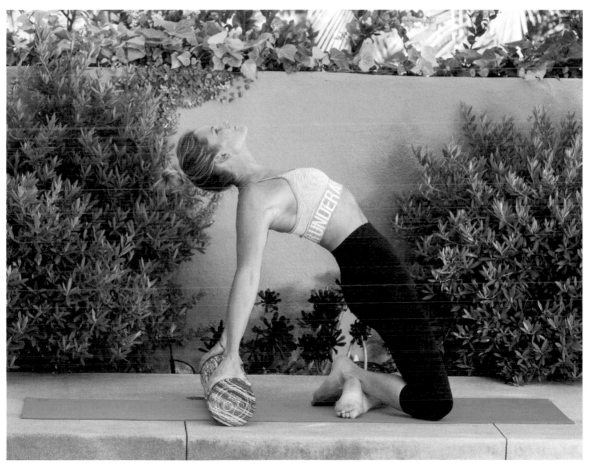

LAUREN ROXBURGH

Inverted Figure Four

Benefits

- Hydrates your connective tissue in your lower back and hips.
- Helps boost collagen and circulation to the face.
- Reduces stress and inflammation to help you glow.
- Inverting the body brings fresh oxygenated and nutrient-rich blood to the face. This also aids sleep.

Lie down on the mat and come to a bridge position, sliding the roller under your hips/sacrum. Hold both ends of the roller to stabilize yourself. Bend and lift your knees, and then cross your right ankle over your left knee, creating an inverted figure four. Keeping the roller stable, inhale as you roll your hips to the right while keeping your ribs and shoulders grounded and stable. Exhale as you come back to the starting position.

Repeat this motion five times on each side, alternating sides.

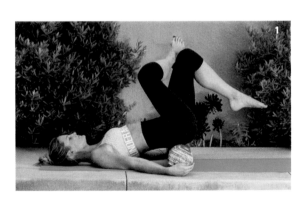

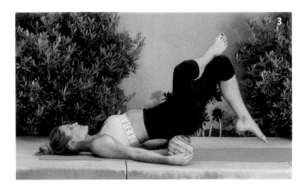

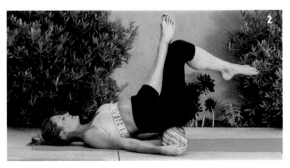

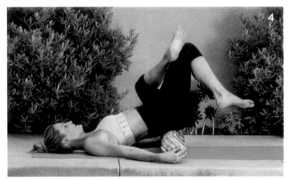

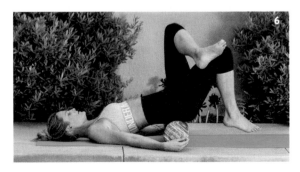

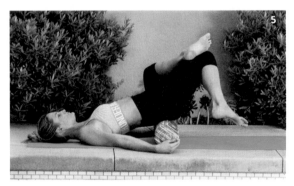

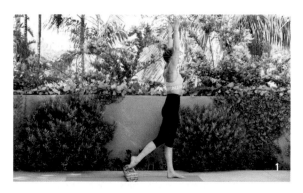

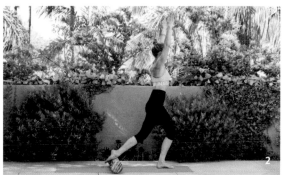

Rolling Lunge

Benefits

- Enhances digestion and elimination.
- Promotes healthy abdominal organ function.
- Balances the pelvis and helps you stand and move in proper alignment.
- Creates length and balanced tone in the abs.
- Helps you calm the nervous system and focus on the present moment.

Stand on your left foot with your left knee slightly bent, and put the top of your right foot on a foam roller behind you with your back leg straight. Raise your arms directly overhead. Inhale as you bend your left knee, keeping the knee over the ankle, and extend your right hip and leg back, pressing into the foam roller as it rolls up your shin until your left thigh is nearly parallel to the floor. Exhale as you use your deep core to pull yourself back up to the starting position.

Repeat this movement eight times on each side.

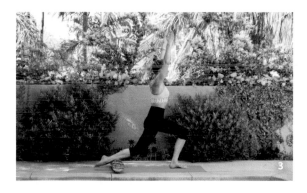

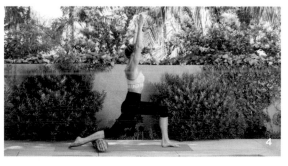

Text-Neck Massage

Benefits

- Melts away tension and stress in the back of the neck.
- Aligns the head and neck into graceful posture.
- Tones the muscles of the neck, face, and throat.

Lie on the roller with your spine supported from your tailbone to the base of your skull (the tight area where your skull meets your neck). Reach your arms long by your sides, with the palms up to open and expand the neck, throat, shoulders, and chest. Inhale deeply as you reach your arms up overhead and exhale as you turn your head to the left, and then inhale as you turn your head to the right.

Repeat this move, turning your head from side to side eight to ten times.

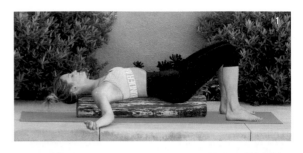

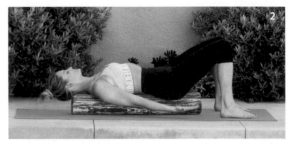

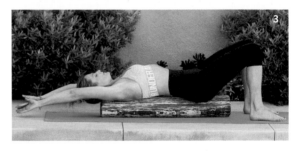

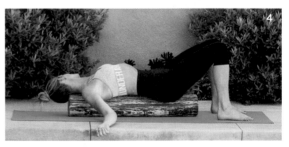

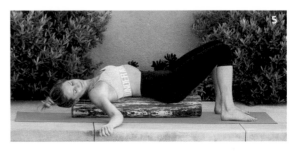

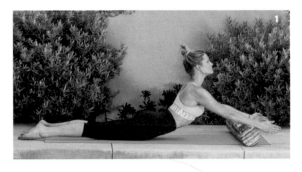

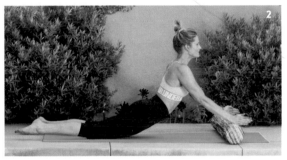

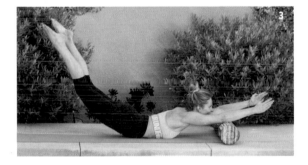

Rolling Swan Dive

Benefits

- Promotes improved digestion.
- Eliminates toxins to improve glow.
- Banishes bloat to flatten the belly.
- Builds strength and sculpts the arms, upper back, booty, and backs of the legs.

Lie belly-down on the mat, with arms stretched in front of you and the roller placed underneath your elbow joints, thumbs facing up. Reach your heels away from your heart to feel oppositional energy and decompress your spine. Inhale and roll the roller toward your wrists, extending the spine and lifting as you roll your shoulders back (taking care to keep your glutes relaxed the entire time so you don't jam your low back while lifting up). Be sure to pull your abs up and in to support your back and elongate the front of your body. Exhale as you quickly dive down and reach your legs up and back behind you.

Repeat this movement eight times.

More Detox Boosters

Two less common detox methods that we've tried are dry brushing and colonics, both of which can be incredibly effective (and perhaps less intimidating than you might think).

DRY BRUSHING

Like foam rolling, dry brushing is a lymphatic system stimulator that we're big fans of. For the ins and outs of the practice we turn to GOOP friend, osteopath, and pain expert, Vicky Vlachonis.

Vicky Vlachonis
ON HOW TO DRY BRUSH

We know that dry brushing is an ancient practice invented in Greece and that it's long been popular in Europe. What's the basis of the practice and why is it still relevant today?

With its 17 square feet of surface area, skin is our largest cleansing organ, akin to our lungs and kidneys. Dry brushing stimulates lymphatic drainage, moving nutrients from the blood into the cells and removing toxins. Your lymphatic system, which is responsible for about 15 percent of the body's circulation, transports white blood cells that help rid the body of toxic materials. Even blockages on the surface of the skin can cause congestion throughout the lymph system, and dry brushing is one of the most effective ways to ensure that the system stays active and clear. Dry brushing can also serve as an emotional release if you're truly present while doing it. As you brush your skin, release all fear, anger, or resentment—any negative emotion at all. Send those harmful thoughts all out of your mind as the dead skin falls from your body.

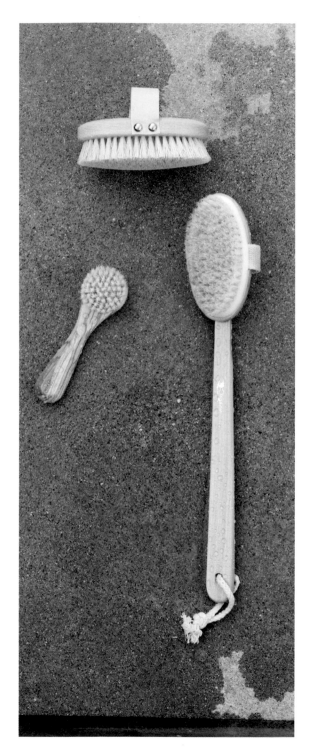

Beyond its effect on the lymphatic system, does dry brushing have any additional benefits?

When you dry brush, you increase your circulation and shed dead skin cells. Another beautiful bonus: Brushing stimulates the production of collagen and elastin fibers, which help support skin as it ages. (But please note: Never do dry brushing on your face; instead, use a wet, soft loofah with some facial cleanser.) I find that dry brushing wakes up my skin and my psyche in ways almost nothing else does!

How do you do it?

1. Start with a natural bristled brush specifically designed for dry brushing. Be warned: Your skin may be very sensitive to dry brushing at first, so go gently.

2. Work the brush in circular movements, starting with the soles of your feet, working upward, and always in the direction of your heart. (When stimulating circulation and the lymph system, you always want to be brushing in the direction of venous and lymphatic flow.) Proceed in the order below.
   - Soles of feet
   - Tops of feet
   - Calves
   - Thighs

3. Now move to the back. Remember to brush in the direction of the heart, alternating sides, in the order below.
   - Buttocks
   - Lower back
   - Sides
   - Lower abdomen
   - Upper abdomen
   - Chest (in a figure 8 motion)
   - Upper back

4. Stop there, and then start on your arms.
   - Fingers
   - Palms
   - Backs of hands
   - Forearms
   - Elbows
   - Upper arms

5. Once you're done, your skin should feel soft and alive and ready for a shower.

6. Visualize any negative feelings being washed away, circling down the drain. After your shower, do a self-massage with oil or cream. You can treat your shower as a mini meditation to prepare your mind for the day.

ARE COLONICS A GOOD IDEA?

Colonics are one of the most debated detox methods. Simply put, during a colonic, your colon—the approximately five-foot long, final segment of your digestive tube—is filled with water and then flushed out repeatedly, with the goal of leaving it fully hydrated and clean. The colon is naturally responsible for both important absorption and elimination in the body. It's the last place where nutrients and water from food are absorbed into our circulation, and it gets rid of what is not absorbed of the foods we eat, as well as bloodstream waste, sending it all out with the feces. Some argue that colonics are necessary to assist with this elimination process because the colon is overloaded with modern-day toxins, but others maintain that the colon is naturally capable of cleansing itself and that colonics can cause damage. Dr. Junger explains.

LOSING YOUR C-CARD

While there are colonic virgins at GOOP, we also have some tepid fans as well as hard-core enthusiasts. Some staffers get a colonic after every flight, and in advance of every detox, while others make it more of an annual or very-special-occasion event if faced with extreme constipation. It sounds way worse than it actually is. There are different types—gravity colonics can be more intense, while a closed loop system is very gentle. You will lie on your side, covered up, and insert a tube up your butt (yep), and then a technician will slowly fill your colon with warm water. When you hit capacity, they reverse the flow and you start to actually see (through the glass) as waste begins to leave your system. Much of it is mucus, and not that visible. After a colonic (they last about 30 minutes), you might leak a little water, though we've never heard of anyone having an actual accident. Some people feel slightly better post-colonic, while others feel incredibly relieved.

Dr. Alejandro Junger
ON COLONICS

Is the colon able to cleanse itself or do we need colonics?
Of course our colon can clean itself. It is designed for that, and it really works well when the right conditions exist. The problem is that most of us create the wrong conditions inside and outside of our colons, and the self-cleansing ability of the colon is something that is affected early on. Stress, processed foods with lack of fiber or excess simple carbohydrates, foods with antibiotics and other chemicals, dehydration, lack of exercise or simple movement, magnesium depletion, artificial sweeteners, and a host of common medications are some of the factors that have most people walking around constipated.

I see articles by closed-minded physicians and other health care practitioners criticizing colonics, saying that the body knows what to do and does not need any help. But they are only correct if they are talking about colons that are functioning the way they were designed to, which means that the people who own them are living in the way that they were designed to live, nature's way. This is not the case for people living a modern life. In these cases, colonics become a very useful tool to correct many of these dysfunctions.

You've told us in the past that most of our intestinal flora—trillions of bacteria that support detoxification, digestion, immune system regulation, etc.—lives in the colon. What keeps these bacteria working? How does a colonic affect our intestinal flora?
There is a growing awareness of the many benefits of a healthy intestinal flora, now referred to as the microbiome. These bacteria live in our intestines and thrive when the right conditions exist. They pay rent by helping us digest food, detoxify, train the immune system, regulate the nervous system, and defend us against other invaders. For the reasons mentioned above, most of us have an unbalanced flora. Constipation does not help, and the lack of elimination keeps toxic waste lingering in our intestines, further damaging the intestinal flora.

A colonic is a way to begin to correct this situation. Yes, if things were functioning normally, and the intestinal flora was healthy, a colonic may wash a lot of these bacteria away. But if our colon is backed with waste, getting it out will wash away bad bacteria and will improve the conditions for the good ones to reproduce and colonize the large intestine. Taking probiotics (or food for bacteria),

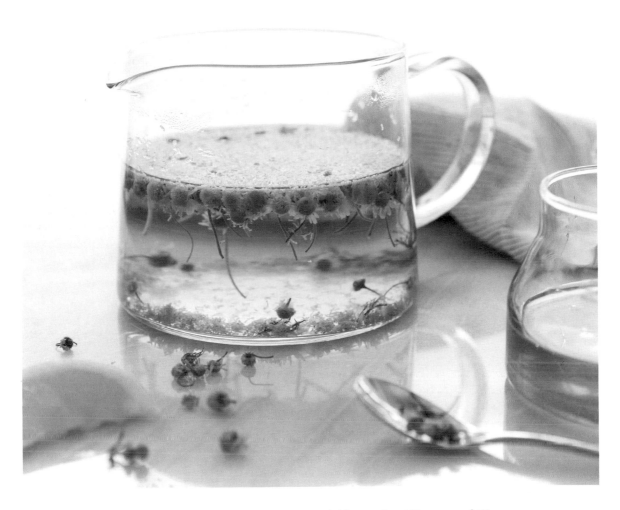

eating fermented foods, and making sure we consume lots of fiber will help restore the intestinal flora after a colonic.

Are there any additional benefits to a colonic? To our gut or otherwise?
There are some specific cases in which colonics using ingredients other than water can further help certain conditions. For example, coffee enemas stimulate the liver and gallbladder, helping release bile and sand, and preventing gallstones.

All in the Name of Detox

Incorporating some of these next-level detox methods into your life—along with clean eating—can go a long way. Because unfortunately eating well (and smart) isn't always enough when our body is faced with the pervasive amount of toxins in our world today—hidden (or not) in all manner of sources. So drink water, sweat it out, burn fat, and stimulate your lymphatic system to keep things moving.

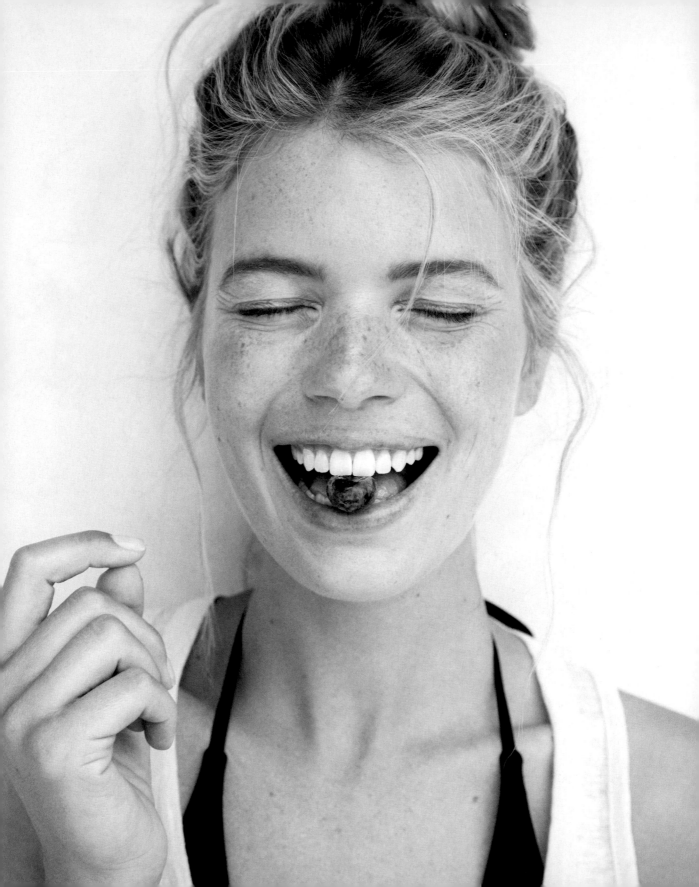

3.

Beauty Superfoods vs. Sapping Foods

A Special Class of Foods

All foods are not created equal. Some foods, we know, are more nutritionally dense than others—packed with more vitamins, minerals, antioxidants, healthy fats, and so on. But foods such as blueberries, acai, and salmon seem to pop up everywhere you look, promising a range of benefits, from preventing heart disease, diabetes, and cancer to enhancing beauty. These foods have been dubbed *superfoods* by the media, but at GOOP, we get that the category is essentially a marketing term. There isn't a medical definition, or a set standard for deeming a food a superfood, and nutritionists—no surprise—don't always agree with what is perhaps liberal labeling on the part of food companies.

But we also really like the name *superfoods*. Because it's true that some foods are super. We love that there are foods that can boost our immune system internally, and visibly boost our health externally—lending a much-appreciated lift to our skin and hair. In this chapter we're going to explore the biggest pro-health, pro-beauty foods

(and supplements)—and see why they're so crazy powerful. And we're also going to pick out the foods that are decidedly less super—the ones that sap our hair, our glow, our energy—while identifying some better alternatives.

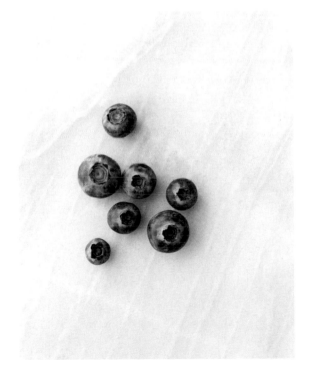

Undeniable Superfoods

While you don't need to eat turmeric at every meal, incorporating more superfoods into your diet is never a bad idea. For us, a superfood is a food (or ingredient) that supports the health, growth, and maintenance of the body in a way that is clearly superior to similar foods/ingredients—and that can actually make us feel and look better. So, if essentially all vegetables are good for us, to be classified as a superfood a vegetable needs to be packed with exponentially more vitamins/nutrients/phytochemicals that are significant to our well-being. Superfoods are thus the foods that do the most for you. On a scale of empty calories on the left to energy dense on the right, superfoods are all the way to the right.

There are also a few common beneficial properties that many superfoods share—from being packed with a particularly powerful vitamin or mineral, to being rich in the healthy fatty acids known as omega-3s. Here are our lists of favorite superfoods, with an eye toward beauty, and the major reasons:

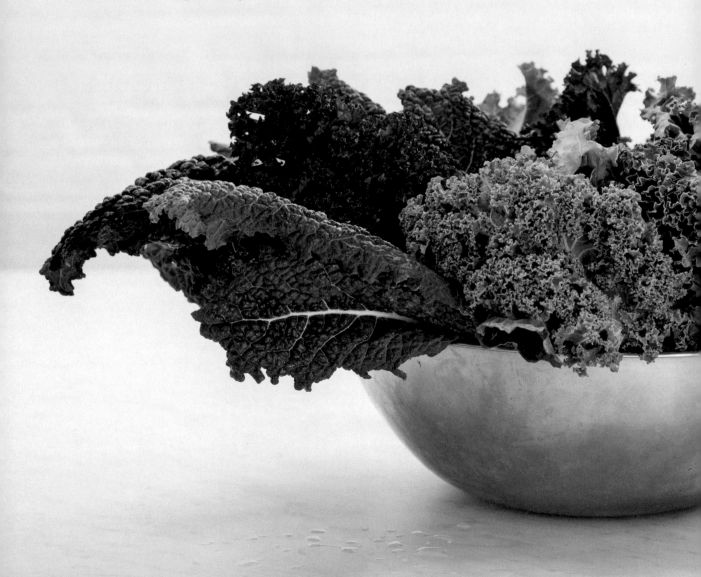

FOR BEING RICH IN ANTIOXIDANTS

Over the course of the average day, we are all exposed to free radicals, which are the highly reactive compounds that form when oxygen interacts with certain molecules that are found in everything from the food we eat to the air we breathe. We'll talk more about free radical damage in Chapter 4 and how to minimize your exposure (see page 117), but in essence, free radicals damage cells by stealing electrons in a process called *oxidation*. The classic example is to cut open an apple—after being exposed to the air, the apple slowly browns, in much the same way our skin eventually ends up wrinkled or spotted by age. Adding antioxidants (vitamins A, C, and E are the most common ones)—the way you'd squeeze lemon on the apple slice to keep it from browning—stops or slows some of those aging, damaging reactions. Here are some of our favorite antioxidant-rich superfoods:

- **Acai:** A popular recommendation for healthier, fresher-looking skin.
- **Blueberries:** Particularly useful for toning down inflammation, which is thought to be the primary cause of skin aging.
- **Dark, green vegetables** such as kale and collard greens: Rich in vitamins A, C, K, and even calcium and iron—great for your immune system. (You're sure to see kale, in particular, on a lot of detox menus—it's also rich in fiber.)
- **Green tea:** Rich in antioxidants called polyphenols—good for warding off inflammation as well as free radicals.
- **Pomegranate seeds:** Skin-damage-fighting vitamin C, numerous other antioxidants, plus fiber make these a skin—and health—essential.

FOR HAVING A WEALTH OF OMEGA-3S

Fat has gotten a bad rap during many nutritional fads and trends, but pretty much every nutritionist today agrees that we need certain kinds of fat in our diets—fats that build cells, produce hormones, give us energy, and allow us to absorb fat-soluble vitamins (A, D, E, K). And the queen of these good fats is omega-3 fatty acid. Omega-3s are also hailed for the effect they can have on our skin—true radiance boosters that help skin keep its moisture. Our top omega-3 superfoods:

- **Olive oil:** Also a source of anti-inflammatory polyphenols.
- **Salmon:** A great source of protein and vitamins (D and B), as well as omega-3. Buy wild-caught salmon if you can to avoid contaminants that occur when fish are farm-raised and to get the maximum nutrients.
- **Walnuts:** An easy snack to pack, plus you don't have to eat many to receive the omega-3 benefits.

FOR BEING ALL-AROUND DYNAMOS

- **Avocados:** They make everything taste better and are loaded with a host of nutrients—oleic acid, lutein, folate, vitamin E, monounsaturated fats, and glutathione (to name a few).
- **Beans:** A particularly healthy energy source for everyone, and very helpful for vegetarians in particular. By eating a variety, you get good doses of B vitamins, calcium, potassium, and folate.
- **Chia seeds:** So small, but packed with the goodness of omega-3 fatty acids, antioxidants, and minerals.
- **Chickpeas:** A lot of benefits (fiber, complex carbohydrates, protein) with no drawbacks.
- **Cruciferous vegetables:** Great source of essential minerals and vitamins, and also a great source of protein and fiber.

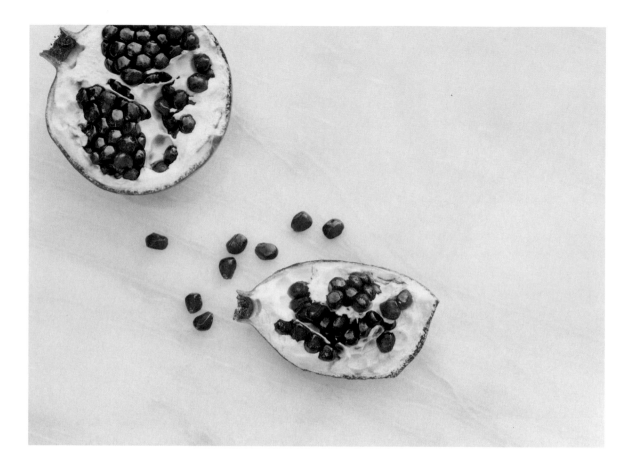

- **Lemons:** Somewhat of a beautifying, detoxifying, health-promoting secret weapon, the key to alkaline-balancing diets, and wonderful for the skin. They contain phytonutrients that help skin retain its elastin and steady collagen, along with the antioxidant bioflavonoid quercetin, which helps regulate the body's histamine response, reducing inflammation and alleviating allergies.
- **Spinach:** Chock-full of nutrients to the point that Dr. Junger has recommended that we eat spinach at nearly every meal "to help protect and support health from head to toe."
- **Turmeric:** An excellent go-to spice containing curcumin, an effective anti-inflammatory agent.

There's a lot of buzz around turmeric right now, and for good reason. The spice is a powerful anti-inflammatory, not to mention antioxidant. It boosts immunity and is especially effective when combined with black pepper.

As you can see, our lists are pretty diverse, and hardly obscure, making it easy to work some superfoods into your diet—whether you're in the midst of a set detox, eating clean, or even having a splurge day. For beauty-boosting superfood recipes that we rely on when we want to look our best, turn to page 106.

Vitamins, Minerals, and Simplifying the Supplement Aisle

It goes without saying that we need vitamins and minerals to maintain our health—inside and out. And while we would ideally get a majority of these through a well-balanced diet, sometimes it's essential to take vitamin and mineral supplements to fill nutritional gaps.

The big difference between vitamins and minerals is that vitamins are organic compounds (meaning they contain carbon) that are broken down more easily, for instance, in food preparation and when cooking. Minerals are naturally occurring inorganic solids (meaning they've never been alive and are not made from plants or animals). Vitamins are either water-soluble (C and the eight Bs) or fat-soluble (A, D, E, K). Minerals are categorized as major/macro if they are present in the body in greater amounts (like calcium, magnesium, sodium, phosphorus) and trace/micro if the body requires very small amounts (like iron, copper, zinc). Each vitamin and mineral plays a certain role in the upkeep of our bodies, and as a rule, when we're deficient in one arena, things break down—manifesting in everything from brittle nails to dry skin, bruises, digestive problems, and disease.

Dr. Frank Lipman, founder and director of Eleven Eleven Wellness Center in New York City, has become a beloved GOOP expert, particularly on matters of nutrition. We asked him for some help identifying the vitamins and minerals that boost hair, skin, and nail health—and the supplements that are truly worth taking. Because even if you do have a great, clean diet, supplements can serve as an important safety net—taking into account our much-needed indulgences and those environmental factors outside of our control.

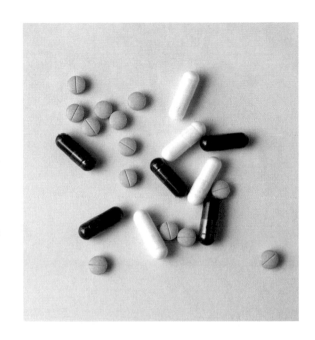

Dr. Frank Lipman's
GUIDE TO BEAUTY SUPPLEMENTS

Supplements are, as the word implies, intended as exactly that: supplements—to an already nutritious diet. They can help your body better deal with stressors and boost your immunity, but no supplement regime can make up for a lousy diet. Think of supplements as your nutritional pit crew, standing at the ready to make those quick adjustments, tweaks, and fixes to your internal engines to get you back out on the road.

While it is safe to take most supplements, the fat-soluble vitamins A and D should be taken only in appropriate doses for what you need and monitored regularly. Most people, especially those of us who don't get regular sun exposure, will benefit from supplementing with vitamin D, but my recommendation is always to get your levels tested first. Once you know where you are, you can take a dose appropriate for you, and then get retested regularly to make sure the levels don't go too high.

BEAUTY-SPECIFIC SUPPLEMENTS

The skin is your largest organ and a window into what's going on—on the inside. Skin issues such as rosacea, eczema, and acne are often evidence that there's an imbalance in the gut. Here are my suggestions for supplements geared toward beauty:

1. Look for a specific hair, skin, and nail supplement, which should include a blend of powerful antioxidants, minerals, and vitamins to help skin cell regeneration, boost your body's own UV protection, and combat free radicals that damage the skin.

2. Fish oil, for its omega-3 fatty acids, as they help protect the skin against inflammation and strengthen skin, hair, and nails.

3. Collagen peptides are a protein supplement that is produced from the collagen-rich connective tissues of animals. Besides promoting gut healing it also promotes healthy, dewy, and glowing skin and prevents early signs of aging (read: fine lines and wrinkles!). It dissolves easily in both cold and hot liquids.

4. Alpha lipoic acid is a potent antioxidant that helps fend off inflammation and protect skin collagen. Take it as a supplement and look for it as an ingredient in your (clean) skincare products as it can help combat signs of cellular aging.

5. Turmeric (and its compound curcumin) has powerful anti-inflammatory effects and can be helpful.

6. Probiotics help replenish your microbiome with good bacteria. Because of the gut-skin connection, any imbalance, infection, or inflammation in the gut can show up on the skin as rosacea, acne, or eczema. Sometimes an antimicrobial formula is necessary to kill the bad guys in the gut and create a balanced microbiome.

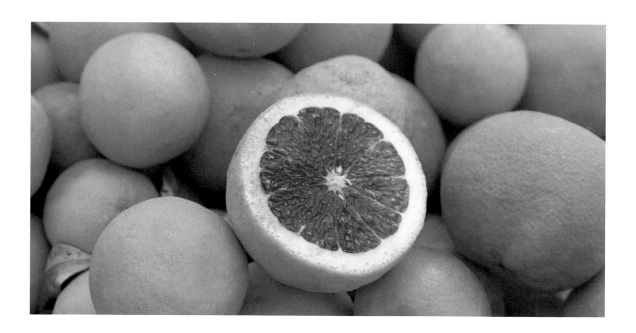

MAKING THE MOST OF NUTRIENTS

Bioavailability refers to the degree to which nutrients can be digested, absorbed, and used by your body. Here are three tips for helping your body absorb more nutrients:

1. Have a little fat with your salad—avocados are great for this—to lend a hand to fat-soluble nutrients. (An Iowa State University study found that eating salad vegetables with some added fat promotes the absorption of health-booster carotenoids.)

2. The raw vs. cooked vegetable debate can get a little dense. We like to keep it simple: Eating vegetables is good for you, and the best way to get the nutrients your body needs is by eating a variety of vegetables prepared in a variety of ways. This is because some nutrients can be lost through cooking (vitamin C, for instance, is sensitive to heat), but some nutrients (like the fat-soluble vitamins A, D, E, K) tend not to be affected, and cooking some vegetables actually makes it easier for you to absorb nutrients (by breaking down the plant's thick cell wall—the valuable mushrooms, for example, must be cooked). One vegetable that tends to be eaten raw a lot but that is actually brilliant when cooked is tomatoes—we like to slow-roast them—as it helps the body absorb the cancer-fighter antioxidant lycopene. And when it comes to cooking veggies, roasting (as opposed to boiling) is great in general as it helps prevent the loss of water-soluble vitamins (like B and C).

3. Whenever possible, shop local and shop organic—for reasons explained on page 96, the produce at the farmers' market is going to contain more nutrients than fruits and veggies that aren't organic and/or have come from afar.

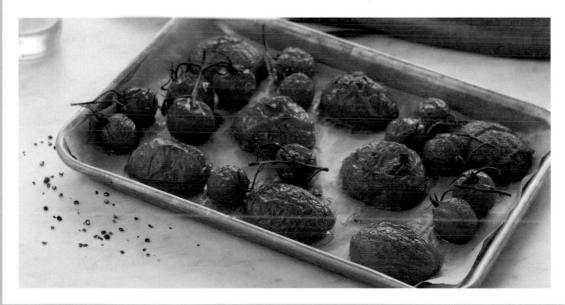

Why Organic Matters— and What Makes Our Food Less Superfood-y

You're probably no stranger to the idea that eating organic is good for you. But the reason is not always so obvious.

For starters, non-organic, processed, and packaged foods are a major source of chemicals and toxins, given that preservatives and coloring agents are added to the food to make it last longer on the shelf and make it look more appetizing. This is possibly your biggest victory from a detox standpoint: Starting with cleaner, more minimally processed foods means your body has less detox work to do off the bat.

Our number two, and a slightly more involved, reason: When you choose organic foods, you're steering clear of another source of toxins— pesticides and herbicides (used to kill weeds) that have been linked to a variety of reproductive and developmental disorders; to brain and nervous system toxicity; to hormone disruption; to skin, eye, and lung irritation; as well as to cancer. The (frightening) truth is that there is still a lot we don't know about how herbicides and pesticides affect our health—such long-term studies are not currently required by the government—but the picture is not a pretty one.

Glyphosate (i.e., the herbicide brand Roundup), for example, is the most commonly and heavily used herbicide—ever—in the world. (In Iowa, to name one place, the U.S. Geological Survey found glyphosate in 60 to 100 percent of the rainwater.) Scientific studies have shown a link between occupational exposure to glyphosate and B-cell lymphoma. And in 2015, the World Health Organization labeled it a "probable human carcinogen."

(There is also a strong correlation between the autism epidemic in the United States and glyphosate usage—pointed out by MIT research scientist Stephanie Seneff. Again, not causation, just correlation—and eerie.)

It is, however, true that herbicides are an important scientific innovation, and that they've been advantageous in some ways for both farmers and the general population. But the problem largely lies with how we've been grossly overusing (and misusing) them to keep up with the ascent of genetically modified organisms. GMOs are organisms whose genetic material, or DNA, has been altered by transferring advantageous genes from one species into another in a way that would not and could not occur naturally. One could argue that husbandry is an ancient practice—that farmers have always modified seeds and come up with new hybrids—but GMOs are problematic because almost all of them (90 percent of the ones in rotation) are engineered to be herbicide resistant. Whereas farmers traditionally only sprayed herbicides for a week or so at the beginning of crop cycles, with GMOs, a farmer can spray as much and as often as desired without worrying about crop damage. And since 1996, when GMOs came onto the scene, herbicide usage is up by more than 527 million pounds, which is *a lot*.

We also know from conversations with Gary Hirshberg—who has been shining a light on the situation—that usage of insecticide/Bt toxin (bacteria used as pesticide) has nearly doubled since 1996. Hirshberg is the chairman and co-founder of the consumer rights initiative Just Label It, and he holds the same titles at Stonyfield Farm, one of the first organic brands to break into the mainstream. An expert on the current situation, Hirshberg puts it simply: "Using double the insecticides cannot be good."

It's become a vicious cycle—the overuse of herbicides and pesticides has led to pest and weed resistance. Ironically (and entirely tragically), now we need *more* and *stronger* chemicals to fight the bugs and weeds. We're running out of effective options as this precarious system breaks down further. We've essentially been wasting herbicides and pesticides, or, as Hirshberg explains: The strategy has been to pour gasoline on fire. (As talked about in Chapter 1, this is also akin to what's happening with antibiotics—overuse and overdependence render the treatment ineffective.)

Possible solutions to end this cycle are for another day (or book), but as an immediate defense, we know we can avoid the toxic downfall by choosing organic foods. And on a less doom-and-gloom note, when you do choose organic foods—or at least non-GMO foods—you're also getting a lot of added benefits. Because in addition to being free of pesticides and herbicides, organic foods also tend to carry more nutrients—and taste—than their non-organic counterparts. The reason behind this is twofold, and one we've come to understand in great part thanks to environmental journalist Amanda Little.

goop TIP

We're a big believer in transparency: Labels—whether on food or makeup—should tell us what ingredients are included in any given product. Period. To find out more about GMOs, and to support our right to know if we're purchasing and eating GMO food or not, visit justlabelit.org.

In a wide range of studies on the topic, organic fruits and veggies have been found to be richer in nutrients. A few noteworthy studies that Little pointed out to us include the University of California, Davis's 10-year study on organic vegetables. Researchers found that organic tomatoes had nearly double the number of flavonoids—antioxidants that can lower blood pressure and help reduce the risk of heart disease and strokes (not to mention prevent and treat aging in the skin). Another study at the University of Florida found that the concentration of phytonutrients (which help to combat cancer) was up to 25 percent higher in organic produce. And so on. As Little expounds, this can in part be explained by what happens with nitrogen—which allows plants to absorb both water and nutrients—in organic soil. In soil that has been chemically fertilized, the nitrogen level is high and fruits and veggies grow rapidly, which means they don't have as much time to develop nutrients. On the other hand, in organic soil, nitrogen is still released into plants—but at a slower rate, and the fruits and veggies grow at a more natural pace, developing their nutrients. They also avoid soaking up too much water, which happens when there is an excess of nitrogen in the chemically fertilized soil. That extra water results in bland produce on your plate—and less nutrient-dense produce to begin with.

The other piece of the story is more logistical. Conventional (non-organic) produce is typically picked before it's ripe and when it's still hard, so that it can survive the hundreds or maybe thousands of miles to its destination. Since it is picked prematurely (on top of being forced to grow quicker than its natural pace), it never has a chance to reach its optimum nutrient level, which it would normally hit when allowed to fully ripen.

To "solve" this, conventional fruits and veggies that are shipped long-distance are chemically ripened in warehouses. This gives the appearance of ripeness—but not the nutrient punch behind the bright color. Or, for that matter, the taste that develops when fruits and veggies are allowed to ripen naturally in the sun. If you've ever tasted an heirloom tomato from a farmers' market on Sunday, and then eaten a packaged sad desk salad from a nondescript chain on Monday, well…you know the difference.

It's no secret that at GOOP we're certain that eating organic tastes better and is better for you—and long-term, even makes you look better. When your body isn't fighting to detox itself from chemical soups like Roundup, it's dramatically less inflamed, so your skin looks better to begin with;

add to that the increased antioxidants and phyto-nutrients present in ripe, fresh produce, and you see just how powerfully beautifying eating organic truly is. We have also found organic ingredients to be incredibly effective and rejuvenating in skincare and makeup products. More on this—and why what you put on your body is just as important as what you put in it—in Chapter 6.

We get that it can be difficult to find and/or afford an entirely organic stock of produce, though. And it's for this reason that we are fans of the Environmental Working Group's (EWG) Dirty Dozen and Clean Fifteen. Based on an analysis of 35,000-plus samples taken by the U.S. Department of Agriculture and the federal Food and Drug Administration, the EWG puts together a list (which they update yearly)—the Dirty Dozen—of

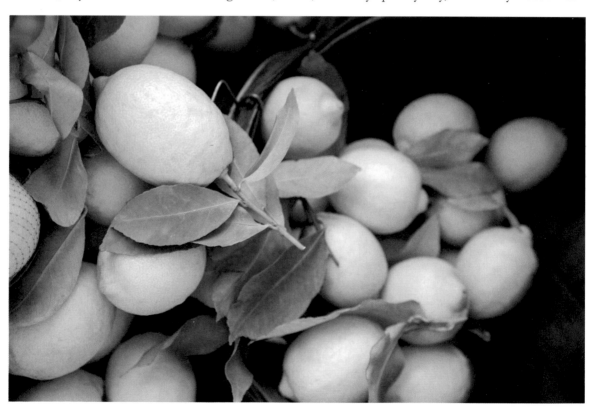

popular fruits and vegetables with the highest pesticide contamination and, therefore, the ones where you have the most to gain by going organic. (In general, this is fruit that you eat the skin of, too, and produce with thin, permeable skin.)

At the same time, if you aren't shopping 100 percent organic, another EWG list offers suggestions on where to go conventional, the Clean Fifteen—i.e., the fruits and veggies that absorb minimal amount of pesticides and fertilizers. For the Clean Fifteen, few pesticides were found on the produce, and when they were, it was a low total concentration.

DIRTY DOZEN
(BEGINNING WITH THE DIRTIEST)

Strawberries ➔ Single samples contained 17 different pesticides

Apples

Nectarines

Peaches ➔ More than 98 percent showed at least one pesticide residue

Celery

Grapes

Cherries

Spinach

Tomatoes

Sweet bell peppers ➔ A single sample contained 15 different pesticides

Cherry tomatoes

Cucumbers

Dirty Dozen PLUS: These don't meet Dirty Dozen ranking criteria but the EWG (and GOOP) thinks they are worth mentioning because they were found to contain trace levels of insecticides that are toxic to our nervous system:

Hot peppers

Kale and collard greens

CLEAN FIFTEEN
(BEGINNING WITH THE CLEANEST)

Avocados ➔ Detectable pesticides were found on only 1 percent of avocados

Sweet corn

Pineapples ➔ 89 percent had no residues

Cabbage

Sweet peas, frozen

Onions

Asparagus

Mangos

Papayas ➔ 81 percent showed no residues

Kiwi

Eggplant

Honeydew melon

Grapefruit

Cantaloupe ➔ 62 percent had no residues

Cauliflower

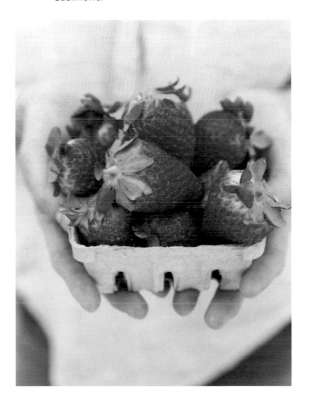

The Bad Guys

There are some foods and habits that really work against our health and beauty goals. And for the most part, the culprits are obvious. But somehow, the workarounds are less simple. How do we, for instance, say no to sugar? With the help of Dr. Frank Lipman, we've found a way.

THE COMMON NEMESIS, SUGAR

It feels almost cliché to talk about sugar at this point. And yet, it's impossible not to because it's so f'ing addictive. Sugar gives you an initial high—it hits the bloodstream almost immediately—and in an effort to process this burst, the body produces insulin to carry the sugar into our cells from the bloodstream. When your insulin level increases, though, your blood sugar level drops. This is the familiar crashing sensation. Followed by a craving for more sugar. And so the series of highs and lows goes, putting extra stress on our adrenals and leaving us anxious, moody (sugar is a mood-altering drug), and exhausted. Awesome.

We also know that sugar is associated with many chronic health issues, such as weight gain, decreased immunity, autoimmune diseases, diabetes, heart disease, and irritable bowel syndrome, along with a host of skin issues, from puffiness, sagging, and wrinkles to breakouts. Sugar works its black magic in a variety of ways but research suggests that one of the ways it threatens our immunity is by inhibiting vitamin C from getting into white blood cells. And via another dark path, sugar stimulates insulin secretion in the pancreas, which triggers the liver to produce triglycerides, which are linked to stroke, heart disease, and obesity. It's a mess.

And sugar is everywhere we turn. If you've watched the documentary *Fed Up*, you might be familiar with some of the sobering stats, like 80 percent of food items in the U.S. have added sugar (i.e., virtually every packaged food on every grocery store shelf—crackers, bread, yogurt, marinades, pasta sauce). A 20-ounce bottle of soda has the equivalent of about 17 teaspoons of sugar. Meanwhile, the American Heart Association recommends women have no more than 6 teaspoons each day.

Sugar also (deceptively) goes by many names. We, too, were once admittedly excited about trendy agave nectar. Which is why we were kind of devastated when Dr. Lipman told us: "Sugar is sugar is sugar. There's really no such thing as a healthy sugar." But, there are still some important differences among types of sugar, and Dr. Lipman has recommended some ways to soothe a sweet tooth. We also wanted to know more from him about the effect sugar has on our skin via a process called glycation—and what we can do about that, too. **Note:** If you've recently killed a major sweet tooth, you might be short on magnesium. As Dr. Lipman explains: "Sugar inhibits mineral absorption, depriving the body of key minerals necessary for health, and depletes the body of magnesium, which is required for proper functioning of every single cell in the human body and essential for calcium absorption and utilization." So consider stocking up on leafy, green vegetables; nuts; seeds; legumes—spinach, pumpkin seeds, and black beans are particularly good sources of magnesium.

Dr. Frank Lipman
ON KICKING YOUR SUGAR HABIT

We know: Sugar is sugar is sugar. But...is any kind of sugar okay in moderation? What are the most suitable alternatives?

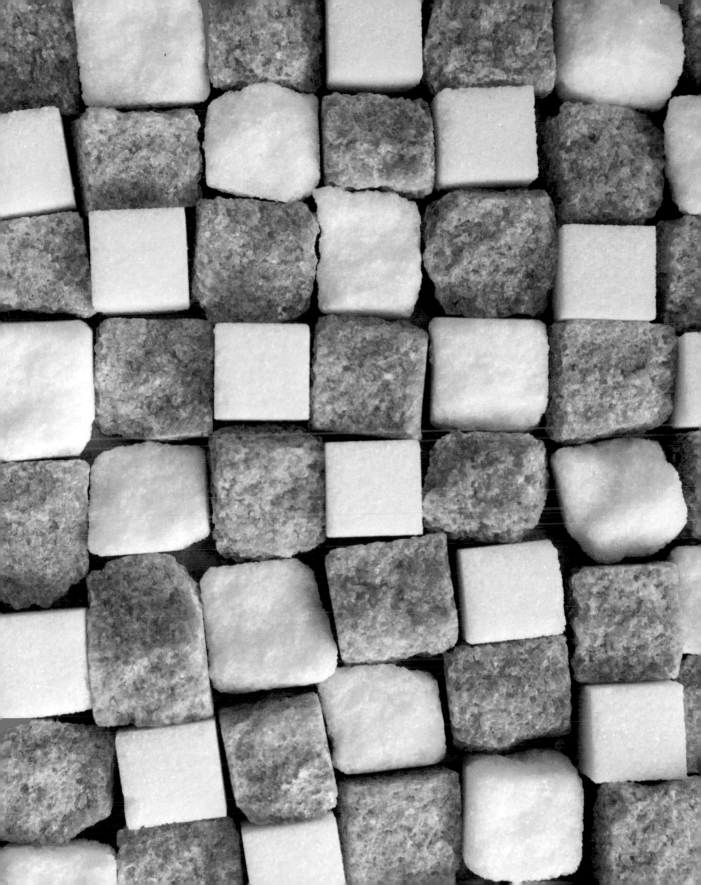

Getting sugar in its most natural whole form—as it is in nature—will always be your best bet. Think real, whole fruits, sweet root vegetables, and winter squashes. If you're looking for a sweetener, stick to the ones nature made. While using dates is a common way to add sweetness to a dish without using any kind of processed, refined sweetener, I don't recommend them as they are extremely high in natural sugar. There are also some sweeteners that won't spike your blood sugar levels as much, and others that have much more nutritional value than the white, refined stuff. Stick to small amounts of raw honey, maple syrup, and palm and coconut nectar for natural sweetness with some added minerals. For a calorie-free sweetener that does not spike your blood sugar levels, try stevia. I recommend looking for an organic stevia (in either powder or liquid form)—and then check the ingredient label. It should not have any other ingredients besides organic stevia. I recommend avoiding Truvia and Pure Via, which are highly processed.

What's the trick to getting over a sugar addiction?
- Fat: Eating enough fat helps you feel satisfied and full for longer, and gives your body fuel to get through the day without constantly reaching for sugar. It also helps keep your blood sugar stable and prevent dips—and sugar cravings.
- Find sweetness, community, and joy elsewhere! Sometimes we reach for sugar when in fact what we're really craving is a hug or a good belly laugh.

When we're having a sugar craving, what should we do?
- Take L-glutamine, 1,000 to 2,000 mg, every couple of hours as necessary. It often relieves sugar cravings as the brain uses it for fuel.
- Hydrate: Dehydration often shows up as cravings for either salt or sugar.
- Find the root cause of the craving. Yes, sugar is indeed addicting, so breaking the cycle can be tough.

However, sometimes the cause of our sugar cravings can be emotional. Whether it's stress induced, related to boredom, or a need for more sweetness in your life—spend some time with your cravings and find the emotional connection so that you can better tackle the cravings when they come up. Maybe a call to your best friend, a walk around the block, or some snuggle time with your loved one is all you need.

Can you take us through glycation and the impact sugar can have on our skin?
Sugar binds to proteins and fats in the body during digestion to create advanced glycation end products, or AGEs, which are free radicals that reduce collagen and elastin in the skin—ultimately causing wrinkles and loss of skin elasticity. Booo! Sugar also feeds bad bacteria and opportunistic yeast in our gut, which can cause inflammation and show up in the skin as acne or puffiness.

Is there anything we can do to combat this skin damage?
Yes. Besides removing sugar and processed foods from your diet, eat an anti-inflammatory diet high in antioxidants from lots of colorful vegetables and some fruits, and eat lots of foods rich in healthy fats such as wild salmon, avocado, olive oil, and coconut.

A NOTE ON BACON

In the fall of 2015 the International Agency for Research on Cancer (IARC)—an independent cancer agency established through a World Health Organization (WHO) resolution—dealt a major blow to America's beloved breakfast meat, bacon. The IARC concluded that there is convincing evidence that processed meat causes cancer. (WHO defines processed meat as "meat that has been transformed through salting, curing, fermentation, smoking, or other processes to enhance flavor or improve preservation." Think: bacon, hotdogs, deli meat, and meat-based sauces.) This research was based on more than 400 epidemiological studies.

In this same report, the IARC also classified red meat as *probably* carcinogenic to humans (including beef, pork, veal, and lamb). As WHO explains in layman's terms, more than 700 epidemiological studies showed "positive associations between eating red meat and developing colorectal cancer," but there wasn't enough evidence to prove causation.

It is not yet entirely clear how eating processed or red meat increases the risk of getting cancer, but as WHO explains it: Chemicals can form during meat processing or cooking that are known or suspected carcinogens. It's also hard to say exactly what might be a safe amount of either processed or red meat to eat, but we're following recommendations to eat them only sparingly—and of course they aren't part of a detox diet—and leaning harder on main-course-worthy vegetables, and fish, chicken, and turkey (see Mix-and-Match Lunches and Dinners beginning on page 14).

ALCOHOL

Speaking of sugar, there's a lot of it in alcohol, which is why a night of drinking can have disastrous consequences on your skin the next day: puffiness, sagging, redness and blotchiness, sallow tone, and dark circles, to name a few. Consistent overconsumption of alcohol has profoundly…unattractive results. Alcoholics who finally manage to quit, for instance, often end up looking as if they're ten to fifteen years younger. But as we all know, even a single night of overindulgence results in serious (if more temporary) un-prettiness.

That said, while it may not be that hard to pass on the dessert menu, it's impossible to imagine days without a glass of wine. We went back to Dr. Lipman for guidance.

Dr. Frank Lipman
ON DRINKING

How does the body process alcohol?
Most alcohol you drink is absorbed through the small intestine and goes to the liver, where it is metabolized by the enzyme alcohol dehydrogenase. This enzyme is interestingly influenced by your gender. In other words, women are more likely to become drunk on smaller amounts of alcohol.

Does drinking actually make people puffy?
Yes, because it dilates the blood vessels.

Are there certain alcohols or drink combinations that are better or worse for us?
Many people seem to overdo it when they drink wine or beer—a typical serving is larger for the amount of alcohol in it, so you end up drinking a lot more. Beer also contains gluten, which I recommend avoiding. Instead of beer or wine, stick with a small amount of clear liquor like vodka or tequila.

Beware of the mixers, though. Choose plain seltzer or soda water rather than tonic, which is loaded with sugar. Sodas and fruit juices are filled with sugar or artificial sweeteners, too, so if you want a little flavor, squeeze a lemon or lime (or both) into your cocktail.

It's often pointed out that red wine contains resveratrol, which has antioxidant properties. Is there a real health benefit to drinking wine?
I believe the biggest benefit of wine is the social setting in which it is consumed. Sharing a drink with family and friends—sitting around the table eating and enjoying your meal and the great company—there are health benefits to that. It's de-stressing and this human connection aspect is so important in this digital age.

How You Look the Next Day— and Years Later

To better understand how these beauty-sapping foods and habits—sugar, alcohol, smoking—affect the way we look, we turn to GOOP contributor Dr. Laura Lefkowitz, who received her MD with honors in OB-GYN, psychiatry, internal medicine, and radiology, before becoming a trusted nutritional science expert and practitioner.

Dr. Laura Lefkowitz
ON SKIN AND HAIR HEALTH

What exactly does drinking/smoking do to our hair and skin?

Although there have been studies saying there is some protective heart benefit from small amounts of alcohol, and you may get a nice temporary flush when you imbibe, when it comes to skin and hair there is absolutely no benefit to drinking alcohol.

Alcohol is perceived by the body as a poison/toxin. When you imbibe, the body immediately revs up production of an enzyme called alcohol dehydrogenase to break down the alcohol. As you drink, the liver is working hard to neutralize this toxin. As the toxin circulates throughout your bloodstream it affects cellular function. The body needs a lot of water to safely break down alcohol and excrete it from the bloodstream through the liver and kidneys without causing organ damage. This effort to protect the liver and kidneys causes dehydration, making the skin appear sallow and wrinkled.

Alcohol stresses the system and causes the release of cortisol, an inflammatory, fat-storing hormone. Alcohol is itself a sugar, and imbibing raises blood sugar levels and the production of insulin, another inflammatory fat-storing hormone. Alcohol impairs judgment, so many will ingest inflammatory foods high in sugar and fats when they are under the influence of alcohol. Alcohol disturbs the natural sleep cycle, preventing the brain from entering deep, restorative sleep, when the body is still and repairs itself. Alcohol causes a restless, dehydrated night's sleep, and without the ability to repair all the cell damage you encountered during the day, you wake up bloated, with under-eye bags and mottled skin.

As far as smoking...where do I start? Cigarette smoke contains more than 4,000 chemical compounds, of which 43 are carcinogens, and over 400 of them toxins. Compounds in smoke cause blood vessels to constrict for up to 90 minutes, causing decreased blood flow to the skin. Every time you smoke you are depriving your skin of adequate oxygen and nutrients for an hour and a half!

When you inhibit circulation, skin cells are starved. They cannot repair themselves or protect themselves from the sun and free radicals; collagen and elastin break down, and therefore the appearance of your skin suffers. The same goes for your scalp. Every time you smoke, you impair blood flow to the hair follicles, robbing them of the oxygen and nutrients that they need to make hair, and you suffer from hair loss and thinning. The change in capillary permeability with every cigarette makes you prone to broken capillaries and veins, which can cause the appearance of broken vessels and dark scarring on the face.

The decrease in blood flow (from constricted vessels) impairs the skin's ability to drain fluid from the face, causing puffiness, bags under the eyes, and sagging skin. Not to mention, every time you take a drag, you're pursing your lips and furrowing your eyebrows. These repetitive motions cause deep lines around the mouth, and vertical lines in between the eyebrows. But it doesn't stop with the inhale, it keeps getting worse. When you exhale smoke, your skin is bombarded with a chemical smoke cloud and these chemicals rest on your skin, clog and congest the pores, predisposing you to blackheads, comedones (pimples), and inflammatory skin conditions like rosacea. Smoking impairs

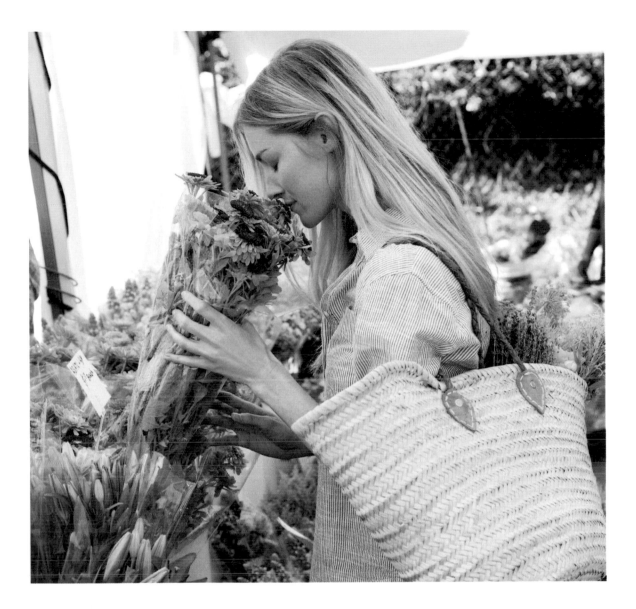

immunity and healing, so if you get cut or have picked at a bad pimple, the skin doesn't heal quickly or smoothly, leading to increased scarring and pigmentation.

Besides the effects on skin and hair, smoking affects every organ system in the body, and smoking cessation is the number one thing you can modify in your lifestyle to radically improve your health, wellness, and longevity.

Maintaining a healthy weight (normal body mass index), eating nourishing foods, exercising daily, getting adequate, consistent sleep, minimizing sugar and alcohol in your diet, and avoiding cigarettes and drugs make all the difference in how you produce and repair cells. You are made up of trillions of cells—the better your cells look, the better your skin and hair cells appear.

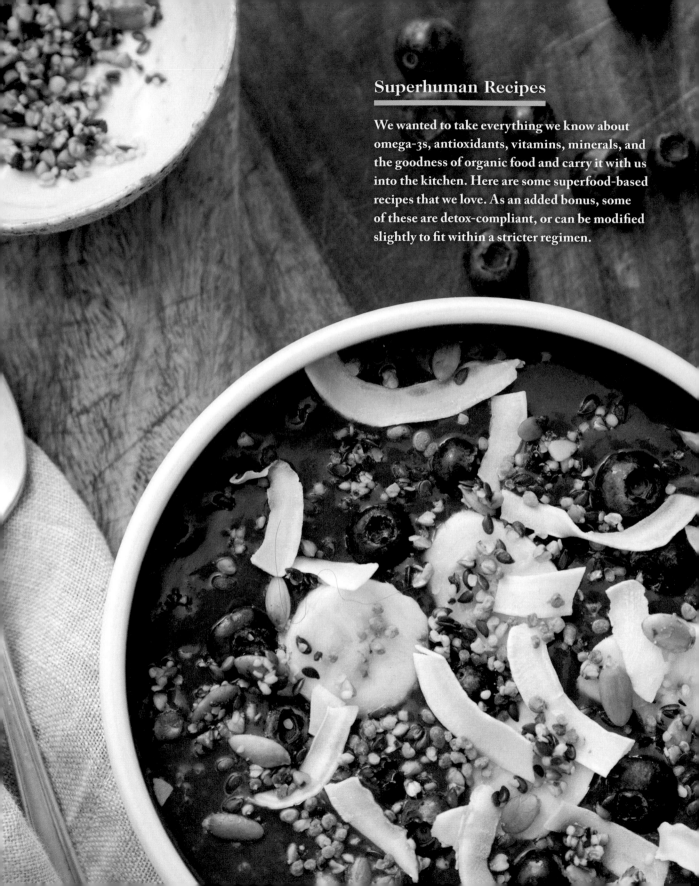

Superhuman Recipes

We wanted to take everything we know about omega-3s, antioxidants, vitamins, minerals, and the goodness of organic food and carry it with us into the kitchen. Here are some superfood-based recipes that we love. As an added bonus, some of these are detox-compliant, or can be modified slightly to fit within a stricter regimen.

Acai Bowl with Bee Pollen

This acai bowl is packed with antioxidants, which are essential for fighting skin-damaging free radicals. The seed mix adds a really nice crunch and is also a delicious snack on its own (but you can substitute with your favorite granola, too). Add a spoonful of almond butter on top for an extra protein boost after a workout.

SERVES 1

FOR THE TOASTED SEED MIX

1 tablespoon pumpkin seeds	½ teaspoon coconut oil
1 tablespoon buckwheat groats	Generous pinch kosher salt
1 tablespoon flaxseed	½ teaspoon honey
1 teaspoon hemp seeds	

FOR THE BOWL

1 (3.5-ounce) frozen acai pack	1 tablespoon coconut flakes
1 banana, cut in half	2 tablespoons blueberries
2 tablespoons coconut water	1 tablespoon bee pollen
1 tablespoon coconut milk, optional	Manuka honey, optional

1. To make the toasted seed mix, heat a small sauté pan over medium heat. Add all the ingredients except the honey and cook, stirring occasionally, for 2 minutes, until nicely toasted. Add the honey, turn off the heat, and stir to combine. Remove the mixture to a plate to cool and crisp up. Once cool, use your fingers to break it up into little pieces.

2. To assemble the bowl, break the acai pack into pieces and combine in a high-powered blender with half of the banana, the coconut water, and coconut milk (if using). Blend on high for 2 minutes, until smooth.

3. Thinly slice the other half of the banana. Transfer the acai mixture to a bowl and top with the sliced banana, 2 tablespoons of the toasted seed mix, the coconut flakes, blueberries, and bee pollen; drizzle over a little manuka honey if you like it sweet.

Grilled Salmon and Avocado Salad, Two Ways

Salmon and avocado are two of the most omega-3-rich foods you can eat, and all that healthy fat not only tastes amazing, but does wonders for your skin and body. Here are two versions of grilled avocado and salmon salad, one with an Asian twist and one with a lovely charred citrus dressing.

Asian Salmon and Avocado Salad

SERVES 2

¼ cup soy sauce (or tamari if on a detox)

2 tablespoons extra-virgin olive oil, plus more for the grill pan

1 tablespoon plus 1 teaspoon rice wine vinegar

2 teaspoons mirin

2 small or 1 large clove garlic, finely grated

1 (2-inch) piece fresh ginger, finely grated

2 (6-ounce) salmon fillets

1 firm yet ripe avocado, quartered

2 handfuls baby spinach, washed and dried

1. Whisk together the soy sauce, olive oil, vinegar, mirin, garlic, and ginger in a glass measuring cup or small bowl. Pour half of the dressing into a shallow bowl, add the salmon, and turn to coat. Marinate for 5 minutes.
2. Meanwhile, heat a grill pan over medium-high heat and brush it lightly with olive oil.
3. Add the salmon and avocado quarters to the pan and grill for 2 to 3 minutes on each side, until the salmon is cooked to your liking and the avocado has nice grill marks.
4. Toss the spinach with the reserved dressing to taste and top with the grilled salmon and avocado.

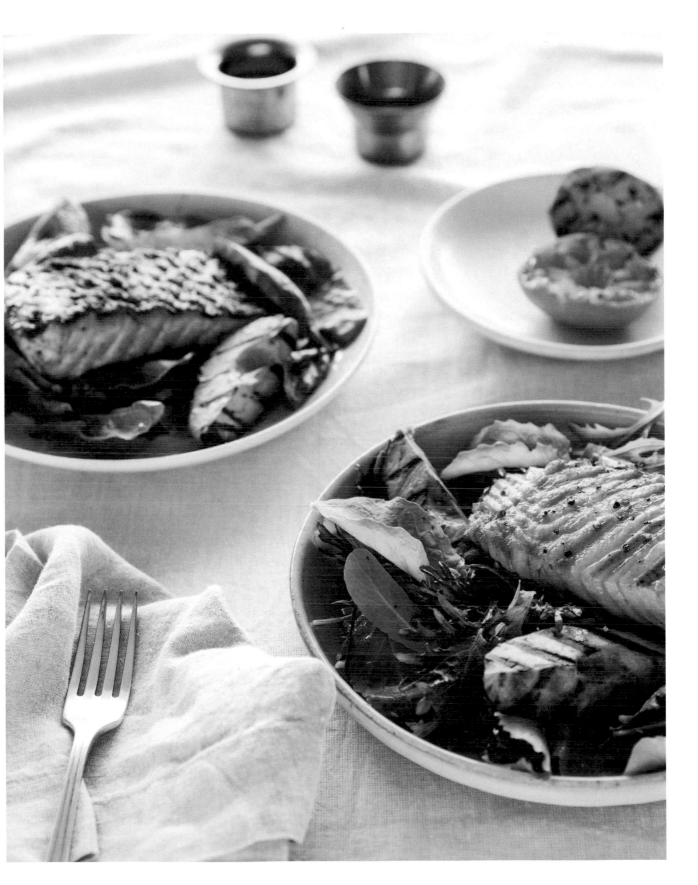

Citrus-Grilled Salmon and Avocado Salad

SERVES 2

2 (6-ounce) salmon fillets

2½ tablespoons olive oil

Kosher salt and freshly ground black pepper

1 medium shallot, cut into ¼-inch slices

1 ripe yet firm avocado, quartered

1 Meyer lemon, cut in half

1 tangerine, cut in half

2 handfuls mixed greens (such as mizuna and arugula)

1. Heat a grill pan over medium-high heat.
2. Brush each salmon fillet with 1 teaspoon of olive oil and season generously with salt and pepper. Toss the sliced shallot with 1 teaspoon of the oil and a pinch of salt and set aside.
3. When the grill pan is hot, add the salmon and avocado quarters and cook for 3 minutes on the first side. Flip to the second side and add the sliced shallot and citrus halves (cut sides down) to the grill pan. Cook everything for another 2 to 3 minutes, until the salmon is cooked to your liking and the avocado and citrus have nice grill marks.
4. Squeeze the grilled citrus over the mixed greens and toss with the remaining tablespoons olive oil, the grilled shallots, and salt and pepper to taste. Place the salmon and avocado over the greens and serve.

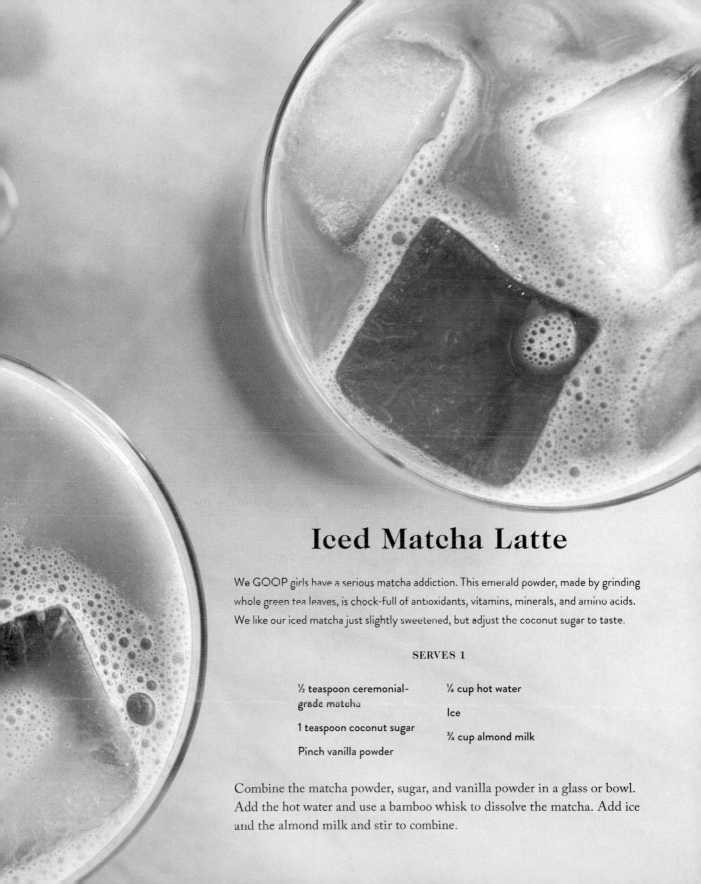

Iced Matcha Latte

We GOOP girls have a serious matcha addiction. This emerald powder, made by grinding whole green tea leaves, is chock-full of antioxidants, vitamins, minerals, and amino acids. We like our iced matcha just slightly sweetened, but adjust the coconut sugar to taste.

SERVES 1

½ teaspoon ceremonial-grade matcha

1 teaspoon coconut sugar

Pinch vanilla powder

¼ cup hot water

Ice

¾ cup almond milk

Combine the matcha powder, sugar, and vanilla powder in a glass or bowl. Add the hot water and use a bamboo whisk to dissolve the matcha. Add ice and the almond milk and stir to combine.

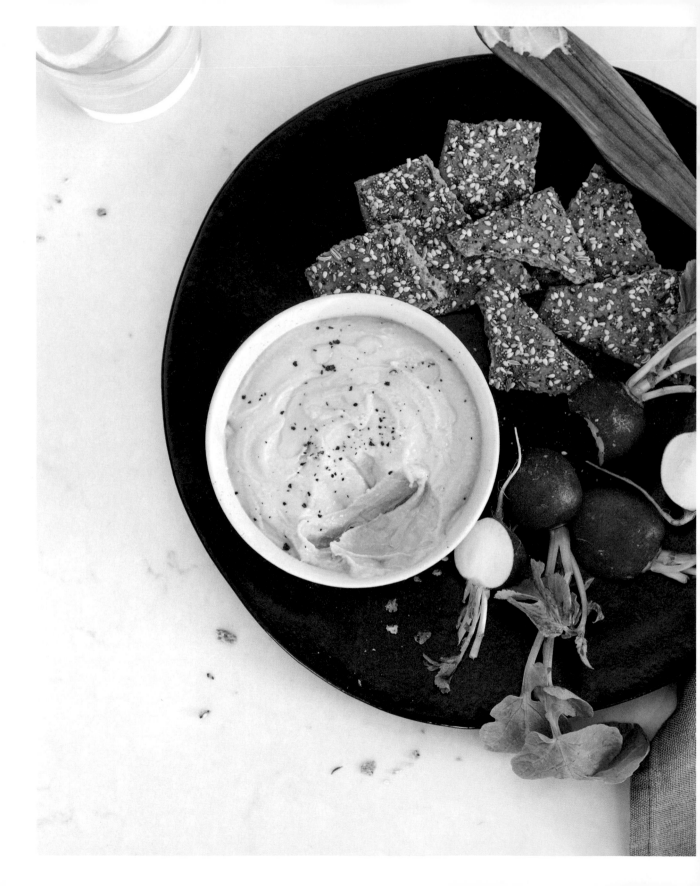

Spinach and Lemon Hummus

Packed with protein from chickpeas, good fat from olive oil, fiber, vitamins, calcium, and iron from spinach, and vitamin C and antioxidants from lemon, this hummus is a serious nutritional powerhouse. It's great with crudités or crackers, spread on a sandwich, or simply eaten with a spoon.

MAKES ABOUT 2 CUPS

1 (14.5-ounce) can chickpeas, drained and rinsed

5 tablespoons extra-virgin olive oil

3 tablespoons tahini

1 cup packed baby spinach leaves, cleaned, dried, and roughly chopped

Zest and juice of 1 medium Meyer (or small regular) lemon

1 large clove garlic, minced

1 teaspoon kosher salt

Combine all the ingredients with ¼ cup water in a food processor and blend until smooth. Add more salt to taste.

Turmeric and Ginger Tonic

Turmeric is one of the most anti-inflammatory ingredients available, so naturally we try to incorporate it into our diets as often as possible. This recipe makes enough for one drink, but we highly recommend making a big batch of the turmeric/ginger infusion and storing it in the fridge.

SERVES 1

¼ cup thinly sliced peeled turmeric (about one 4-inch piece)

2 tablespoons thinly sliced peeled fresh ginger (about one 2-inch piece)

⅓ cup water

1 tablespoon honey

2 tablespoons fresh lemon juice

Ice

Sparkling water

1. Combine the turmeric, ginger, water, and honey in a small saucepan and bring to a boil. Cover, turn off the heat, and infuse for 20 minutes. Let cool, then strain through a fine-mesh sieve.
2. Combine the infused water in a glass with the lemon juice and some ice, then top with sparkling water.

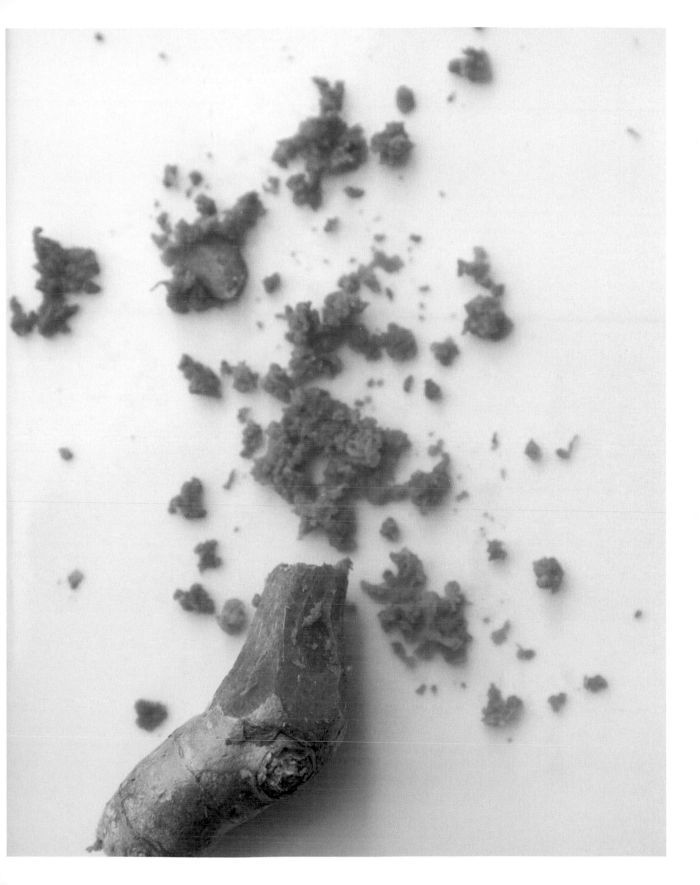

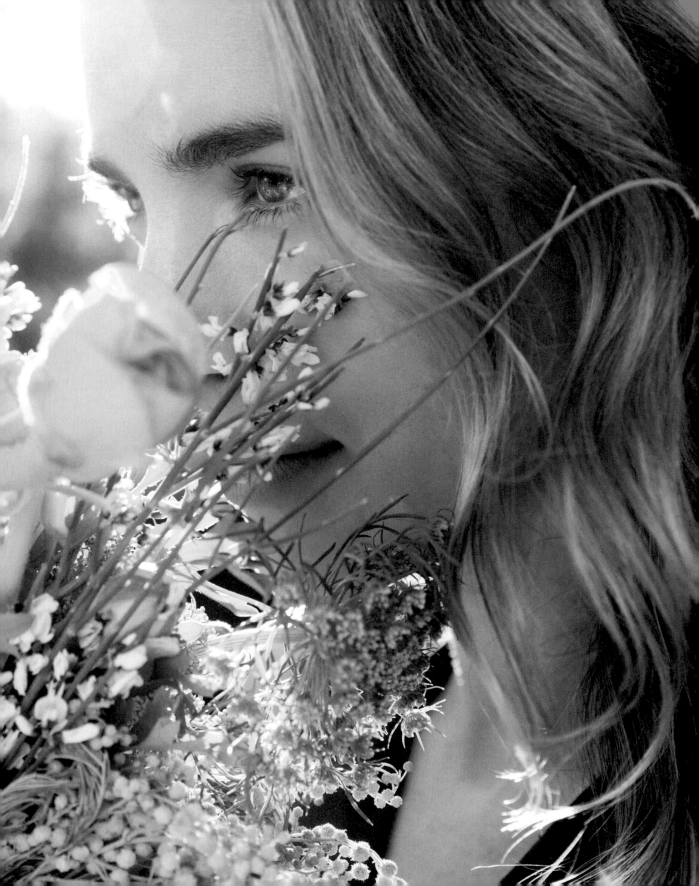

4.
The Impact of the Environment

Compare and Contrast

Compare the skin on the back of your hand with the skin on your butt. If you're over eighteen or so, there's probably a difference. Do it when you're forty, and the difference is going to be dramatic. The environment has an enormous impact on our skin. The cruel trick of it is the lag time between when environmental damage happens—sun exposure, smoking, pollution, exposure to toxins in general—and when it manifests in the mirror.

If the hand/butt contrast doesn't convince you, Google *twin studies and smoking*, and/or *twin studies and sun exposure*. The difference in how fast identical twins age depending on whether they smoke/don't wear sunscreen/drink heavily and all manner of other environmental stressors on skin is visible...and sobering.

Here's the great thing: There's a lot in our environment that we *can* control to limit the development of free radical damage. And even when we can't change the environment we're in, we can still often control its effect on us. And interestingly, commonly known aging factors like sun exposure

and stress aren't always bad for us—on the contrary, they can sometimes be very beneficial.

Maintaining a youthful glow and smooth, supple, plump skin indefinitely is a prospect that appeals to just about everyone. Modulating your environmental exposure to reduce its negative impact on skin is what we're all about at GOOP. From the sun to pollution to ingested or breathed-in toxins, there are beauty-sapping aggressors to be sidestepped; at the same time, the environment is full of opportunities to make ourselves look and feel more beautiful.

Minimize Free-Radical Damage

As we discussed earlier, free radicals have seriously damaging effects on our skin. And certain situations and habits expose us to an unhealthy amount of free radicals, making us more vulnerable to wrinkles and skin spots than we would normally be. You expose yourself to many more free radicals when the sun hits your skin, and when alcohol, sugar, smoke, or other toxins enter your body.

Staying out of the sun, wearing sunblock, not smoking, and not living in the smog of Beijing or Delhi all protect you from some degree of free radical formation. But you can further up your protection against free radicals by consuming antioxidants, and/or applying them topically. Again, vitamins C, E, and A are the most common antioxidants; green tea is packed with them, and cosmetic and food companies are forever combing the globe for new antioxidant compounds in plants (e.g., acai berries, rose hips, arctic cloudberries).

Antioxidants absolutely work and should be part of anyone's routine, no matter your age or skin type. Apply them topically under sunscreen, moisturizer, or makeup (or all of the above if you're a big layer-er). Eat all manner of fruits and vegetables that contain them. Your skin—not to mention the rest of your body—will seriously benefit.

GO INTO REPAIR MODE

Your body—which makes its own free-radical-scavenging enzymes—repairs itself when given a break. Meaning that if you stay out of the sun or wear sunblock, your skin doesn't have to expend as much energy defending itself, and will switch gears and devote itself to repairing the damage that's already occurred. Similarly, stop smoking and your body has more energy to repair damage to the lungs, rather than merely trying to defend itself. So changing your behavior—whether it's being safer in the sun (more later in this chapter) or quitting cigarettes—doesn't just stop the current damage, it starts reversing it. Never mind face creams and even Botox: Quitting smoking and protecting yourself from the sun are the two biggest wrinkle fighters that exist.

Why You Need Vitamin D and Time in the Sun

The only doctors who talk about "safe tanning" are being paid by the tanning-booth industry. But getting enough sun exposure for vitamin D synthesis is a daily process and has nothing to do with tanning.

For a long time, we've been aware of the potential health consequences associated with getting too much sun. But we don't always consider whether we're getting enough, or the right kind, because time in the sun without sunblock is a major source of vitamin D. And we're facing a worldwide vitamin D deficiency that we rarely hear about. A 2014 study published in the medical journal *BMJ* reported that almost 70 percent of Americans and more than 85 percent of Europeans are vitamin D deficient. Other studies have estimated that vitamin D deficiency affects more than one billion people globally—possibly the most common medical condition.

Vitamin D is involved in a multitude of essential body processes. As Dr. Lipman says, "Vitamin D is in a class by itself." Interestingly, it behaves more like a hormone in the body than a vitamin. (It's made in the skin, travels via the bloodstream to your liver and kidneys—where it becomes activated as a steroid hormone called calcitriol—then moves on to your intestines, bones, and other tissues.) It helps build muscle and bone, plays a part in creating hundreds of disease-preventing proteins and enzymes, supports the immune system, has anti-inflammatory effects—it affects more than 2,000 genes in the body. And low levels of vitamin D have been linked to serious health issues like cancer, heart disease, and diabetes. Vitamin D impacts how healthy we are and how healthy we

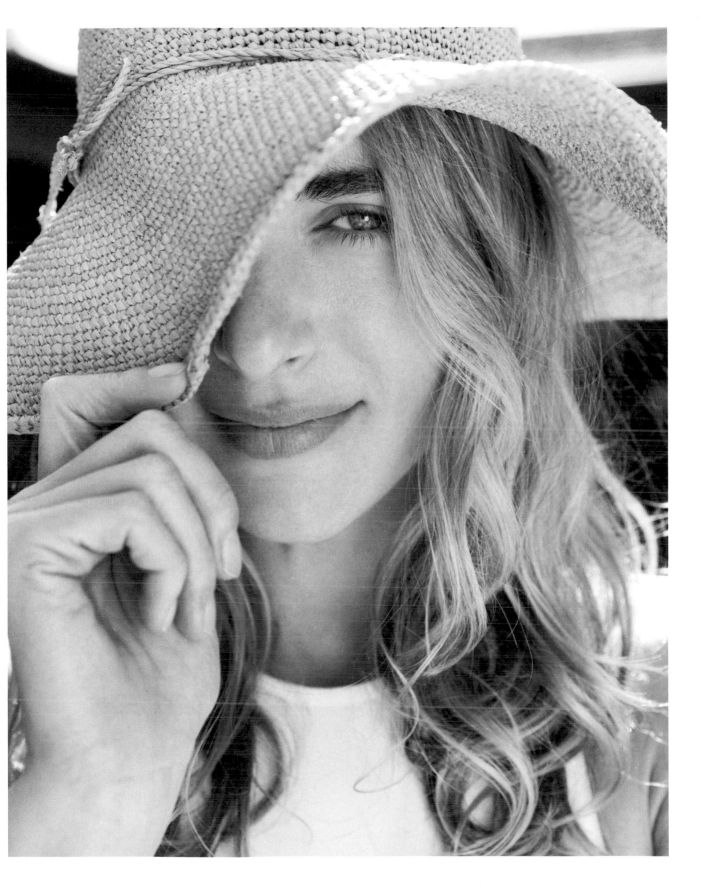

look. We've asked Dr. Lipman to explain how we can be sure we're getting enough—from the sun and otherwise.

Dr. Frank Lipman
ON GETTING ENOUGH VITAMIN D

How much vitamin D do we need, and is it the same for everyone? How often should we have our vitamin D levels checked?

Your vitamin D needs vary with age, body weight, percent of body fat, latitude, skin coloration, season of the year, use of sunblock, individual variation in sun exposure, and—probably—how ill you are.

At least once a year, especially at the beginning of winter, have your vitamin D levels checked. If you are supplementing, I suggest you monitor your vitamin D levels approximately every three months until you are in the optimal range. If you are taking high doses (10,000 IU a day), your doctor must also check your calcium, phosphorus, and parathyroid hormone levels every three months.

In order to keep a healthy vitamin D level, how much—and what kind of—sun exposure do we need?

Be sensible and always avoid sunburn. It's best to build up tolerance by slowly increasing the time you spend in the sun to avoid getting burned. Once you have built up tolerance, the recommendation is about 15 to 20 minutes of direct sunlight on unprotected skin three to four times a week between 10 a.m. and 3 p.m. (To help you monitor sun exposure, pick up a SunFriend device—www.sunfriend.com

If we take a vitamin D supplement, do we still need to spend time in the sun?

I believe getting direct sunlight is important for a lot more than just our vitamin D levels. Sunlight boosts your mood and helps regulate your circadian rhythm—so getting sun exposure during the day can help us sleep better at night. The sun is a source of energy for the whole planet, and getting regular exposure to that warm light is important for our overall well-being.

Can we get a substantial amount of vitamin D from our diet?

It is extremely difficult to get adequate vitamin D from diet alone. Most people need regular exposure to the sun to get enough vitamin D—and most people also need to supplement. Cod liver oil and fatty fish such as wild salmon and sardines contain some vitamin D, but you'd need to eat a lot to get enough for what your body truly needs.

SUN RESPONSIBLY

Ideal sun exposure is short and frequent, but of course, sometimes we find ourselves out in the sun for much longer periods of time than Dr. Lipman recommends. And in these instances, we do need to be smart about how we protect ourselves. The ground rules that we live by (and enforce with our kids where appropriate) are:

- When you're going out in serious sun, sunblock is obviously in order: a physical block, not chemical (see next section on sunscreen vs. sunblock), SPF 30, reapplied obsessively.
- Hats, sun-protective clothing, umbrellas, and plain old shade—deployed in conjunction with sunblock—are a must, and the best protection you can get. Sun-protective clothes and hats have become seriously cute, and they allow you to stay out in sun that would otherwise be too much.
- Dermatologists also recommend restricting beach time to before 10 a.m. and after 3 p.m.; it should be noted that most people also look better cavorting in the waves at sunset, as opposed to high noon.

- You get sun when you're driving, and if you've got an office with a window; UVA rays penetrate glass—so apply sunblock.
- You get more solar radiation when you're in sand, snow, or on the water, because the rays reflect off the surface. You get more at high altitudes because the air is thinner, and you get a huge amount when you fly. So go nuts with the sunblock in these situations, and since all of them are also very drying conditions, stay moisturized, too.

goop TIP

A great airplane bag includes an antioxidant oil or moisturizer, lip balm, but most of all, SPF 30 sunblock—and remember to do your hands as well as your face, reapplying after you wash them.

goop PICKS

Hats are kind of glamorous—especially the two adorable brands Artesano and Hat Attack, which also happen to be amazing at protecting your skin. Even if you're not a hat person, become one for the beach. You'll protect your hair color and your skin, too.

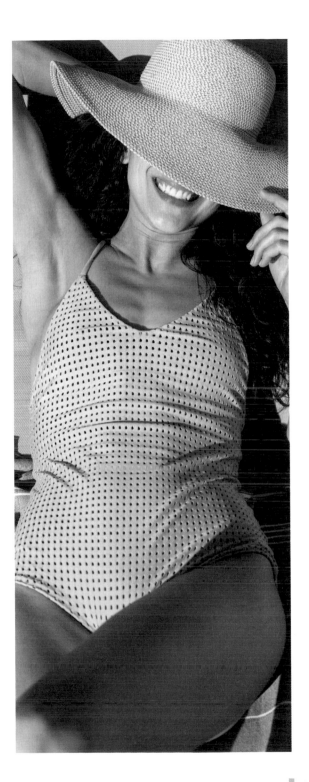

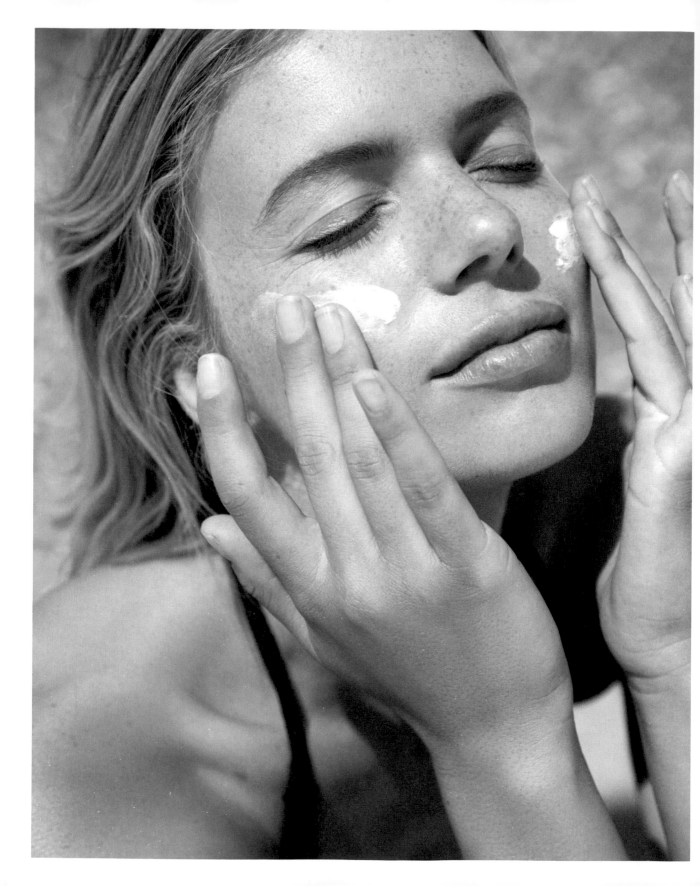

SUNSCREEN VS. SUNBLOCK— FIND YOUR FOREVER-FAVORITE

We've been taught that if we apply sunscreen, we're safe from sun damage—premature aging, cancer, and sunburn. But that oversimplified perspective is dangerously wrong. Chemical sunscreens were originally designed to protect skin from UVB rays—the ones that cause sunburn. But the premature-aging and potentially cancer-causing rays are UVA, not UVB. Today, most chemical sunscreens include some degree of UVA protection—the higher the SPF, usually the more UVA protection, though not always—but they still present problems. Physical sunblocks (also called mineral sunscreens)—titanium dioxide and zinc oxide—are harder to rub in, but a better choice for many reasons, starting with the fact that they block both UVA and UVB.

SPF AND THE LAW OF DIMINISHING RETURNS

The difference between an SPF 4 and an SPF 15, protection-wise, is enormous. The difference between an SPF 15 and an SPF 30 is less so, but still significant. The difference between an SPF 30 and an SPF 50 is vanishingly small; go up to the 80s and 100s and you're just putting extra chemicals on your body for little reason. Most dermatologists agree an SPF 30 is perfect for just about every situation.

Here's why you should choose a physical sunblock:

- Chemical sunscreens absorb the sun's rays; sunblocks physically deflect them by sitting on top of the skin.
- Many chemical sunscreens are known skin irritants; a primary ingredient in sunblocks, zinc oxide, is actually skin-soothing (it's what diaper-rash creams are made of).
- Chemical sunscreens degrade coral reefs (!); sunblock is nontoxic to the environment.
- Chemical sunscreens, avobenzone (the most commonly used one) in particular, degrade in sunlight—it's why sunscreen labels all say to reapply every 2 hours. So that "daily" sunscreen you apply in the morning is probably gone by the time you step outside for lunch. (Some sunscreens now contain stabilizers to make them last longer, but not all.) Sunblock does not degrade in sunlight, so putting some on at 8 a.m. is actually more of the basic shield you're imagining.
- Chemical sunscreen ingredients like oxybenzone, octinoxate (octyl methoxycinnamate), homosalate, octisalate, octocrylene, and avobenzone can contain hormone and endocrine disruptors that are most harmful in small doses, as they mimic our bodies' hormones and thus interfere with everything from our reproductive systems to our metabolism. They're particularly bad for children, whose systems are rapidly developing. Oxybenzone is especially awful, earning an 8 from the Environmental Working Group (EWG), which rates products on their toxicity (1 to 3 being ideal). (There is also some research suggesting that some chemical sunscreens could be associated with skin cancer. According to the EWG, retinyl palmitate, a form of vitamin A, is added to about 18 percent of beach

and sport sunscreens. Although it is an antioxidant that can be used to prevent the skin from aging, it may actually encourage the development of skin tumors and lesions when used on the skin while out in the sun.)

It's Good If You Have to Rub It In

Dermatologists and cosmetic companies shake their heads and explain that women won't use products that take longer to rub in. The ease-of-rubbing-in obsession has brought us our most problematic sunscreen and sunblock products of all: Sprays, which present serious issues when inhaled. Even physical sunblock, in which the ingredients are not toxic—is no good for you when inhaled. Some physical sunblock companies have tried to make their products easier to rub in (and less white and chalky looking) by using nanoparticles of titanium dioxide and zinc oxide, but nanoparticles are too small to be safe, particularly in the case of titanium dioxide—they can enter your bloodstream and have been shown to crop up in brain tissue.

The bottom line: Find a non-nano, physical sunblock you can live with and then…live happily and healthily with it. Sprays are especially appealing when you've got small children to coat before the beach, but don't do it. The extra minutes rubbing in sunblock (and, if you're at the beach, reapplying) are more than worth it, in terms of both actual sun protection and toxic load to you and the environment. And you can think about how fantastic you'll still look in 10 years. Just be sure to apply enough: If you're covering most of your body, the amount you use should equal about a full shot glass.

The Ingredients Checklist

When shopping for sunblock, read the labels, looking out for:

• *Active ingredients:* Mineral sunscreens (i.e., physical sunblock) will list zinc and/or titanium dioxide *only*. Be wary of the term *mineral-based*, which often means zinc and/or titanium dioxide have been mixed with chemical sunscreens.

• *Water resistant:* A sunscreen can only claim to be water resistant if it has undergone a 40- or 80-minute test. If it's not stated clearly on the label, most likely it will wash or sweat off.

• *Broad spectrum:* Important, as it means that the sunscreen blocks both UVA and UVB rays. All physical sunblocks are broad spectrum.

• *Inactive ingredients:* Even if the active ingredients are nontoxic (i.e., mineral), make sure that it's not otherwise loaded with toxins. Red flags include phthalate, fragrance, and anything ending in -paraben or -glycol.

Stress: Friend or Foe?

For a long time we've been intimidated by stress—not entirely unlike how we've come to worry over sun exposure. We've been told it's the reason for gray hair, breakouts, wrinkles, belly fat, anxiety, and unhappiness. Newspapers, magazines, news programs, and health blogs have all proclaimed different iterations of the same headline for years: Stress kills. But we've recently discovered that the story of stress is more complex than we'd been led to believe—and not nearly as grim.

As Dr. Frank Lipman reports in his book *10 Reasons You Feel Old and Get Fat,* acute stress (as opposed to unrelenting, chronic stress—which we admit is not always possible to avoid) actually has a positive impact on our well-being. Acute stress (e.g., a challenging work project, a demanding fitness goal) allows us to keep the two halves of the autonomic nervous system in balance—the sympathetic nervous system (regulates stress response) and the parasympathetic (regulates the relaxation response). With acute stress, the body is energized with adrenaline and other stress hormones to meet the task at hand, to grow, to learn—but then the body can relax, the stress hormones recede before your system becomes inflamed, and other hormones are able to take over. A real-life example: You have a hectic day at work but you get a lot done, leave the office feeling accomplished, and head home for a nourishing dinner with your family, followed by a bit of time to unwind.

As important as it is to find ways to unwind (which we'll do later in this chapter), the way we approach stress initially (and, interestingly, think about it) also matters. Kelly McGonigal, PhD, a health psychologist and lecturer at Stanford University, uses two (fascinating) studies to explain why:

The first study tracked 30,000 adults in the U.S. for eight years. The study asked people how much stress they experienced in the last year and if they believed that stress was harmful to their health. The study then looked at public death records to find out who died. People who experienced a lot of stress in the previous year *and* believed stress was harmful had a 43 percent increase in the risk of dying. This was not true of people who experienced a lot of stress but did not believe it was harmful. This group actually had the lowest risk of dying—lower even than the people who had relatively little stress.

The second study gives some insight into why. Participants in this particular Harvard study were put through a series of stressful tests—some of the participants were taught first, though, to think of their body's stress responses as helpful. Pounding heart = preparing you for action. Breathing hard = getting more oxygen to your brain. The participants who were taught that stress was good were found to be less stressed, less anxious, and more confident. And their physical stress response was different. In a "normal" stress response, your heart rate goes up and your blood vessels constrict (a piece of the link between stress and cardiovascular issues). But participants who thought of their stress responses as helpful? Their blood vessels did not constrict, they stayed relaxed even though the heart was pounding. Get this: Their hearts looked as they might in times of joy or courage. Over the course of years of everyday stress, this biological change alone could change the health of your heart, the whole of your life.

We commonly picture stress as fatiguing, increasing inflammation in the body, releasing too much of hormones (like cortisol) that can run amok—but when our relationship to stress is healthy, we can avoid the pitfalls that make us look and feel…old and exhausted.

How to Unwind and Refresh

Sometimes, despite our best intentions and deepest wishes, stress, anxiety, and crazy schedules threaten to push us to the point of feeling and looking completely drained. And we need to find a way back. The yoga and exercise methods mentioned in Chapter 2 usually help—going to Tracy Anderson classes (see page 67) on the weekends or after work makes our editorial director, Elise Loehnen, infinitely happier. Meditation can be incredibly effective—keep reading for tips on how to begin meditating if it isn't already a practice for you. Sleep, too, plays a big role in keeping us (looking and feeling) sane—more on this in the next chapter. Also key to staying energized: understanding the adrenal system and how to support it.

> # goop PICKS
>
> Meditation apps and online recordings can be helpful when it comes to kick-starting (or strengthening) a practice. Dr. Junger has a free, 5-minute soothing session. Oprah Winfrey and Deepak Chopra offer a 21-day program. And, in the app store, try: Headspace, Simply Being, and—if you're more advanced—Equanimity. (Also, see the section on yoga nidra recordings on page 144.)

ADRENAL FATIGUE AND HOW TO RECHARGE

The adrenals are two tiny glands that sit on top of the kidneys. They help to produce the hormones that regulate the fight-or-flight reactions, adrenaline, and noradrenaline. Dr. Junger likens the adrenals to the power strip into which our organs are plugged for energy—like an iPhone and its charger into a socket. When the adrenals aren't at 100 percent, neither are the body's organs. Neither are we. Adrenal fatigue can negatively impact everything from our immunity to the health of our hair and skin. Dr. Junger explains how we can fortify ourselves.

Dr. Alejandro Junger
ON REJUVENATING THE ADRENAL SYSTEM

What causes the adrenal system to stop working properly? In a nutshell, it is the unnatural way in which we live that causes the adrenals to get exhausted and to not be able to perform their important functions effectively. One of the most important functions of the adrenals is the fight-or-flight reaction. Under natural conditions, these reactions are necessary every so often, but most of the time the adrenals should be on standby. But these days the fight-or-flight reactions are triggered all day long, and even at night. Someone cuts you off while driving, you miss the train and are going to be late for work, you remember a bill you are behind on, you get bad news about something important, someone treats you unfairly...and the list goes on and on. Stress keeps the adrenals working nonstop, and like any organ forced to do that, they get exhausted. On top of it, lots of us don't get enough sleep, which is when the adrenals should recharge. And to make matters worse, many of us don't get the necessary nutrients to keep the adrenals functioning properly, either.

What does adrenal fatigue look and feel like? What about skin and hair health?
Lack of energy, weakness, lack of mental clarity, difficulty concentrating, bad moods, cravings for stimulants, thinning hair, frequent infections, difficulty healing, and weight gain are all very common ways in which adrenal fatigue manifests.

Do changing cortisol levels play a role, and how we do ensure that our bodies are producing the right amount?
The adrenals are the ones producing cortisol, so adrenal fatigue is not caused by changing levels of cortisol. Adrenal fatigue is the cause of these shifts. In order to produce the right amount of cortisol, we need to reduce the stress (constant fight-or-flight conditions mentioned previously) that we put on the adrenals.

Can we revitalize the adrenals?
Good sleep and rest, restorative yoga, good nutrition, meditation, and exercise are all ways to reverse adrenal exhaustion.

Are there ways through diet or lifestyle that we can proactively protect our adrenals and ourselves when we are going through a particularly difficult, anxiety-prone time?
Yes. All the things I mentioned, when done in a regular, consistent way, not only help revitalize the adrenals, but will prevent them from getting exhausted to begin with.

THE MINDFUL REBOOT

One of the most compelling ways to manage stress and recharge is through meditation. Although not fully mainstream (yet), pretty much every week or so, we hear about another GOOP friend who has picked up meditation and now swears by it—and science has been backing up the wide and varied benefits of the practice. Studies have shown that meditation decreases negative emotions like anxiety and depression, as well as physical pain.

A piece of the science behind meditation, as explained by pain expert Vicky Vlachonis, is this: Brain scans show that meditation reduces activity in the area of the brain that processes pain (primary somatosensory cortex), and simultaneously increases activity in the areas responsible for regulating pain and emotion. Meditation thus makes pain hurt less, and helps you to react in a healthier way, emotionally and physically, to the pain that is present.

Below, Vlachonis reveals how meditation—along with a few other methods, tips, and tricks—can allow us to reboot when we need it most: when we're tired or worried, under the weather, or have that headache that just won't go away.

Vicky Vlachonis
ON MEDITATION AND MORE SELF-HEALING

What's the optimal way to meditate, and to begin a practice of doing so?
Beginning a new ritual can sometimes be tricky—*one*, it could be unfamiliar territory, or *two*, you're overwhelmed by adding yet another "task" to your already full daily agenda. However, the beauty of meditation is that you only need 12 minutes daily and it can be done almost anywhere—you'll learn this once you've fully blossomed in your practice. The best way to begin your new practice is to place its time slot before another essential ritual, like brushing your teeth or taking a shower—so set your morning alarm 15 minutes earlier!

HOW TO MEDITATE:

1. Sit up straight with your chest tall and open. You can even sit against a wall for support and proper posture control.

2. Close your eyes softly.

3. Place your hands on your knees, palms facing up. This could be with your legs crossed or straight—whatever feels more comfortable for you.

4. Take deep breaths—in through your nose and out through your mouth. Allow your breaths to be louder than your thoughts. Focus on your breath.

5. Relax your lower jaw. Drop your tongue from the roof of your mouth.

6. Set an intention and be fully present.

7. Talk to yourself about your intention. For example, if your intention is forgiveness, you could repeat something along the lines of:

   I forgive _____ for upsetting me.
   I release all anger and resentment.
   I will not allow negative emotions to
      hurt my body.
   I forgive myself.
   I am taking charge.
   I am grateful.
   I send all my love to _____.

8. Focus and visualize blood flow throughout your entire body. Begin at the bottom of your feet and move up your body. Proceed in the order below.

   - Bottom of feet
   - Top of feet
   - Ankles
   - Back of calves
   - Front of calves
   - Back of thighs
   - Front of thighs
   - Pelvic floor
   - Sacrum (at the base of the spine)
   - Lower back
   - Lower abdomen
   - Stomach
   - Ribs/diaphragm
   - Chest/lungs
   - Heart
   - Front of shoulders
   - Back of shoulders
   - Back of neck
   - Front of arms
   - Back of arms
   - Front of hands
   - Back of hands
   - Front of neck
   - Throat
   - Face
   - Top of head

9. Place your left hand over your heart, your right hand over your diaphragm, and finish with three deep, cleansing breaths. Your heart should feel fluid—like a wave flowing in and out.

What are some of the (mind and body) rejuvenating benefits of meditation?

As I shared in my book, *The Body Doesn't Lie,* meditation is a miracle that makes it possible for you to control your body and your health with your mind. A meta-analysis of 47 studies and over 3,500 subjects released in the *Journal of the American Medical Association* showed that meditation has been definitively proven to decrease anxiety, depression, and pain. Research at UCLA has found that just 12 minutes of meditation a day can give you younger cells and a younger brain. Who doesn't love younger? Previous research has also found that meditation reduces stress hormones and blood pressure while it simultaneously increases focus, concentration, memory, contentment, immunity, blood sugar control, and even the size of your brain. These effects can enhance every aspect of your life, as well as help with all pain, no matter where, how often, or how intensely you feel it. So not only can meditation improve the inside of your body, but it can also improve your appearance by releasing stress, anxiety, and depression—all factors in premature aging.

Can you explain self-healing trigger points, and how we can use them to alleviate pain or give us a boost?
Your body has all the tools it needs to manage your pain—you just need to learn to tap into those internal self-healing mechanisms. One of the most efficient ways is to use your own fingers to trigger a soothing release.

Following principles used in acupuncture, reflexology, and Chinese medicine, gently manipulating your own self-healing trigger points can help relieve some of your most stubborn pains. These points help you tap into energy meridians in the body that have specific therapeutic effects on the corresponding organs of the body, as well as release muscular tension, stimulate circulation, disperse accumulated toxins, and bring oxygenated blood throughout the body.

To release each point of tension, apply gentle pressure with your thumb, holding it flat, and moving it slowly in a circular motion for 10 seconds. (Note: Trigger point release is not massage; your hands should not be spread out.) As you apply the pressure, slowly breathe in through your nose and say to yourself, *I allow my body to release anger, frustration, heat, and inflammation. I move forward.* Then breathe out through your mouth, feeling the pain moving out of your muscles, and repeat: *I am balanced. I am grounded. I let go.* Repeat the full cycle three to five times, or until you can feel less resistance, that the muscle isn't as tight and your thumb can go deeper. You can incorporate trigger point therapy throughout your day—when you first wake up, before you go to sleep, and any time during the day that you need release.

Remember, everyone's pain is unique and different. Please always consult your physician, especially if you are pregnant, your pain is acute or intense, or if your symptoms are combined with fever and abdominal discomfort. Here is one really good trigger point to try:

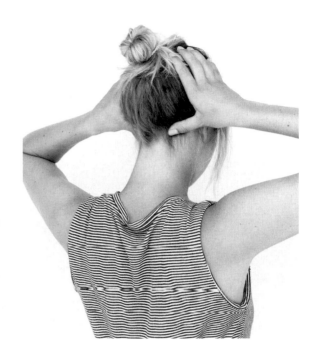

Where it is: Count four to five fingers from the back of your ear, aiming for your hairline at the base of your skull. Use your left hand for the left side (and vice versa). Apply gentle pressure with your left thumb. When you've located the correct spot, you will feel a dip and a tender point.

What it does: This point is very versatile—most of us instinctively rub this spot because it makes us feel emotionally and physically better so quickly. This point increases the blood supply to your brain, face, and middle ear, helping you think more clearly and confidently. It also relieves tension headaches and sinus issues and helps lessen insomnia, fatigue, and vertigo. Use it to quickly wipe away fear and confusion, help you make tough decisions, and to feel rooted in your own power.

What are other worthy ways to unwind?

Essential oils are powerful tools to induce relaxation—not only because of calming scents like bergamot, ylang-ylang, and rose, but also because they remind you to breathe. You might be thinking, *I don't need to be reminded to breathe,* but I can almost guarantee that you do—we all do! How many times throughout the day do you actually take deep, cleansing breaths? Probably not many, if any at all! Using essential oils can trigger deep breathing, as you smell the oils. Deep breathing, also known as diaphragm breathing, is when you inhale through your nose to fully fill your lungs and exhale deeply through your mouth. Breath is linked to our autonomic nervous system. Deep breathing activates your "rest and digest," the parasympathetic nervous system, helping your body relax and unwind.

Beauty World

When it comes to how we want to look and age, the way we interact with and account for the environment makes a big difference. Just as eating clean and exercising supports our body's detox processes, there are steps we can take to avoid problematic environmental factors and moves we can make to help our body's natural ability to repair the damage caused by the ones we can't avoid. For us, it boils down to being smart in the sun, using stress to motivate and prepare us rather than deter us, unwinding when we inevitably run into a wall despite our best intentions, fortifying our bodies with every manner of health and beauty booster (e.g., bring on the green tea)—and getting enough of the biggest beauty booster of them all, sleep (next up).

TAPPING INTO EARTH

Earthing (or grounding, as it's sometimes referred to) is the idea that we get healing benefits from touching the earth—walking barefoot outside or using conductive systems when indoors to transfer Earth's electrons from the ground to your body. It sounds a little cuckoo at first, but it happens to be grounded in research, and we can't help but be charmed by it. An article in the *Journal of Environmental and Public Health,* which reviewed the research on earthing, reported that the act has been found to "promote intriguing physiological changes and subjective reports of well-being." These positive changes seem to have the ability to impact the body in a variety of ways—from helping with stress and pain management to reducing inflammation. (The seemingly best explanation for the anti-inflammatory effect, for one, is that when grounding, the earth's negatively charged antioxidant electrons enter the body and neutralize the positively charged free radicals where the body is inflamed.) So, consider taking a barefoot walk the next time you're in a grassy park or on the beach—after all, there's not much to lose.

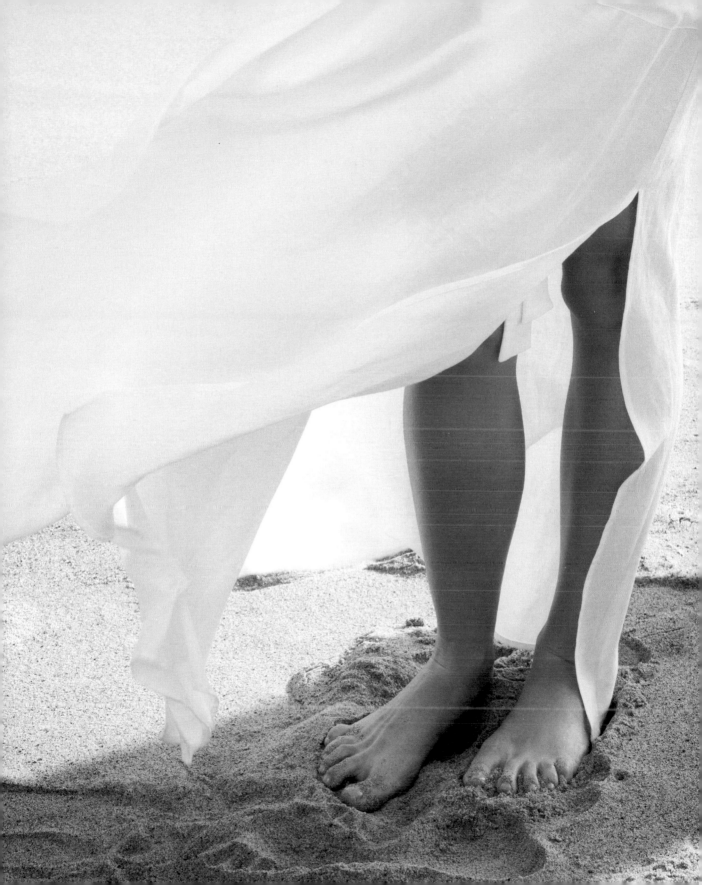

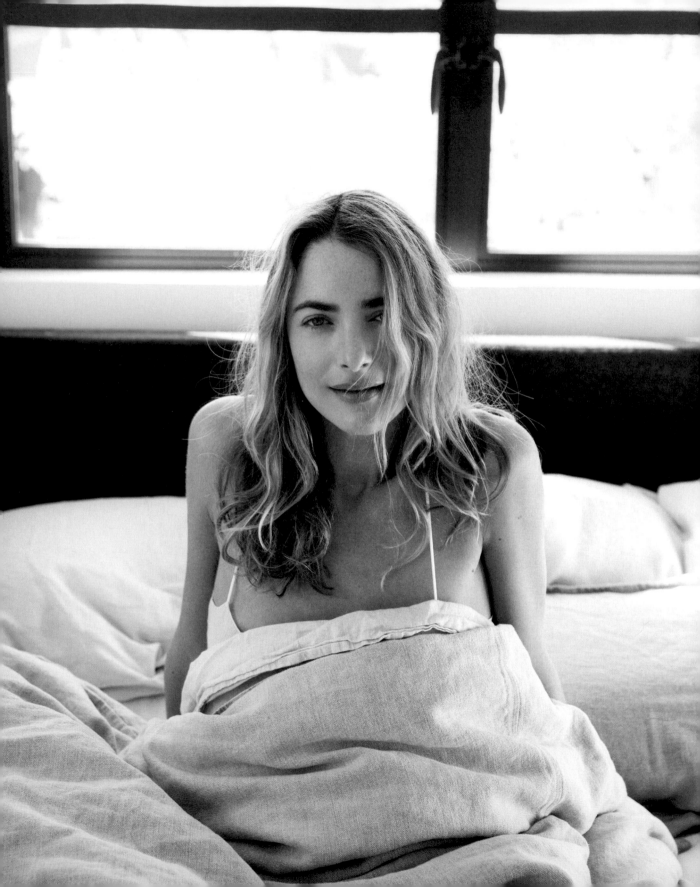

5.
Sleeping Soundly

Why We Seriously Need Sleep

We all know that we need sleep—in the same way that we understand that exercise is good for us. But in reality, when we're busy and there just doesn't seem to be enough hours in the day to get everything done, our sleep time is often the first thing that gets compromised. It's easy to rationalize staying up an extra hour to finish work, to watch one more mindless episode after a *long* day, to finally do the kids' laundry. In his book *10 Reasons You Feel Old and Get Fat* (not getting enough sleep is #7), Dr. Frank Lipman reports that America is having a sleep crisis: Between 50 and 70 million Americans have some trouble sleeping, and several million Americans take prescription sleep aids. "Trouble sleeping" is perhaps so common and pervasive that we don't even think of it as a problem. It might be hard for us to wake up, or we wake up feeling tired, or we need a Diet Coke to get us through the afternoon, or we're too wired when we get in bed to doze off, or we toss and turn throughout the night—but we don't necessarily consider any of these circumstances real problems. Just the way it is.

Although it often seems like no big deal to skimp on sleep—there's always coffee, *I'll sleep in on Sunday*—the truth is that it's a really big deal. And our sleeping hours should really be one of the last elements of our lives that we shortchange. Dr. Lipman explains that lack of sleep is linked to a host of unwanted conditions, including:

- Unsettling your metabolism and hormonal balance, leading to weight gain (more coming on why and how).
- Negative moods.
- Impaired memory and brain fog.
- Leaky gut—gut walls are repaired during sleep.
- Inflammation—increasing the likelihood of chronic disease.
- Decreased immune function, and even shorter life span.

And it goes without saying that poor sleep is terrible from a beauty perspective. Although there are beauty tricks that really do make a difference—we'll talk waking up with tired eyes later in this chapter—there's no comparable substitute for good sleep in terms of how well rested you'll feel and look. That's because sleep is a magical time for your body—it's when some of the body's most important repair and revival work happens. Again, we turned to Dr. Lipman to fill us in on what happens to the body when we're asleep:

- The secretion of human growth hormone (HGH)—"a natural fountain of youth" with major anti-aging effects. Some people even inject doses of it, although Dr. Lipman doesn't recommend it, especially when you can get it naturally through sleep (and also, side note, through intense exercise).
- Overall hormonal balance—you need enough sleep to produce the right amount of a variety of hormones, including the sex hormones.
- Muscle repair—working out naturally breaks muscles down, and the work of repairing and growing them takes place when you're sleeping.
- Parasympathetic nervous system work—the system also shines during sleep hours, meaning bedtime is an important time for your body to heal aches and pains.
- Immune support—quality sleep is important for staying healthy and warding off inflammation and chronic disease.
- Vital brain activity—key amino acids and other biochemicals that your brain uses when under stress are restored during sleep. Also, the glymphatic system, which removes toxins from your brain, is only active when you're asleep. Plus you consolidate memories when you sleep—which is significant for processing, storing, and retrieving information while awake.

Dr. Lipman
ON WHY WE GET FAT WHEN WE DON'T SLEEP

How does sleep, or lack of it, affect our weight?
Lack of good sleep affects our weight because it disrupts our metabolism and hormonal balance in a number of ways, and they all reinforce each other. For instance, lack of sleep is a stressor...stress stimulates cortisol...and cortisol cues your body to retain fat. Excess cortisol also disrupts your insulin response, which further cues your body to retain fat. And just as it throws your insulin out of whack, when you don't sleep enough you don't produce enough glucagon. And just as insulin cues your body to store fat, glucagon tells your body to burn it. So not enough sleep means you don't make enough glucagon to keep that fat burning.

We often hear that we should be getting 7 to 9 hours of sleep—is that true?
Yes, that's true; most research has shown we need 7 to 9 hours of sleep a night. If you are feeling irritable, anxious, and/or depressed, if you get easily frustrated, if you are suffering from a loss of mental clarity, an impaired memory, or a decreased ability to tolerate physical and emotional stress, a weak immune function, or a tendency to gain weight and a hard time losing it, you may not be getting enough sleep.

If we know we are inevitably going to be running low on sleep during a busy time at work/in life, is there something we can do to otherwise keep our metabolism and weight steady?
Yes: Cut out sugar, meditate, exercise, and keep your microbiome healthy and balanced.

HORMONAL SLEEP

As mentioned already, part of the reason sleep is so important is that we need it to maintain healthy, balanced levels of our most essential hormones. We asked our resident hormone advisor, Dr. Laura Lefkowitz, to tell us more.

Dr. Laura Lefkowitz
ON WHY "BEAUTY SLEEP" IS REAL

How does sleep or lack thereof play into hormone levels? Not getting enough sleep is almost a badge of honor in modern society, one bad lifestyle factor that I believe is becoming far too comfortable. Some people even boast about their ability to function on very little sleep. Sleep is not a waste of time. Sleep is vitally important to good health. During sleep the brain rests and processes the day's thoughts, learning, and activities. During sleep the body repairs itself and detoxifies from all it is exposed to during a long, busy day. Before electricity, we were awake in daylight hours, and slept when it was dark. Today, many people are in bed only 4 to 6 hours per night on a regular basis and are not getting restorative sleep. Now, with electricity, you can work any hour of the day. When sleep is poor in quality and quantity, hormone output is affected.

The two major pathways by which sleep affects the release of hormones are through the autonomic nervous system and the hypothalamic-pituitary axis.

Autonomic Nervous System

The body has two opposing autonomic nervous system states. The first is called the parasympathetic nervous system, which is our state of rest and calm. The second is the sympathetic nervous system, our fight-or-flight state. This system activates your body for stressful situations, such as raising your breathing and heart rate so you can run away from danger.

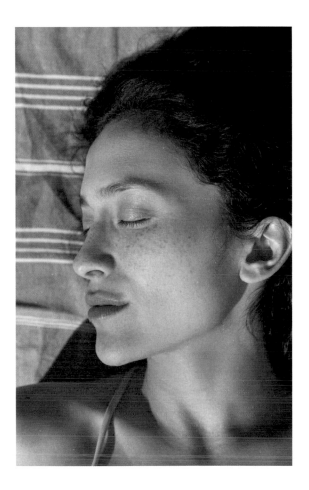

Most hormone-secreting organs are sensitive to changes in the sympathetic nervous system. During deep sleep, the sympathetic nervous system activity should be decreased, as you safely rest. Sleep deprivation is associated with higher sympathetic activity and an increase in insulin and cortisol secretion (both fat-storing, inflammatory hormones).

Hypothalamic-Pituitary Axis

The hypothalamus and pituitary gland are very important glands located in the brain that start many of the hormone cascades throughout the endocrine (hormone) system. The pituitary is often called the "master" endocrine organ

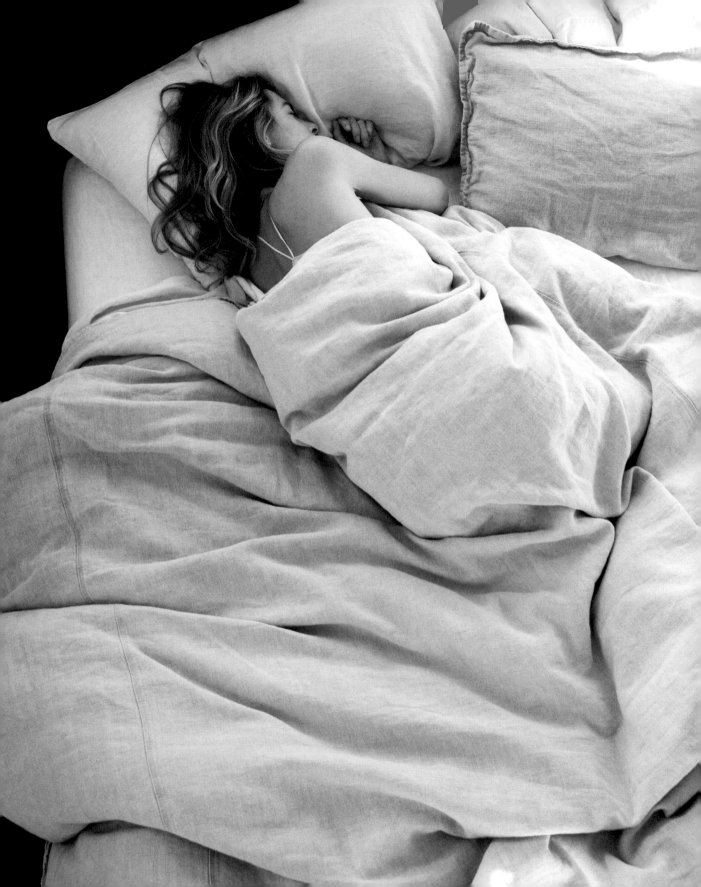

because it controls the secretion of many hormones in peripheral glands throughout the body, e.g., the thyroid, ovaries, adrenals. This hypothalamic-pituitary axis is markedly influenced by sleep. During adequate states of sleep, hypothalamic-pituitary factors are activated or inhibited to keep the body in sync. Sleep deprivation can alter the appropriate activation/inhibition and cause hormonal imbalances.

The following hormones are affected by sleep deprivation:

- **Cortisol:** An abdominal fat-storing hormone that causes inflammation in the body and raises blood sugar levels in order to have energy when sleep is deprived. Chronic sleep loss causes elevated cortisol levels and the development of insulin resistance, a risk factor for obesity and diabetes. Chronically relying on your adrenal glands to produce cortisol to keep you functioning on inadequate sleep can also lead to adrenal fatigue.

- **Free thyroxin (FT4):** The main hormone produced by the thyroid that increases metabolic rate and affects growth and development. Sleep deprivation causes an increase in circulating thyroxin in order to keep the metabolism humming to get through the day in a sleep deprived state. Chronic elevated blood levels of thyroxin from sleep deprivation make the brain think there is too much thyroxin in circulation. This causes a negative feedback loop on the pituitary gland, leading it to decrease production of thyroid-stimulating hormones to quiet the thyroid gland down, but over time this suppression can cause decreased thyroid function and hypothyroidism.

- **Human growth hormone (HGH):** A hormone that plays a role in muscle health, how our bodies store fat (especially around the abdomen), brain function, the ratio of high-density to low-density lipoproteins in our cholesterol, and bone density.

Normally there is one big HGH pulse after sleep onset. With chronic sleep deprivation the normal single HGH pulse splits into two smaller pulses, one before sleep and one after sleep. This is a problem because our organs are now exposed to HGH for an extended period of time, which, because HGH has fat-storage anti-insulin-like effects, adversely affects glucose metabolism, causing obesity and diabetes.

Recent studies in humans have shown that the levels of hormones that regulate appetite are profoundly influenced by sleep duration. Sleep loss is associated with an increase in appetite that is excessive in relation to the caloric demands of the extended wakeful period.

- **Leptin:** An appetite suppressant hormone, released by fat cells, that signals satiety to the brain and suppresses appetite. Leptin production is dependent on sleep duration. Studies in humans have shown that sleep deprivation causes a decrease in blood leptin levels, so with less sleep you feel less satiated by the food you eat, causing you to overeat, gain weight, and further aggravate insulin resistance and glucose metabolism.

- **Ghrelin:** An appetite stimulant hormone that is released in the stomach and is also dependent on sleep quality and quantity. Sleep deprivation causes a rise in ghrelin levels, causing increased hunger and appetite, especially for foods with high carbohydrate contents. This is a nasty combination with lower leptin levels and a decreased ability for achieving satiation from your meals, so you overeat, specifically glucose-dense foods that need insulin to be processed, which causes weight gain and further aggravates insulin resistance and glucose metabolism, leading to diabetes.

Sleep loss therefore alters the ability of leptin and ghrelin to accurately signal our caloric needs and could lead to excessive overeating, especially when food is in abundance.

All these disturbances in hormone function caused by inadequate sleep cause a metabolic shift in the body's ability to metabolize sugar, even with normal insulin levels, and puts everyone at risk for insulin resistance and type 2 diabetes.

If we look one step further as menopause approaches, changes in sex hormones can affect sleep more than during any other period in a woman's life. The declining levels of estrogen affect sleep quality before you are in actual menopause. Hot flashes and irritability can happen on and off throughout the decade before menopause hits, causing wakefulness throughout the night and poor sleep quality.

Once you've actually made it into menopause, hot flashes should disappear and sleep issues should settle down, but perimenopausal women may struggle with sleep disturbances for years.

Clearly, sleep is not only for the brain but essential for the entire body. Sleep is not a waste of time. If you want to age gracefully, with a slim waistline, glowing skin, and lush hair, you must prioritize getting 7 to 9 hours of sleep every day of the week. Before all the scientific research, the old saying, "You must get your beauty sleep," could not be truer.

More Is More

When you look at all the cons of lack of sleep and the pros of getting good sleep, our best advice is pretty obvious. *Get more sleep. Get higher quality sleep.* But how do you do it without adding hours onto an already stretched day? When time is a premium commodity, there's actually a lot that is still under our control when it comes to maximizing the rest you *can* get in.

Diet and exercise can play a huge role in getting the most out of your precious shut-eye. By minimizing the amount of energy your body needs when it comes time to repair, you set it up to be efficient and focused on what systems need the most attention. By eating clean, decreasing your toxic load, supporting your gut and adrenals, exercising, and unwinding, you've done most of the important work during the day—allowing the body to dedicate its sleep hours to the tougher stuff. Living a detox lifestyle is a great step toward maximizing your sleep hours—digestive issues, hormonal inconsistencies, and mental and physical hurts could be standing in the way of your sleep. Clearing yourself of these problems through detox may help you fall asleep faster and stay asleep longer.

Still, there are even more useful methods for getting more and better sleep. We asked Dr. Rafael Pelayo of the Stanford Center for Sleep Sciences and Medicine to help us understand how.

Dr. Rafael Pelayo
ON SLEEPING RIGHT

What are the biggest culprits of sleep deprivation?
I think the biggest culprit is people not making sleep a priority in their lives. People view sleep as an inconvenience. They'll get sleep whenever they can but they make other things more important. So if they have other things to do, they'll just get a little less sleep. I think that stems from the fact that our sleep needs are variable. If you ask someone how much sleep she should get versus how much she actually gets—everybody has two numbers in their heads. For example, "I like to get 7 hours of sleep but I can get by with 5." Everybody knows the minimum amount of sleep he or she needs to get by. And people tend to start off with good intentions—*I'm going to get 8 hours of sleep*

tonight—but then things come up, and we end up getting as little sleep as possible. So we are just getting by, but not doing as well as we possibly could.

Can you explain the concept of sleep debt?
There's a misunderstanding that many people have about sleep: that they can somehow catch up from 5 days of sleep deprivation in a 2-day weekend. But that's not how the brain works. People tend to think about sleep in terms of the amount of hours we sleep, but sleep is also modulated by something called the circadian system.

If you normally sleep 8 hours a night, but one night you skip sleep completely, the next day, you're 8 hours behind. But you're not going to be able to sleep 16 hours in a row. The brain won't let you, for one, because the circadian system—which predicts dawn and dusk—will wake you up. (This is how you get jet lagged and why people have trouble adjusting to Daylight Savings Time—the brain is anticipating dawn and dusk from the previous night.)

We should pay our sleep debt back, though. If you deprive yourself enough, you will fall asleep when it's not safe to do so—for example, at the wheel. The power of sleep is so intense that it puts you down even though you're not safe to fall asleep. Sometimes we fall asleep for a few seconds—little micro-sleeps—and we don't even realize it. When people are in a very light sleep (called stage one), they will often swear to you that they are awake. You've probably seen this if you've ever sat through a boring PowerPoint presentation—a co-worker's head drops, you know she's asleep, but when you nudge her the first thing she says is, "I'm awake, I'm resting my eyes!"

To actually pay the sleep debt back, you often really need to change your lifestyle in order to get enough sleep. And we've seen this work in studies. There are a few tests we use to measure sleep debt and the process of paying it back, like the Maintenance of Wakefulness Test and the Mean Sleep Latency Test. And we see sleep scores improve as people get extra time to sleep. But it's not just about the score—as people pay the debt back, they feel better, are more alert, tend to be less grumpy, feel sharper, their memory is better, they're a little less forgetful, less irritable.

What should we know about the difference between REM and non-REM sleep, and the stages of sleep?
From what we can tell, the brain has three different states: awake, asleep but not dreaming (which is non-REM), and asleep and dreaming (which is REM).

Non-REM sleep makes up the majority of your night's sleep, and can be broken down into: light sleep (stage one), intermediate sleep (stage two), and slow wave sleep (stage three). Non-REM sleep is what we think of as really resting—slow breathing, slow heart rate. Our heart rate is slowest during slow wave sleep—this is when it's the hardest to wake up. During slow wave sleep, the growth hormone surges. (This is when little kids grow.) This is also when abnormal behaviors like sleepwalking occur.

REM sleep is characterized by rapid eye movement and dreaming—REM takes up about 20 percent of sleep on average, and dominates the last third of the night. When you're in REM sleep, the brain is active. If I look at your brain waves when you're awake and when you're in REM, they look pretty much the same. The difference is, when you're awake, you can move your muscles and you're engaged with the outside world. During REM, you're disengaged, and the brain sends a signal to the spinal cord not to move your arms and legs, thereby paralyzing them. In contrast to non-REM, your heart is also very active in REM sleep. If you have a sedentary lifestyle, your peak heart rate is actually when you're dreaming, in REM. (This is the sleep stage that's associated with having a heart attack in your sleep.)

All stages of sleep are important, and play roles in our learning processes. For example, REM is associated with learning new sequences. And non-REM with comparing your old thoughts to your new thoughts from the day.

Should adults be napping?

Yes. Napping is like snacking. If you don't get enough food from your regular meals, a snack is a good thing. But if you're skipping meals, snacking isn't going to be good. Napping is a way of getting extra sleep. If you normally get 8 hours of sleep, but you only get 5 one night, then it would be healthy to take a nap. But if you're having trouble sleeping at night, and napping during the day—that's not healthy.

There's also a smart way, or time, to nap. Our body temperature is 98.6°F on average but it actually fluctuates during the day a bit. When your body temperature dips, we get sleepy, and when it climbs we feel more awake and alert. Our body is very sensitive to temperature—think about how it's more comfortable to sleep in a cool room than a hot room. And we all get a little drop in our temperature in the afternoon, around 2 p.m. on average. That's why people get a little sleepy after lunch. They blame it on their lunch, but that's not really the case; breakfast and dinner don't make you tired. Knowing your temperature drops in the afternoon, that's when you want to plan a nap.

What can we do to be better sleepers?

We sleep best when we feel safe, when there's serenity in our lives. But we often lack serenity. And while we can fall asleep under any circumstance if we're sleep deprived enough, this often means we're sleeping in spurts—not good enough. So one of the things we do with a lot of our patients at Stanford is create an environment of serenity in the bedroom—make their bedrooms sanctuaries. We want people to look forward to sleeping. You shouldn't view sleep as a chore—it's not that you have to sleep, it's that you get to sleep. It's a reward—you earn this nice place to sleep, it's a place and a time to enjoy.

SLEEP TIPS WE SWEAR BY

At GOOP we know how hard it is to make sleep a priority—maybe tomorrow we'll all be less busy?

So, we've collected our favorite sleep-enhancing tips:

- Try to go to sleep and wake up around the same time as often as possible, letting your body get into a steady rhythm. Consistency matters—and is superior to trying to "make up" for lost sleep all in one long slumber. As Dr. Lipman says, "A regular sleep rhythm reminds the brain when to release sleep and wake hormones, which in turn affects all the other hormones, ultimately affecting our overall health."

- Speaking of rhythms, get in sync with the sun's schedule. Spend time in natural light during the day. This sounds obvious, but a lot of us spend entire days inside, at our office desks. The body has long taken its sleeping and waking cues from sunset and sunrise. And despite all our modern inventions and how different our days (and nights) look now, we aren't turning over this evolutionary fact any time soon. (This is the reason some people—somewhat jokingly—trace modern issues with sleep to Thomas Edison, inventor of the light bulb.)

- Staying with the light/dark theme, make sure your bedroom is completely dark. In order to fall asleep, the body produces an essential hormone called melatonin that makes us drowsy. And the body knows to produce melatonin when it can't see any light. So having a dark bedroom is important—even with eyes shut, a bright light (be it your partner's reading light or city streetlights) can be disturbing. Eye masks can come in handy for this.

- Unplug at the end of day: If you're watching TV or working on your laptop until bedtime, that blue light from the screen signals to your body that it should still be up and alert, making it harder to fall asleep once you've called it quits. And if you find yourself checking email at 3 a.m. when you wake up to pee, you're not alone. Keeping your cell phone on the bedside table is never good for sleep. The light (or noise) of phones going off while you're sleeping—even if brief—can interrupt the body's production of melatonin. If you can't rest unless it's next to you, modify the settings to emit less light during evening hours, and put it on the "Do Not Disturb" setting, so that it doesn't ring or vibrate.

WI-FI-FREE ZONE

Preliminary research has suggested that the radiation from cell phones and Wi-Fi signals could be detrimental to our health (and particularly so for children), linking it to changes in brain metabolism and to cancer. For that reason, experts on this front recommend limiting your exposure to cell phones and Wi-Fi—which sounds like an entirely unrealistic order when our daily lives require us to be constantly plugged in. And yet, nighttime presents a suitable opportunity to check out. The easiest option is probably to turn off your Wi-Fi router and devices before bed (or switch your cell to airplane mode). A step up, and ideal for getting the best shut-eye, would be keeping the bedroom entirely free of electronic and digital equipment, and thus blue lights as well as electromagnetic fields.

- Stay away from caffeine later in the day. Everyone's tolerance level is a bit different but if you're having trouble falling asleep, caffeine might be the culprit. There should be no surprise by this point: Caffeine

can fatigue your adrenals, increase cortisol in the body (associated with waking up, not falling asleep), and increase your heart rate—all making sleep difficult. A carefully set detox can provide a really good baseline for figuring out how well your body processes caffeine, if the latte is worth it, or when your cutoff time is for a cup. After you detox, try reintroducing caffeine in small amounts (maybe you have a green tea one day, a small coffee in the morning another day), and see how your body and sleep are affected.

- Resist midnight snacks to prevent the digestive process from disturbing your sleep. In order to allow the body to really cleanse overnight, Dr. Junger recommends keeping a regular 12-hour fasting window—so if you finish dinner at 8:30 p.m., you shouldn't eat breakfast until after 8:30 a.m. the next day. This is because the body doesn't go into deep detox mode until about 8 hours after your last meal, and then it needs about 4 more hours to do its job. If you are eating late at night, opt for something without sugar, which can jolt you at the worst time. Sugar is part of the reason that alcohol, which might seem like a means to falling asleep, isn't the best solution—as your body processes the alcohol, it can disrupt your rest.

- Avoid sleeping pills/aids, which have a lot of undesirable side effects: addiction, agitation, sleep-walking, drowsiness (during the day), dizziness, and more. Many sleep aids are anticholinergic, meaning they suppress the REM (rapid eye movement) phase. And they might not actually give you all that much more sleep! Dr. Lipman points to an NIH analysis, which found that sleep meds (compared to placebos) reduce the time it takes to fall asleep by a little under 13 minutes on average—increasing total sleep time by approximately (and only) 11 minutes.

Sleep Rituals

Nighttime routines aren't just for calming unruly toddlers. A natural set of bedtime rituals can help guide you into more relaxed, restful sleep. A good start is to look back at the unwinding and stress-balancing methods from Chapter 2 and Chapter 4. Incorporating these as part of your natural routine—cardio, yoga, meditation, self-healing trigger points—can help the body to find better balance and better rest at night. Here are some great additional sleep-time rituals.

BATH HEAVEN

A bath is like slow food for the mind and body. Taking a bath is an especially amazing way to end the day—it has a calming effect that lasts beyond the moment you step out of the tub. And it actually helps signal your body that it's time to sleep. While a bath is an ideal way to warm up on cold winter days, when you get out of the tub, your body actually cools slightly—and this lowered body temperature helps put you to sleep.

There's hardly a wrong way to enjoy a bath, whether you like to have music in the background, or just a little peace and quiet. We recommend adding body oil to the bath—as opposed to conventional "bath oil" or a bubbly product—to combat the bath's drying effect on the skin. Conventional bath oils are typically made with surfactants (super-drying detergents), which help the oil disperse more evenly but do not help you in the moisturizing department. They actually deplete the moisture in your skin. Instead, use your body oil in the tub—and if there are oil droplets left on the surface of the water, rub them into the skin for extra moisture. Also, many body/bath oils have aromatherapeutic scents (lavender, jasmine,

rose, or chamomile, for instance) that can further encourage sleep.

THE 3-MINUTE FOOT MASSAGE

A basic 3-minute foot massage can also be pretty life changing. A spa visit is an undeniable luxury, but a self-massage (or one given by a friend/lover, or to a loved one—including your kids) is undervalued in terms of making a difference in overall well-being and especially in sleep. You don't need to know reflexology or have any training. Just grab a tub of cream—think moisturizing, thick, textured—that has a scent you love. (See the sleep-inducing aromatherapeutic scents recommended for baths. Foot-specific creams tend to have an almost medicinal smell, so if you don't love them, use a body cream, which is of course suitable for the feet, too.) Creams that work in antioxidants and omega oils get major bonus points—you'll find many in the GOOP shop, where all our creams are obsessively nontoxic, not to mention beautifully indulgent.

Massaging your feet (or someone else's) even for just 3 minutes will make anyone's night better, and their next day happier. (Obviously, it also helps relax the muscles in the feet, and eases any aches from being in heels for an evening or on your feet all day.) It creates a real grounding sensation, which may help relieve some of the mental tension from the day, and prepare you for truly restful sleep.

INDULGENT PILLOWCASES

Tuck yourself between the thick linen sheets at La Colombe d'Or in the south of France and the air rustles with the supremely relaxing scent of lavender. Spritzing your sheets with a combination of essential oils and water is an ancient practice worth

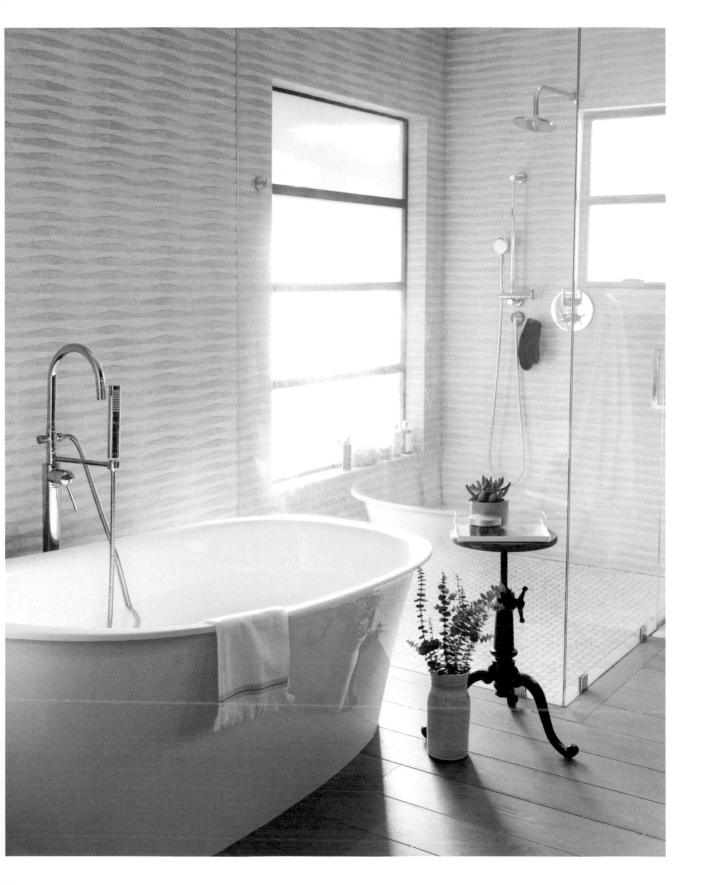

reviving, both for its sleep- and relaxation-inducing powers and just knowing that you've taken the time to make your environment a little bit luxurious, to make yourself feel extra cared for.

PSYCHIC SLEEP

Yoga nidra, which means "psychic sleep," is an ancient practice that can be highly restorative—a single session (between 20 and 40 minutes) is said to be equivalent to hours of sleep. You aren't actually sleeping during a session, but you're meant to get close—to be talked down to the moment when your body is still enough to sleep and yet your mind is still awake. The goal is to quiet the conscious mind in order to tap into the potential of the subconscious. The overall effect is deeply relaxing.

If you're interested in giving it a try, and we recommend you do, you can find recordings of yoga nidra meditation online—we've listened to Kirit Thacker, the head of yoga at Ananda, the very luxe and very authentic Ayurvedic spa in India. The more you practice yoga nidra, the easier it becomes to conjure the sensations requested (hot and cold, feelings of lightness and heaviness). And although you can do a session at any time, it's an ideal right-before-bedtime ritual—particularly if you struggle with a restless body while attempting to fall asleep.

SUPREME BEDDING

The ultimate beauty sleep would be going to bed forty-five years old and waking up forty. While this is still a fairy tale, copper-infused pillowcases are hailed for their ability to reduce wrinkles—a claim that is supported by two small studies in the *Journal of Cosmetic Dermatology* and the *International Journal of Cosmetic Science.* Researchers found

that copper-infused pillowcases made a difference within weeks. The pillowcases are also thought to help the skin's natural renewal process (collagen production, enhanced elasticity, and so on)—which has made some dermatologists vocal proponents. Copper's antimicrobial properties could also help tame breakouts, a great bonus for hormonally troubled skin of all ages. Although the idea of a copper pillowcase might sound strange, the copper is infused into ultra-soft, satiny fabric.

goop PICKS

Ananda, an Ayurvedic spa in India, is the real deal—a trip there will leave you feeling lighter, more relaxed, and with valuable lessons learned that will help you take better care of yourself at home. Not surprisingly, our list of other beloved wellness and detox retreats is fairly long. *For a spa-centric trip that incorporates other exercise and nutrition*—to name a few—we like Cal-a-Vie, Chiva-Som, Kamalaya Koh Samui, Mii amo, Golden Door, Rancho La Puerta, and Ananda. *For a more intense bootcamp-like experience or hardcore detoxing,* we like Pritikin (focused on weight loss and changing eating habits), Ann Wigmore Natural Health Institute (focused on a restorative diet), Sirona Therapy Spa, The Ranch at Live Oak, The Ashram, and We Care. *And for a clinical, medical-minded approach to wellness,* check out: Espace Henri Chenot, SHA Wellness Clinic, Grand Resort Bad Ragaz, Lanserhof Lans, and VIVAMAYR.

Beating Jet Lag

Jet lag is essentially the body's way of saying it is totally confused. The body's melatonin level normally rises at night, when it gets dark, and falls in the morning as it gets light. But when you fly across time zones, it's easy for your body to get out of sync with nature's clock, especially if the daylight patterns are different from your usual time zone. Traveling (while it is certainly an awesome privilege in most instances) can really mess up your sleep schedule and be exhausting. There are some ways to make overcoming jet lag easier so that you can land feeling, and looking, fresher and less tired. (And we've tried all the ways, as it seems like more often than not we're heading off on a red-eye to a business meeting or press event that we actually want to look our best for.)

One tip is to bolster your immune system before you fly. It's all too easy to come down with something when you're stuck in close quarters with so many other people for many hours, breathing recycled air. So, eat well and hydrate in the days leading up to your flight. Pack food to bring with you—see our travel salads on pages 52–56—this way you don't get stuck eating something that's going to upset your stomach mid-flight, or leave you craving sugar in the air. You can also give your immune system a boost by adding vitamin C packets to your water right before takeoff. (Hydrating when you fly can feel like a nuisance—especially if you're in the window seat and have to climb over your seatmates every time you head to the bathroom—but it goes a long way toward feeling better when you land.)

Packing a good flight bag can make all the

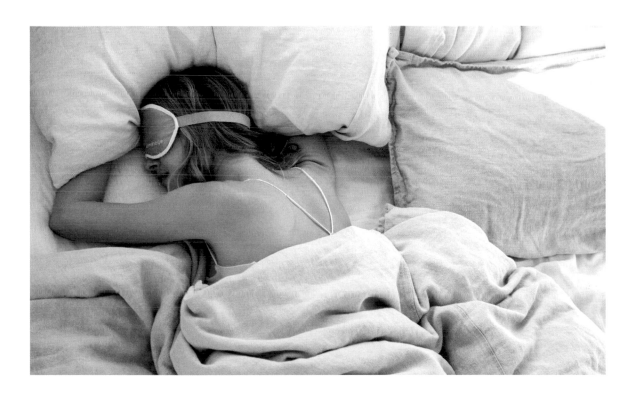

difference, even after you've landed. Think lip balm and moisturizer to keep your lips and skin from becoming dry; and travel towelettes are nice for refreshing and making everything a little more hygienic. (You can use them to wipe down the tray table, too.) Ward off germs by spraying a bit of colloidal silver in the air around your seat. As GP says, it can be worth the few odd glances.

Falling asleep on a plane, or staying asleep, in particular, can be nearly impossible. For this reason, a great flight bag also includes the tools that are going to help you get some rest if you're flying through the night. (At GOOP, we created our own flight pack with all the TSA guidelines in mind.) Must-haves include an eye mask, headphones, and powerful earplugs to block out plane noise. Also consider getting in a dose of magnesium and/or melatonin to help your body relax and prepare for sleep.

For more specifics on how to best adjust to new time zones, we turn back to Dr. Pelayo.

Dr. Rafael Pelayo
ON CROSSING TIME ZONES

What does jet lag do to our bodies to make us feel so wiped out?
Your body secretes hormones at certain times of day, and your brain expects different hormones to be at work at certain times. For example, cortisol, a stress hormone, rises in the morning when you're about to start your day and face the world. The growth hormone is produced at night. This is all controlled by the endocrine system, and the timing of these hormones helps your brain know whether it's day or night—based on the previous day and night. But when you travel, all of a sudden you're awake when your body is supposed to be asleep, or vice versa. So

your behavior is out of sync with your body's hormones and the endocrine system. And the end result is that you just don't feel right. You can function, but you're not at your sharpest; you have a malaise, your thinking is a little fuzzy, you might get a headache or a stomachache; your body is out of sync with itself.

It takes about 3 to 5 days to get over jet lag—and the more time zones you skip, the more severe the jet lag will feel. There are ways of minimizing jet lag, but no matter what we do, our brains aren't meant to take such huge shifts—3, 6, 12 hours if you go abroad—in our schedules.

How are we affected differently depending on which direction we are traveling?
The circadian system is the part of the brain that deals with biological activity around the 24-hour cycle. More specifically, there's a little piece of tissue behind the eye, where the optic nerves crisscross, called the suprachiasmatic nucleus (SCN), that helps coordinate all the various biological rhythms of the cells in our bodies. The SCN measures time and acts like a conductor—letting all the cells in the body know what time the sun is expected to come up tomorrow based on when it came up today.

A quirky thing about this clock in our head is it's not a 24-hour clock; it's about a 24-hour-and-10-minute clock. It overshoots. (This is true for almost all of us, although a few people do have clocks that are a bit shorter—these people tend to have a hard time staying up late.) We also get a surge of alertness in the evening that's modulated by this conductor, too. And because of this it's always easier for you to stay awake later than it is to go to bed earlier. Let's say your normal bedtime is midnight—it's going to be easier for you to go bed at 2 a.m. than 10 p.m.

If you apply this to jet lag, it makes more sense that we are affected differently depending on which direction we are headed. If you're going east, you are going to a shorter day—you have to go to sleep earlier. Going west, your day is extended, you get to stay up later—easier because you are adapting to prolonging the day. A friend of mine taught me this saying about traveling: *East is a beast and west is best.* It's true, but when you're doing really long trips, making big jumps in time, you're going to get messed up in either direction.

How do we use this knowledge to our advantage when it comes to planning our travel and tackling jet lag?
To start, think about which way you're traveling, how long you will be spending at your destination, and the purpose of your trip.

If you are going somewhere for more than 5 days or so, you may want to begin adapting to your destination's time zone before you leave. You do this in 15-minute increments—so if you were going to New York from California, you would go to bed 15 minutes earlier on the nights leading up to your trip, as practical and possible. But, if you're only going to be away for a few days, it's best to keep your local time zone, and deal with the jet lag while you're away.

Either way, you want to keep in mind five critical moments to better plan your trip and manage the jet lag:

> 1: The time you usually get up.
> 2: The time you usually go to bed.
> 3: The time you are most awake—generally 2 hours before you fall asleep, when your temperature rises.
> 4 and 5: The two times you are the sleepiest—generally around 2 p.m. and 2 hours before you wake up, when your temperature drops.

Figure out what those times are for yourself in your local time zone, and plan accordingly (as much as you can) in your destination time zone. For example, if you're scheduling a business meeting, do it when you're normally most alert in your home time zone—about 2 hours before your usual bedtime. Avoid a meeting when it's just after lunch in your local time zone—if you're sleep deprived, catch a nap during this time if you can. If you can't nap, plan to exercise—a good way to chase away sleepiness and help you sleep better at night. The same logic applies if you're a tourist—don't plan a sedentary bus tour when your body is going to be sleepiest; you want to do that when your brain is more active.

You can also use light or darkness to help you change time zones, although it is difficult to make big changes in a short amount of time just relying on light. For instance, you'll see people wear sunglasses on the plane to signal to their bodies that it's night and to help get some sleep. And then, when you land at your destination, it's a good idea to take in some bright light during the day to help you reset your clock. Usually, if you want to adapt quickly to your new environment, try to get as much light in the morning at your destination as you can. But if I'm traveling to New York from California for a short trip, and I want to actually avoid getting on NYC time since I'll be back in California so soon, then I want to minimize my light in the morning.

For short trips during which you don't really need to adapt to a new time zone, depending on the purpose of the trip, I also recommend that people attempt to do activities in their local time zones as much as possible—particularly when you're visiting a city that is busy around the clock. For instance, if you're traveling east, maybe you become more of a night person during your trip. If you're heading west, check out the sunrise.

What are other tricks for adjusting quicker?
Avoid alcohol and stay hydrated. Also, there are four variables that regulate our rhythm—I use the acronym, *SELF:* social interactions, exercise, light, food. If you control these four variables, you can control your body's rhythm. For example, you can time your meals during your trip to adjust your rhythm.

The problem is that it can be difficult to manipulate the body's rhythm and make big shifts on short trips. This is why some people might consult a doctor about taking medication to help with sleeping or staying awake for a short trip that requires them to be alert and on, particularly if there is nothing they can do about their schedules. (You can of course use caffeine to help you stay awake, but some people are very sensitive to caffeine.) The medication won't replace sleep but it can help. Note that you never want to mix alcohol with sleeping pills—and you should be especially careful when traveling alone and taking sleeping pills.

Look Alive

Jet lag, plain old busy-woman-lack-of-sleep, a night of overindulging with cocktails (sugar inflammation!), and allergies can all wreak havoc on the eyes. Waking up to see puffiness, redness, or dark circles in the mirror is never a welcome sight. Here's what to do about it:

- **Cold:** Useful for taking down some of the puffiness, just as it's used to reduce various kinds of swelling. Some people like to keep eye cream in the fridge, but it doesn't really sustain coolness. A more effective option is refrigerated, reusable gel-filled eye masks. Or, improvising, really anything that can stay cold lightly pressed onto the eyes for a few minutes, like thick cucumber slices.
- **Moisture:** As any makeup artist will tell you—apply eye cream (or regular moisturizer) under your eyes before doing anything else makeup-wise. Even if you have oily skin—the skin under your eyes doesn't produce oil like the skin on your nose and cheeks. Moisturizing under the eyes plumps up lines, smoothes, and rejuvenates. (And even if you don't have particularly tired eyes, it's a good idea to put moisturizer under your eyes every day—you'll need less makeup if you do.)
- **Massage:** Simply smoothing in eye cream helps to temper puffiness, but you can do even more with a sonic device around your eye area.
- **Eye drops:** Not a long-term strategy but key when you need to do away with redness quickly.
- **Antihistamines:** If allergies are the cause, stopping some of the reaction and inflammation can make a noticeable difference.
- **Concealer:** See page 234 for application tips—but the key is to pat, not rub. And for the darkest of circle days, smooth on a thin, pen- or sponge-applicator-type concealer first, then go in with a thicker, pot-type concealer, dabbed on with a brush and patted to blend, over the top. It sounds like too much product, but use sparingly and it will be precisely the opposite of too much product: Natural-looking, invisibly un-circled under-eyes.
- **Pop:** To draw attention away from your dark circles, line your eyes lightly, and give your eyelashes a coat of mascara (more tips in Chapter 11). Deflection does work.

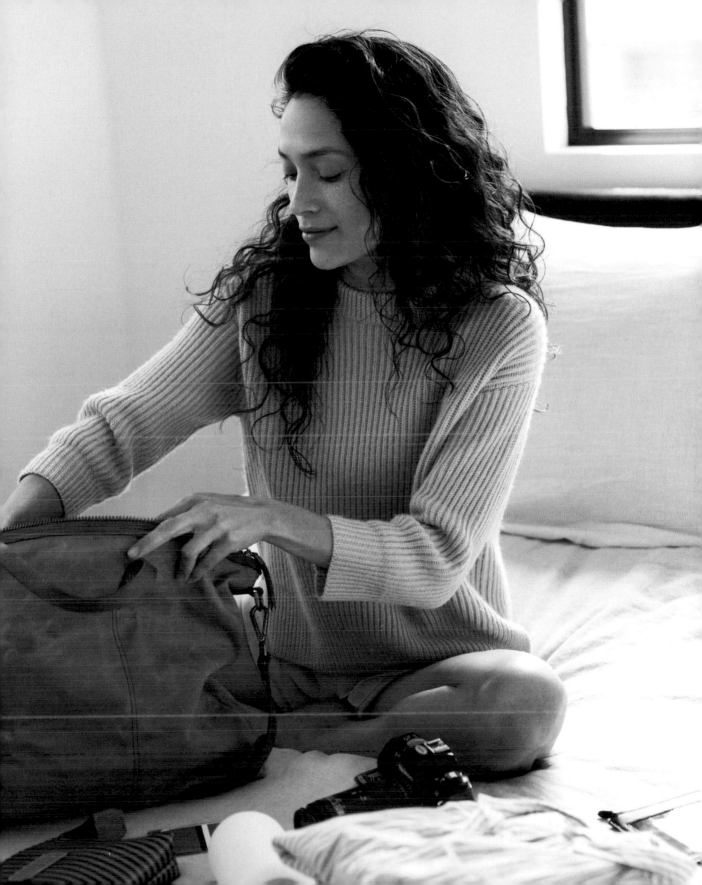

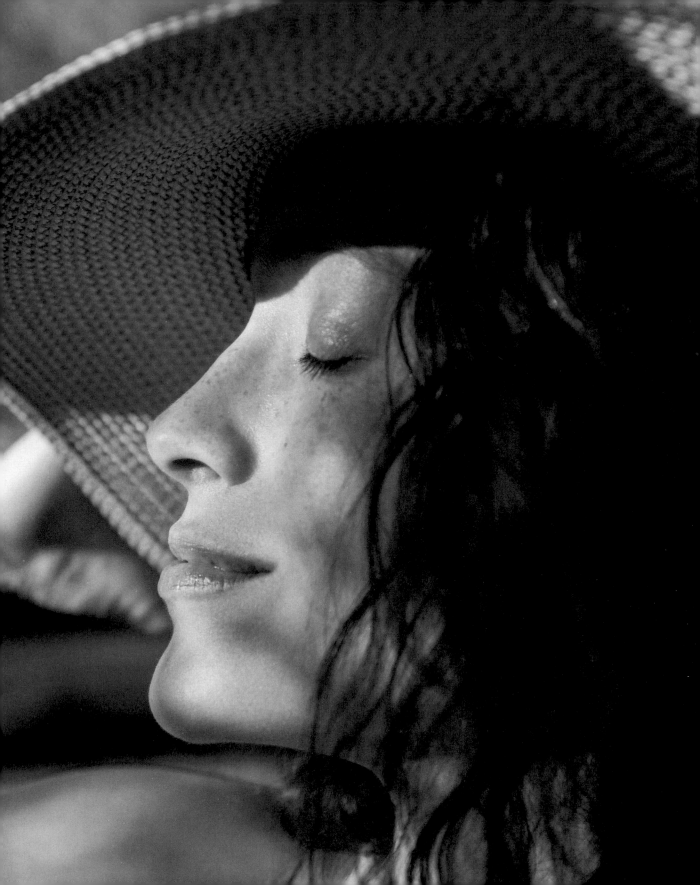

PART 2

Your Clean Beauty Routine

What you put into your body (food, water) and the way you treat it (detox, exercise, sleep) is the foundation for beauty. Internal (eating antioxidant-rich veggies) and external (applying an antioxidant-rich cream) factors are constantly interacting with one another to influence the way we ultimately feel and look. So, while the second part of the book focuses more on the topical treatments, ingredients, and products we use in the name of beauty, you'll see additional overlap with internal methods and tips. And also that we enforce a similarly strict standard of GOOP clean on the topical as we do on the internal—we believe it really works, and that it's incredibly important given that there aren't safe government or industry standards for the products we put on our bodies every day.

In the following chapters, we've culled together everything we've learned as we've cleaned up our own beauty routines, along with expert recommendations for treating varied skin and hair issues, and pro styling tips that make the perfect cat-eye or beachy wave entirely DIY-doable. In other words, everything you need to look your best—always.

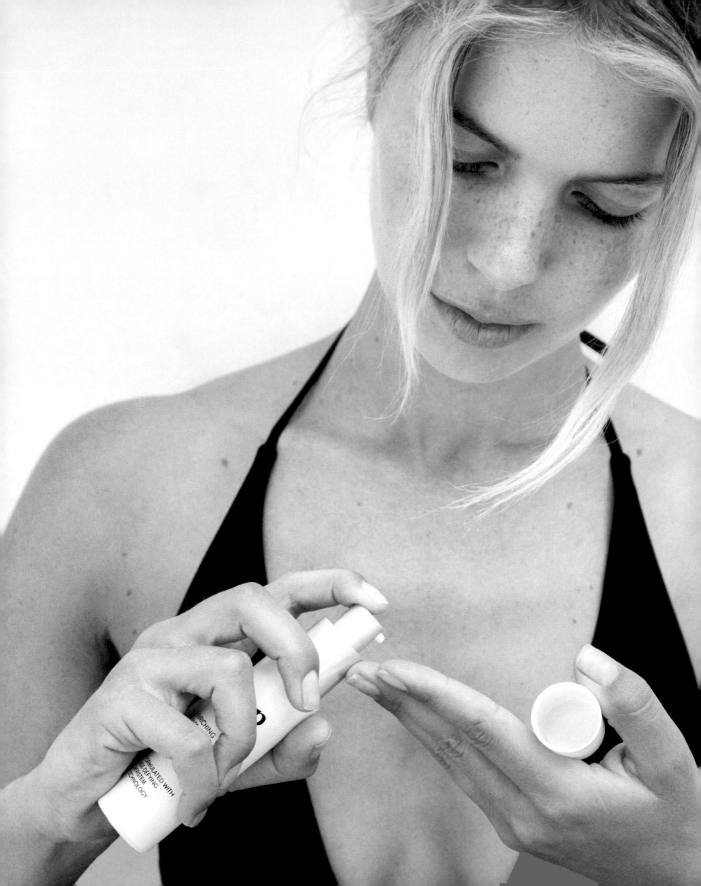

6.
What's in a Product

It's Not So Innocuous

The beauty industry is essentially unregulated—cosmetics companies can legally put all manner of toxic and even known carcinogenic ingredients into the products we use every day, and the kicker is, they don't even have to list them on the label. As a result, our medicine cabinets, shower shelves, and makeup bags are often, unbeknownst to us, crammed full of harmful chemicals. You consume any lip product you wear, from gloss to balm to full-on lipstick. And eye products like liner and mascara go directly into your eyes with each wear (brush the mascara on, blink, and you've applied mascara to your eyeball). You inhale perfume, and just about anything you use in the shower, from body wash to shampoo. Your skin—the body's largest organ—absorbs what we put on it: lotions, creams, and oils of all ilk, for face, body, and hair, across the board. The list goes on: your foundation, your conditioner, your foot cream, the mousse for your hair, the polish for your toes, eye shadow, antioxidant serum...all of it.

Another startling fact: Ingredients typically used in cosmetics are often found in human tissue—for example, those used in antiperspirants/deodorants were found in breast tumors in a 2004 study published in the *Journal of Toxicology*. Even more harrowing: Tests done on the umbilical cord blood of newborn babies have produced staggering statistics on the amount of synthetic chemicals that babies inherit from mothers and our environment. One Environmental Working Group study found a total of 232 toxic chemicals in umbilical cord blood, while another found 287 different industrial chemicals and pollutants—180 of which are known to cause cancer in humans and 217 of which are toxic to the brain and nervous system.

Corporations making products with trace amounts of toxins in them argue "the dose makes the poison." Perhaps true, if those trace—or even not-so-trace—amounts didn't add up: Think of the number of basic personal care products you use in a day, from hand wash to lip balm to lotion to shampoo. The dose of toxins we end up being exposed to—never mind their potential and untested interactions with one another—is far larger than what's in that individual swipe of body cream or spritz of hair spray. Plus, some of these toxins—which we'll discuss in more detail—can actually be even more potent in tiny doses.

Whereas the FDA regulates the food industry, it doesn't exercise power over the personal care industry. Without government regulation, most beauty brands are free to use—and do use—an alarming number of ingredients that are harmful to our health, without any warning to consumers. The FDA requires cosmetic labels to include a list of some, but not all, of the ingredients in a given product. But legally, any ingredients considered trade secrets do not have to be listed on a product label—namely, those ingredients that make up the label terms *fragrance, perfume,* and *flavor.* Unfortunately, these proprietary "ingredients" often serve as Trojan horses—companies pour thousands of toxic ingredients into them, and never have to mention any of them on the label.

Putting this huge transparency issue aside for a moment, there is also the fact that the FDA doesn't actually have the authority to approve, or disapprove, cosmetic product labeling. That's left up to the manufacturers and distributors. And, as the FDA states on its own Q&A page: "With the exception of color additives and a few prohibited ingredients, a cosmetic manufacturer may use almost any raw material as a cosmetic ingredient and market the product without an approval from FDA." Along with no power to police what's in products, the FDA also has no power to recall products that are known to be toxic or unsafe.

It doesn't seem possible that today, in the United States, it is perfectly legal for companies to use undisclosed ingredients that are known to be toxic—even ones classified as carcinogenic—in our beauty products. But it's true. The federal government has not passed a law to regulate the personal care industry since the 1938 Food, Drug, and Cosmetic Act—which included just a couple of pages on cosmetics and largely left the industry to its own devices. Today, the personal care industry is still allowed to regulate itself through their Cosmetic Ingredient Review, but even their own recommendations of restricted ingredients are not enforced. To put our (broken) system into perspective: The European Union has banned or regulated more than 1,300 ingredients in personal care products. The U.S. has banned eleven.

The results of our non-regulation: Carcinogenic dyes that the FDA bans from food are still used in beauty products in the U.S. The colorants used in lipsticks are often contaminated with heavy metals like lead, aluminum, and cadmium (a groundwater contaminant that's another known carcinogen and has been found in breast cancer tumors). Then there are the chemicals classified as endocrine disruptors—found in everything from soap to shower gel to perfume. Endocrine disruptors are extremely tiny in form, which might make them sound harmless—how dangerous can just a small dose of chemicals in just a little dab of concealer be? But it's their small size that makes endocrine disruptors so devastating—it allows them to mimic our hormones. To get an idea of the micro-ness of your natural hormones themselves, imagine your body as an Olympic-size swimming pool: The amount of hormone swimming around in your pool isn't even a teaspoon; it is smaller than a few grains of sand. Endocrine disruptors confuse our body's hormone signals, throw off the production levels of our hormones, and force our hormones to do harm—wreaking havoc on our endocrine systems and possibly leading to severe, long-term health damage, from reproductive issues and birth defects to metabolic problems and cancer. This is particularly worrisome for little ones, whose systems are still developing.

The potential health consequences of endocrine disruptors largely refute the claim that a little bit of a toxin is okay. *But even if* trace amounts of toxins were "safe," it's very easy to underestimate the amount and number of toxins that you are actually ingesting and absorbing from personal care products. Even if you don't wear foundation or lipstick regularly, most of us wash our hair at least every other day, apply moisturizer or lotion, deodorant, and so on. When you start to track the different products you apply, even the most basic routine adds up. An Environmental Working Group survey found that the average woman uses twelve products containing 168 unique ingredients every day. One hundred and sixty-eight ingredients! The number of known toxic chemicals used in personal care products is startling—as is the number of unstudied, untested chemicals for which the long-term health effects remain unknown. And possibly worse: We know little about the long-term effects of using multiple products and being subjected to many mixes of chemicals in combination with all the other pollutants and toxins to which we are exposed daily.

The lack of regulation in the cosmetics industry puts us all at a disadvantage when we're walking down the store aisles. But we don't have to wait on the government to change the market, or even rely on the government to help us make informed decisions about what products we put on our bodies. Consumers have enormous power to directly influence the quality of products that companies sell—something we've seen proven by the expanding organic food movement. When consumers understand what's actually inside processed food, or conventional shampoo, they are moved to ask

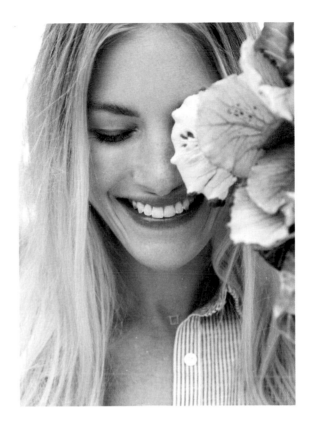

and fight for—and pay for—better options. And, although the vast majority of beauty products available still contain toxic ingredients, new, innovative companies are springing up and elevating our options. In truth, clean (nontoxic) personal care products—makeup in particular—didn't start off as all that exciting or good-looking, but thanks to the work of creative, conscientious companies and brilliant green chemists, the natural landscape is transforming every day. So, you can now get a great scent, soft hair, even a smoky eye, without using any toxins. (More on how later in this chapter.)

But perhaps the most salient point is that you should be able to choose the products you want to use—clean or not—based on real, valid information. So, here's what we've learned…

What's in a Label

As with any product that you're putting in or on your body—whether it's food or a face serum—it's obviously a good idea to carefully read the label, including the list of ingredients. With beauty products, it's particularly important to look past empty marketing promises. Since the personal care industry isn't regulated, companies can get away with a galling amount of greenwashing. In general, this is what we keep in mind when shopping:

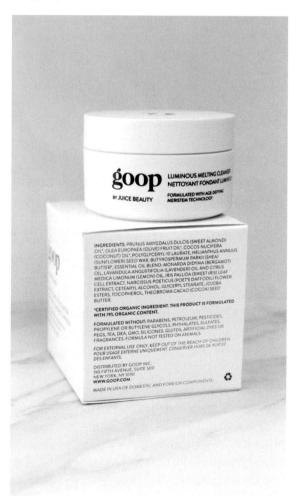

- Don't count on appealing, safe-sounding label terms (e.g., *natural, green, eco, nontoxic*) alone—such label declarations are meaningless because there are no legal standards for them.
- There are various private standards—again not regulated by the government—for personal care

BUT— IF IT'S "ORGANIC"?

A slight exception to the all-but-unregulated norm is USDA-certified organic products. The FDA does not define or regulate the term "organic" for personal care products. But if a beauty product contains (or is made up of) agriculture ingredients that meet the USDA's standards, the ingredients can be labeled organic. In order to carry the USDA Organic seal, a product must contain at least 95 percent organically produced ingredients (excluding water and salt). Below that threshold, beauty products can't carry the USDA seal. Products that contain at least 70 percent organic ingredients can be labeled "made with organic ingredients," and at less than 70 percent, the specific ingredients that are USDA-certified organic may be identified on the product's information panel.

Another rigorous standard to note is the California Organic Products Act of 2003 (COPA), which mandates that products sold in California cannot be labeled as organic if the formula isn't at least 70 percent organic in composition. Our GOOP by Juice Beauty skincare line is certified by COPA.

products. If you're not familiar with a particular seal on one of your products, or a certification that a brand lists on its website, and its standards, dig for information. One valid certification that you can rely on for endorsing only nontoxic products is the Environmental Working Group's EWG Verified.

- Be on the lookout for red flags—mainly missing essential ingredients. You might have seen beauty products labeled *preservative-free*, but any product that contains water requires preservatives. So, if a product containing water claims to be preservative-free, yet doesn't require immediate use or refrigeration, ask for more info. It could be that an ingredient came to the formulator already preserved, which isn't mentioned on the label. Often toxic preservatives are attached to ingredients like aloe so they don't have to be disclosed in ingredient lists. (Or they're put into the "fragrance" category on the label, that corporate hide-whatever-you-want loophole.)

- People often say that you shouldn't use products with long ingredient lists or those containing ingredients that you can't pronounce. But this isn't a valid statement when it comes to beauty products. (And it's also probably not a realistic rule to hold yourself to, as many sophisticated products have lengthy ingredient lists.) Chemical names can sound complicated even when the chemical itself is neither complicated nor harmful—not everything that is synthetic is toxic to us. And even the chemical names of more commonplace, and entirely harmless, ingredients can sound complicated on the back of a label. (For instance, coconut oil is *Cocos nucifera*. Vitamin E is tocopherol.) Increasingly, clean beauty brands are also listing layman's terms next to the formal names of ingredients, which can help when you're trying to decipher a label.

DO WE NEED TO WORRY ABOUT PRESERVATIVES?

Like many classes of ingredients, preservatives are neither inherently good nor bad for us. But they are necessary. As with our food, preservatives are added to beauty products that contain water in order to protect us against microbes. Not surprisingly many have been found to be toxic, as preservatives are meant, by design, to kill bacteria. (Two particularly worrisome toxic sub-classes of preservatives are parabens and those that release formaldehyde—more coming on both.) Finding nontoxic preservatives that do their jobs effectively is not easy. But there are brands in the clean beauty space that are working hard to find alternative preservatives, and raw materials suppliers are coming up to meet this goal. This is the major challenge to be tackled in the future of nontoxic beauty. Already, though, there are some suitable, safe preservatives being used in beauty products—for example, sodium benzoate, which is a food-grade preservative, and phenoxyethanol. We allow both types of preservatives in products in our clean beauty shop—they are both nontoxic and wonderfully effective.

- Another widespread misconception is that the ingredients in nontoxic beauty products are all vastly different from those used in traditional beauty products. This has in part contributed to a general reluctance to use "natural" beauty products—there is a common belief that natural products just won't work. But the truth is that often a lot of, or all of, the active ingredients in a given nontoxic beauty product are the same as the active ingredients in its conventional counterpart, which aren't actually toxic to us. (For example, hyaluronic acid, AHAs, essential oils, and butters are all perfectly safe, and appear in both clean and conventional products.) So there is plenty of overlap between the ingredient labels of nontoxic and conventional products. What's often different is the extra stuff—the added scent, the absorbency or stickiness quality, the preservative used, a certain experiential element, like texture, that's been added. And it's largely this extra stuff—which is often toxic in traditional products—that innovative clean beauty brands have found nontoxic alternative forms for.

- If you're unsure of whether a particular product or ingredient is cause for concern, look it up. The EWG has a helpful database called Skin Deep (ewg.org/skindeep; also available as an app) where you can look up brands, products, and ingredient information.

Not in Our Vanities

Like with every detox category, we don't think of perfection as the goal. Just goodness. With that in mind, these are the ingredients that we like to keep out of our daily routines, and the ones you won't find in the GOOP shop:

PARABENS

Function: Preservative.
Problem: They are endocrine disruptors, and, as reported by EWG, parabens have been found in human breast tissue.
What you'll see on the label: A variety of ingredi-

CLEAN ENOUGH TO EAT

You'll sometimes see beauty brands refer to ingredients in their products as "food-grade ingredients." The idea is that the ingredient—whether it's avocado oil or a preservative—would be safe for you even if it were on your dinner plate. Although we don't plan on eating anything from our medicine cabinet with a fork, we do look for preservatives, in particular, in beauty products that have been declared by the FDA as safe food additives. We end up ingesting a lot of the ingredients in our personal care products, so it's a big plus to smooth something into your skin that you know wouldn't be harmful to eat.

---

ents ending in *paraben*, e.g., butylparaben, isobutylparaben, methylparaben, propylparaben.

FORMALDEHYDE RELEASERS

Function: Preservative.
Problem: Formaldehyde is a known carcinogen. It's also associated with asthma, neurotoxicity, and developmental toxicity.
What you'll see on the label: You'll never see formaldehyde on a label, although it's in makeup, hair, body, and skincare products. What you'll see are the names of the chemicals that are added to product formulas, that release formaldehyde. (When added to water, these chemicals slowly decompose, forming molecules of formaldehyde.) So, look for: 2-bromo-2-nitropropane-1,3 diol (Bronopol), diazolidinyl urea, DMDM hydantoin,

imidazolidinyl urea, sodium hydroxymethylglycinate, quaternium-15.

PHTHALATES

Function: Plasticizers make products pliable, help fragrance stick to skin, and nail polish to nails.

Problem: They are endocrine disruptors associated with birth defects.

What you'll see on the label: Stay away from dibutyl phthalate (DBP), diethylhexyl phthalate (DEHP), diethyl phthalate (DEP).

FRAGRANCE

Function: Scent.

Problem: This is a tough one to swallow. But it's on the list because, as mentioned, "fragrance," a trade secret, prohibits transparency. A loophole in the Federal Fair Packaging and Labeling Act explicitly exempts fragrance ingredients from the list of cosmetic ingredients that need to appear on product labels. When the International Fragrance Association finally published a list of the ingredients generally used in formulas, it totaled 3,000. The scary truth is that we can't really know what's in a product that contains fragrance. But what we do know is that fragrances are commonly made up of a toxic mix of chemicals, often added to get the fragrance to stick to your skin (i.e., phthalates), or as solvents or colorants. (One example of a solvent ingredient is methyl cellosolve, associated with neurotoxicity and development toxicity. Another, butoxyethanol, is associated with skin, eye, and respiratory irritation. Still another, resorcinol, a colorant, is associated with skin irritation and organ toxicity.) When the Campaign for Safe Cosmetics and the EWG analyzed seventeen name-brand perfumes, they found thirty-eight undisclosed chemicals—fourteen on average

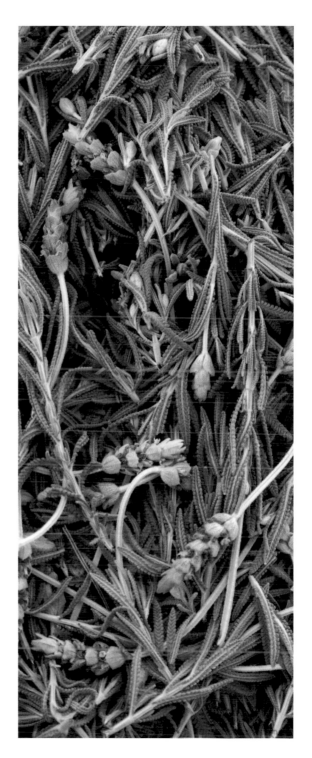

per brand. A total of twelve different hormone-disrupting chemicals were found in the seventeen products, with an average of four in each. Sixty-six percent of the discovered unlabeled ingredients had never been assessed for safety. And EWG reports that fragrance ingredients are now found in human fat. Eerie, yes, but it makes sense, as toxins are generally lipophilic and live in our fat. **What you'll see on the label:** Fragrance, perfume, parfum, flavor.

goop TIP

Landing on a nontoxic perfume that applies, lasts, and smells like a conventional one takes some doing. But smelling fantastic without conventional perfume ingredients is both easy and pleasurable. Scents made with essential oils—like bergamot, lavender, lemon—can be gorgeous, complex, feminine, sexy...some are even more exquisite than conventional perfumes. Even those of us who might not be ready to toss all our perfume bottles can still cut down on other products that use fragrance, and therefore that source of toxic load. That's because there are fragrance-containing products that are generally easy enough to swap out for suitable non-fragrance alternatives. Conventional soaps, skin creams for both face and body, shampoos, conditioners, laundry detergent, and hand sanitizers all commonly contain fragrance, which we don't miss when using the nontoxic versions.

EDTA

Function: Binding, stabilizing ingredient.
Problem: It's admittedly not always clear if an ingredient is harmful to us or not. (In part because so many ingredients in personal care products are not tested.) Available research suggests that EDTA could be toxic to our organs, so we avoid it.
What you'll see on the label: Ethylenediaminetetraacetic acid (EDTA), calcium disodium EDTA, disodium EDTA, tetrasodium EDTA.

1,4-DIOXANE CONTAMINATION

Function: 1,4-dioxane itself doesn't have a specific function. It's a by-product that's created through a process called *ethoxylation*, which occurs when ethylene oxide is added to other chemicals (which often serve as surfactants or emulsifiers, thickeners, solvents, or softeners) to make their effect on our skin less harsh.
Problem: 1,4-dioxane penetrates the skin and is linked to a host of health issues, including cancer, organ and respiratory toxicity, and skin irritation.
What you'll see on the label: You won't see 1,4-dioxane on a label, but certain ingredients are likely to be contaminated with 1,4-dioxane, and you're most likely to see them in your suds and bubbles products, like shampoo or a foaming face wash. Look for: compounds that include PEG or polyethylene glycol in the ingredient name (for example, PEG-8); compounds that include *laureth* in the ingredient name, like laureth-7 and sodium laureth sulfate (SLES); and ingredients that include the word *ceteareth*.

ETHANOLAMINES

Function: Surfactants.
Problem: Associated with inhibited fetal brain development, hormone disruption, allergies, skin toxicity.

What you'll see on the label: Ethanolamine (ETA), diethanolamine (DEA), cocamide DEA, mono ethanolamine (MEA), triethanolamine (TEA).

CHEMICAL SUNSCREENS

Function: Sun protection.

Problem: They are endocrine and hormone disruptors—plus severe skin irritants—linked to a variety of health concerns. (We went further into depth on these in Chapter 4.)

What you'll see on the label: Chemical sunscreen ingredients are used in products beyond sunscreen—you'll find them in moisturizers and creams, and the same chemicals are sometimes included as fragrance ingredients. Avoid: avobenzone, benzophenone, homosalate, octinoxate, octisalate, octocrylene, oxybenzone.

OTHER INGREDIENTS WORTH BLACKLISTING

- Benzalkonium chloride: a preservative and surfactant connected with severe skin, eye, and respiratory irritation and allergies.
- Butylated hydroxyanisole (BHA) and butylated hydroxytoluene (BHT): used to extend a product's shelf life—and linked to cancer and hormone disruption.
- Coal tar: the colorant in mascara, eyeliner, hair color, and anti-dandruff agents, coal tar ingredients are known carcinogens that are the by-product of petroleum combustion.
- Hydroquinone: a skin lightener associated with cancer, organ toxicity, skin irritation.
- Methylisothiazolinone and methylchloroisothiazolinone: preservatives linked to allergies, skin irritation, and neurotoxicity.
- Thimerosal (mercury): a preservative associated with neurotoxicity, and organ and developmental toxicity.
- Toluene: a solvent known to damage the immune system and linked to human reproductive toxicity.
- Triclocarban and triclosan: antimicrobials associated with aquatic toxicity and human reproductive toxicity, not to mention antibiotic resistance.

Bad Hair Days

Hair dyes, hair straighteners, and perms are some of the biggest toxic beauty perpetrators—and for many women, GOOP staff included, the most important components of our beauty routines. We'll go through hair health and tips in more depth in Chapter 7, but here's a snapshot (based on data from EWG):

- Hair dyes often contain coal tar ingredients (e.g., aminophenol, diaminobenzene, and phenylenediamine, often more toxic than those in mascaras and liners, which are bad enough) linked to cancer, and many are already banned in Europe. PPD is in practically all hair color formulas, and is linked to bladder cancer, non-Hodgkin's lymphoma, and autoimmunine diseases like rheumatoid athritis. Resorcinol (also used in fragrance products) is toxic to our immune systems and may irritate skin. Resorcinol has also been found to disrupt thyroid function in animals. Although the U.S. government regulates resorcinol exposure in the workplace, it does not restrict its use in hair products. Other toxic chemicals used in hair dyes (some of which we've already covered) include: toluene, lead acetate, and ethanolamines. In general, lighter dyes are less toxic than darker ones. The truth is, nontoxic dyes that are both entirely safe and as effective in terms of results as the toxic ones don't yet exist.
- Chemical hair straightening treatments and perms typically use very harsh ingredients to permanently change your hair's shape—most are toxic. To stiffen the hair, some hair straighteners (including keratin treatments) use formaldehyde—which is a known carcinogen, as mentioned before, and neurotoxin. The nontoxic alternative for straightening or curling is of course heat treatments, which damage your hair and often involve toxin-filled styling products. (More on this in Chapter 7.)

That said, few people who color their hair—70 percent of American women do, and the women in the GOOP offices almost directly reflect that statistic—are willing to give it up. (And if you fall into that category, too, there are of course still plenty of other meaningful ways you can pare down on the toxins in your routine.)

For a whole section on hair color processes, see page 174.

Clean Beauty Guru

For a better understanding of what goes into making a clean beauty product that is free of all the toxic ingredients that conventional beauty companies persist in using, we turn to Karen Behnke, founder of our partner Juice Beauty, a California-based company that has been innovating in the nontoxic and organic space for more than a decade.

Karen Behnke
ON GOOD, GORGEOUS, CLEAN BEAUTY

At Juice Beauty, you use food-grade preservatives—can you explain what that means, and why you choose those? What are the limitations?
Food-grade preservatives are ones that have been recognized by the FDA as safe to use in food products. They help prevent microbial growth, keep products fresh so you don't have to refrigerate them, and help create a solid shelf life. Common food-grade preservatives that we use in small amounts include radish root, vitamin E, potassium sorbate, and sodium benzoate. I guess the limitation is that we have a 2-year shelf life instead of 3 to 5 years—but that's just fine with us. We don't mind manufacturing all the time so we have a constant stream of fresh products. After a customer buys a personal care product and opens it, it should be thrown out within a year anyway.

At Juice Beauty, we constantly review and test the latest natural and safe preservatives so we can stay on the cutting edge. With our very first products in 2005, we were paraben-free, which was pretty much unheard-of

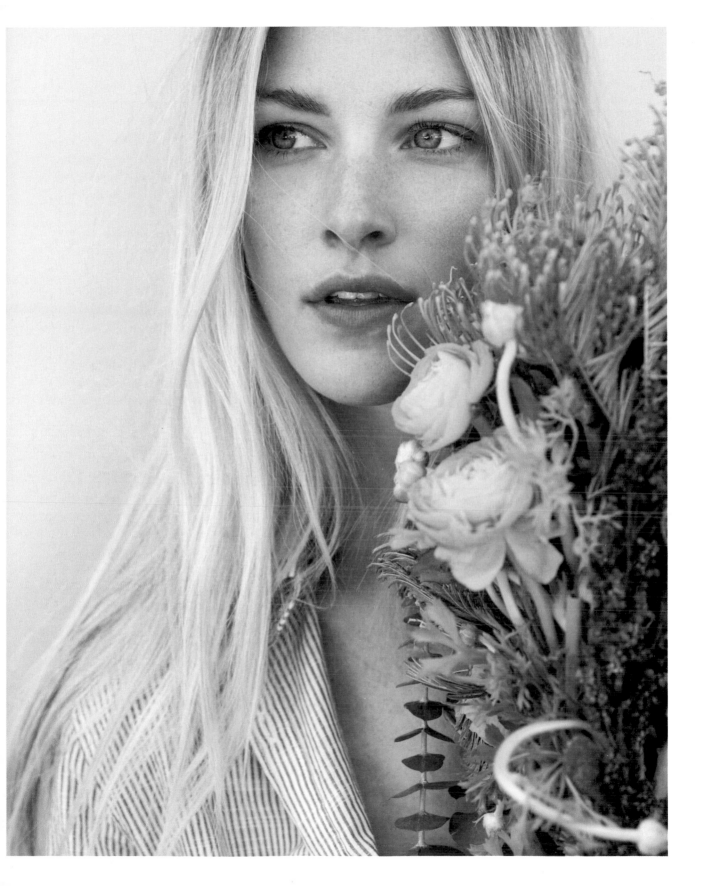

at the time. I'd researched preservatives and found that many of these chemicals can be absorbed through skin—that measurable concentrations of six different parabens were identified in biopsy samples from breast tumors, and that those particular parabens correlated closely with the patient's use of personal care products.

The problem with many of these preservatives is that they mimic estrogen and can disrupt the endocrine system, which can lead to an increase in certain cancers. It's hard to ignore research that is coming out of solid universities like Tufts and the University of California, and the Breast Cancer Fund. Once I read this research, I knew we had to take a leap into trying something very unusual for personal care products—food-grade preservatives. My theory was simple: If it worked for food that one ingested—why not moisturizers, and why not give it a try? This hunch proved to be successful and here we are years later with many safely preserved products.

Many conventional beauty products contain plasticizers—what's the function of silicone, microbeads, and other emollients in beauty products? How do you achieve the same results with alternative ingredients?

Can you imagine competing against tiny little smooth plastic-like particles that roll over your skin, feeling rather luxurious? It was truly a challenge to try to replace the silicones and dimethicones and plastic microbeads widely used throughout the beauty industry in skincare, makeup, and hair care. Despite their amazing initial "slip and feel," silicones can build up on the skin and scalp and actually lead to dull skin and oily hair. Juice Beauty uses natural emollients like organic shea, jojoba, and grape seed, as well as plant-derived ingredients to help improve slip and feel, and provide amazing hydration. In our newly launched Phyto-Pigments makeup collection, we worked with really new, cutting-edge ingredients like luscious alkanes derived from coconut to enhance a smooth makeup application and increase makeup wear. We also used silica minerals

(*not* to be confused with silicones!) to help blur the look of fine lines and wrinkles.

Of course microbeads, widely used in beauty products, are awfully toxic as they wash off into our lakes and oceans, where our fish eat them, and then we, in turn, eat the fish. Sherri Mason, PhD, professor of chemistry at the State University of New York at Fredonia, sailed with a research team to collect data on the prevalence of the plastics in the Great Lakes. They dragged a fine-mesh net in the waters to snag anything bigger than a third of a millimeter. What they found was astounding. Her tests showed, on average, 17,000 bits of tiny plastic items per square kilometer in Lake Michigan, and up to 1.1 million plastic particles per square kilometer in Lake Ontario. At Juice Beauty we use dissolving jojoba beads that roll wonderfully and exfoliate, and then eventually dissolve, thus not harming the planet. We also use grape seed, which is resveratrol-rich and luxurious, in place of these types of microbeads, which have fortunately now been banned.

How pervasive is petroleum in beauty products, and why is it problematic? What's the work-around for Juice Beauty?

Petrochemicals are incredibly pervasive in beauty products; so many common ingredients are derived from them. A huge health concern with petroleum products is that they can generate 1,4-dioxane, a substance known to potentially contribute to some cancers. It's also a kidney toxin, neurotoxin, and a respiratory toxin, not to mention a leading groundwater contaminant. The Environmental Working Group (EWG) found that an alarming 22 percent of all conventional personal care products contain unsafe levels of 1,4-dioxane. EWG also found that "these trace contaminants in petroleum-based ingredients often readily penetrate the skin...and their presence in products is not restricted by government safety standards."

Some of the common ingredients in beauty products that are petrochemical-derived include:

- Paraffin wax
- Mineral oil
- Toluene
- Benzene
- Anything with *PEG* (polyethylene glycol)
- Anything with *DEA* (diethanolamine) or *MEA* (ethanolamine)
- Butanol and any word with *butyl:* butyl alcohol, butylparaben, butylene glycol
- EDTA (ethylenediaminetetraacetic acid)
- Any word with *propyl*—isopropyl alcohol, propylene glycol, propyl alcohol, cocamidopropyl betaine
- Parfum or fragrance—95 percent of chemicals used in fragrance are from petroleum. This one word can contain many, many chemicals that don't need to be listed and are likely endocrine disrupters.

And the other problem with petroleum is that there have been a few international conflicts going on over petroleum—it would be nice to limit our addiction to it.

Instead of petroleum, Juice Beauty uses ingredients like organic coconut oil, olive oil, jojoba, and sheas that not only help the skin retain moisture but provide nutrients as well.

How does Juice Beauty make products without using phthalates?

Phthalates are chemicals that have been linked to endocrine disruption, developmental and reproductive toxicity, and possibly some cancers. In cosmetics, phthalates have been used in nail polish to reduce cracking, hair sprays to reduce stiffness, and as a solvent for fragrances. Phthalates can also be found in some plastic packaging, with the concern that it can leach out of the plastic. Juice Beauty uses essential oil blends or aromatic extracts, never artificial or synthetic fragrances. We also use packaging that does not contain phthalates or leach, and conduct tests to check for these issues.

The Super-Beauty Stuff

Finding a new brand of laundry detergent or hand soap that isn't toxic and that performs as well as a conventional brand isn't all that hard. But our skin, hair, and makeup products tend to be more personal, and the thought of trading them in for cleaner products is a tougher sell. In theory, of course, no one wants to be exposed to chemicals in conventional beauty products—but women rely on high-performance lipstick, hairspray, and anti-aging creams because they want to look better; it's a primal human urge for most of us. And for a long time, that meant toxins—because it was only conventional beauty products that could fight dark circles, smooth dry skin, give you that subtle glow as if you weren't wearing makeup at all, create a true, red lip, and so on.

But a small subset of revolutionary cosmetic companies, along with new advances in technology and chemistry, have changed this. There are now natural beauty products with vibrant colors that are bright and dark, natural makeup that is genuinely sheer. There is natural makeup for your everyday, barely-there look, and your night-out, red-lip look. We became familiar with the exacting process behind designing elevated, entirely nontoxic makeup when GP collaborated with Juice Beauty on its collection of clean makeup. They used the high-performance, conventional products that GP relies on for the red carpet as the benchmarks for how well Juice Beauty's natural products would need to perform—not easy to accomplish.

For example, to create "carbon black" used in conventional mascara and eyeliner, companies typically combust heavy-duty petroleum products or coal. Used in tires, inks, films, and plastics, carbon black is classified as possibly carcinogenic in humans and is proven to be carcinogenic in animals. To get the same level of pigment toxic-free, Juice Beauty figured out how to use natural pine resin instead. This took years of experimentation—as Juice Beauty founder Karen Behnke says: "Pine resin isn't exactly a 'normal' ingredient for mascara so it's all new for our scientists—or for any scientist." Similarly, the team developed plant-derived phyto-pigments that are extracted with carbon dioxide, thereby avoiding the hexane or acetone that is usually required to extract vivid colors.

The obvious beauty of shopping a trusted, clean brand is that you don't have to spend the time and energy dissecting and worrying over every label. Which is why we only stock clean products in the GOOP shop. But what's equally noteworthy about great nontoxic beauty products is that not only do they eliminate the bad stuff, they often contain a lot of the really good beauty-boosting stuff.

---

goop TIP

Here's a cool health-and-happiness-boosting bath/shower tip—try rubbing essential oil blends into your torso before showering or bathing to maximize benefits (say, a wake-up blend in the morning or a more relaxing one for evening). We love the Alchemy oil concoctions from Naturopathica.

A Mani-Pedi Manifesto

The nail salon is a good example of how toxic the world of personal care has conventionally been, and also how much better it can be going forward. A lot of salons and nail polish brands are cleaning up their acts—great for all of us who get regular pedicures, and very important for the health of salon workers. Still, many salons and polishes are more toxic than is safe. Here's what you should look for:

- At a minimum, use polish that is *3-free*: no phthalates, no formaldehyde, no toluene. These are three things you don't want to inhale or touch. All polish was once made with these ingredients and now most are not.
- Even better, though, is *5-free* polish, which also cuts out formaldehyde resin and camphor. There are beautiful 5-free options, and 5-free is the GOOP standard. Beyond that, a lot of the ingredients that companies draw attention to excluding were never used in nail polish to begin with. (It's great to see nail polishes continue to become cleaner, but there is unfortunately some greenwashing going on.)
- When it comes to nail polish removers, choose *non-acetone*. Acetone—still used in conventional brands—is very toxic (it's essentially paint thinner) and very drying, too. It can also leave a (toxic) residue on your nails when finished. Non-acetone removers work, although they do take a bit longer. Hold the remover over the nail longer before you swipe away. Or, manicurist tip: Use tinfoil to hold a remover-soaked tissue over your fingers.

SAFER SHOWER

As mentioned briefly in Chapter 1, filtering your water is a worthy household upgrade. Tap water can contain dangerous chemicals, such as lead, disinfection by-products (often called DBPs), chlorine, and if you live in a rural area, possibly arsenic and nitrates from fertilizer runoff. Exposure to these chemicals has been associated with short-term issues like upset stomachs, and severe long-term effects ranging from bladder cancer to birth defects. You can look at the annual safety reports that your local utility sends, which tell you the level of contaminants in your water and whether they are within the legal limits set by the EPA. Countertop filters and pitcher systems are handy for the kitchen. But water experts—like research analyst Paul Pestano and water filtration authority William Wendling—also recommend shower filters. For the cleanest rinse, look for a carbon shower filter.

You also breathe in—and absorb through your skin—the ingredients in your body wash, soap, shampoo, conditioner, scrub, and anything else you use in the shower, so clean beauty products are particularly important here. Some GOOP Clean Beauty Shop bestsellers: shampoo and conditioner from Lavett & Chin, Rahua, and Grown Alchemist; scrubs from Ila and French Girl Organics; body wash from Grown Alchemist and Rahua.

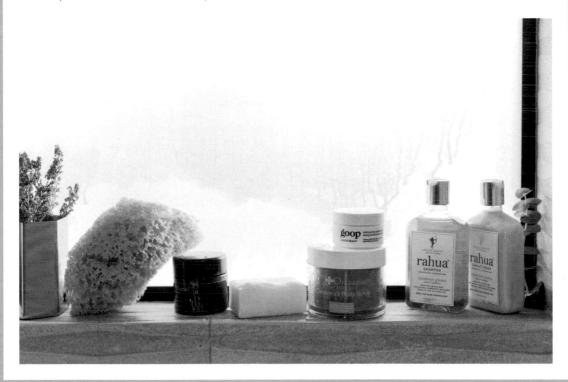

If You Want to Do More

From a personal standpoint, cleaning up your product routine feels good, doesn't require beauty sacrifices, and is totally worth it for your health. Zooming out, though, there is undoubtedly a bigger issue at play: The lack of regulation and transparency in the personal care industry leaves us (and our children) vulnerable to being exposed to harmful chemicals every day. The toxins we've described are scary and all too present in the conventional products we buy regularly. But what's really maddening is that we're being denied the right to know what's in our products and to choose whether or not we want to use those ingredients.

On top of that, we're forced to wade through layers of greenwashing and marketing that have no legal backing, which can lead us to think we're making a clean, healthy decision for ourselves or our family when we are not. When we sit down to enjoy a pizza and martinis with friends—real life calls for real allowances—we understand the choices we are making. The same should be true for the beauty products we put on our bodies. With valid information, many women might change their daily moisturizer, find a nontoxic shampoo for the kids' shower, or only spritz perfume on certain occasions. Regardless of what our individual choices may be, we should be afforded the ability to make those choices.

If you're like us, you probably once assumed that the government regulated everything, including the cosmetics industry. And you might have friends who think that. Tell them. Tell them to tell their friends.

The more interest we take in this important issue, the more we spread the word, the more change we will see. We've already begun to see some of the impact we can have. By supporting clean products and brands with our wallets, consumers have proven that there is a viable market for nontoxic beauty (as there is for organic food), and we're seeing the rise of the first groundbreaking nontoxic beauty brands. And we've even seen some changes in major corporations that are finally removing some of the most known harmful toxins from their products. At the political level, we've seen some steps in the right direction, too. The state of California, for one, has its own Safe Cosmetics Act. Manufacturers/packers/distributors that are selling products in California are required to provide the California State Cosmetics Program with a list of all cosmetic products that contain any ingredients known or suspected to cause cancer, or developmental or reproductive harm. The program then makes this information available on their website (cdph.ca.gov/programs/cosmetics).

And yet, we clearly have a long way to go. To take more action, check out the Campaign for Safe Cosmetics (safecosmetics.org). And pass this information on.

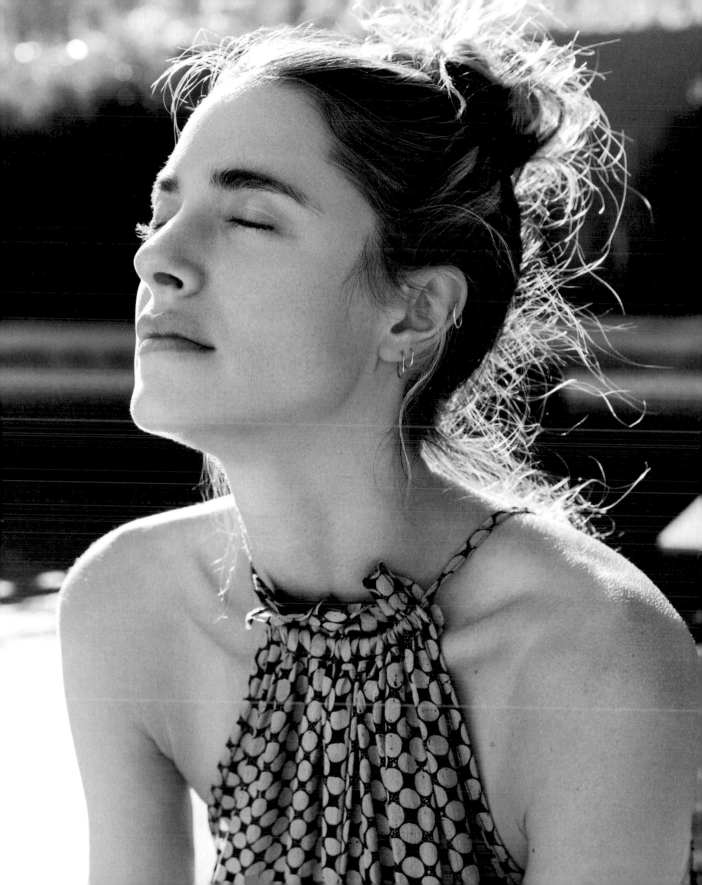

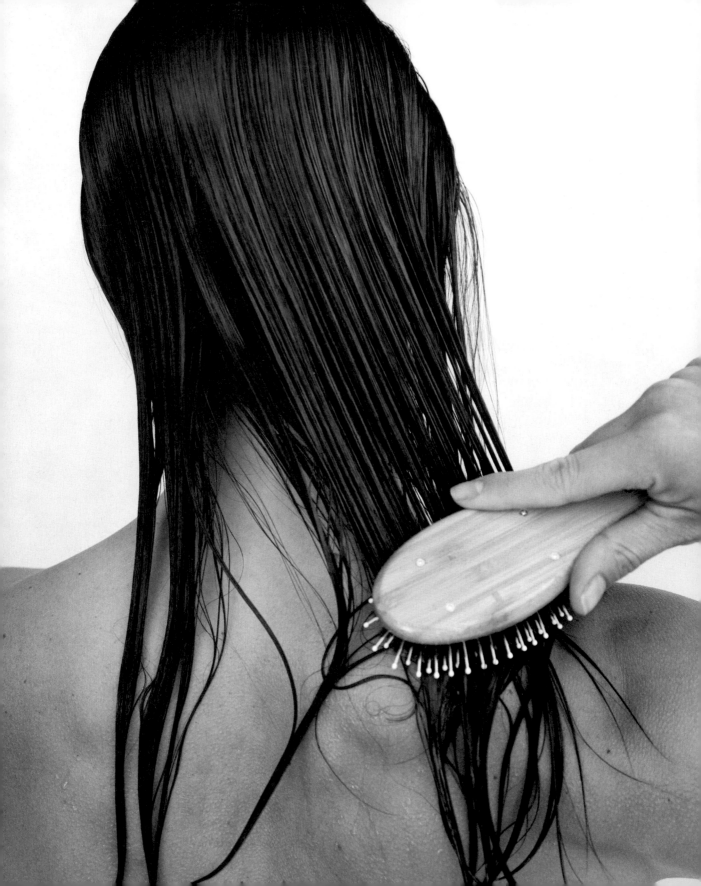

7.

Ultimate Hair Health

The Nuts and Bolts of Shiny, Bouncy, Healthy Hair

Healthy hair looks and feels fantastic—maintaining it, or regaining it, involves an as-minimal-as-possible routine, along with diet support. Heat styling, coloring, chemical straightening or curling, chlorine, sun exposure, and even just plain cleansing take a toll on hair; mitigating the damage will keep your hair looking its best.

A brilliant stylist who knows you and your hair also makes a huge difference. You'll know you've found the right person when he/she *doesn't* criticize your previous stylist's work and instead focuses on you—really looking at you, asking you questions about your lifestyle, what you like, how you care for your hair.

The right cut should make it so your hair needs a minimal amount of styling to look good. Getting there should be a collaborative process: Bring along pictures of cuts you love, to give your stylist an idea of what's ultimately going to make you happy. Pictures of yourself in different hairstyles are also incredibly helpful. A great stylist will take

all of your input, along with what he/she sees and knows, and come up with something you love.

Maintaining the look you have the day you walk out of the salon—whether you have fresh color, a new cut, or just a blowout—is the bigger challenge. Whether your hair is oily, dry, or in between, focus on washing it as little as possible. A conventional routine involves a powerful, highly lathering shampoo that foams impressively because it's full of detergents. Detergents—otherwise known as surfactants—lift dirt and oil out of your hair, but they also strip it of all its natural oils (which give hair shine, flexibility, and softness) and they strip hair color like crazy, so it fades more quickly and becomes brassy. In addition, harsh surfactants can irritate the skin on your scalp. After the shampoo strips down, the rest of a conventional routine is about building back in softness, shine, and texture—and invariably involves more frequent coloring for the 70 percent of women who dye their hair.

Getting oils back into your hair is difficult, and making it stay there is a temporary proposition at best. Conditioners coat the hair with oils and/or silicones that make it easier to manage, and feel and look temporarily softer and shinier. Depending on the formula, most of those go down your shower drain. Conditioning masks and oils, especially if applied with heat, encourage more moisture into the hair shaft, but even the intensive, hours-long oil treatments famous in India—which do result in a dramatic increase in elasticity and shine—last only a few weeks, max.

The more natural oils you can preserve to begin with—by shampooing less, and/or using non-detergent shampoo—the healthier and shinier your hair will be. This is true even for oily hair: Stripping oil from your scalp completely can cause your skin to produce more oil than it normally would, so harsh formulas can actively make the problem worse. For seriously oily hair, dry shampoo can absorb some of the oil without stripping it, and give you at least an extra day before you need to cleanse.

Styling products further re-texturize hair on the surface, whether it's shine, volume, softness, piecey waves, or any other desired effect. Their benefits can fade within hours (as in the case of most volumizers, for instance), or last until the next shampoo (industrial-strength hairspray will stay stuck to your hair until you wash it out). Once you start a routine of going easier on your hair in the shower, you'll hopefully find that you need less help in the shine-and-softness department, not to mention with frizz and split ends, but many people will still want to use their beloved stylers—if something gives you a great hair day, who's going to go without it?

Most hair stylists advise building in styling products while your hair is still wet: Add anti-frizz serums or thickening lotions before you blow-dry and the results will be dramatically smoother and sleeker than if you blow-dried alone; mousse builds in more volume and bounce than a simple blow-dry can ever achieve.

Once your hair is dry, more stylers—from heat tools to products—can also make a huge difference in the way your hair looks. They can also be damaging, and it's important to note that very few styling products are nontoxic, and most are full of plastics, artificial dyes and fragrances, preservatives, and more. The fewer you use, especially sprays that end up being inhaled, the better. There are a few good hair-styling brands in the clean beauty space and they are worth seeking out.

goop PICKS

Our all-time favorite clean hair styling products: Lavett & Chin makes a great Sea/Salt Texturizing Mist for perfect day-at-the-beach waves. Reverie's RAKE styling balm holds a look softly in place and adds bounce.

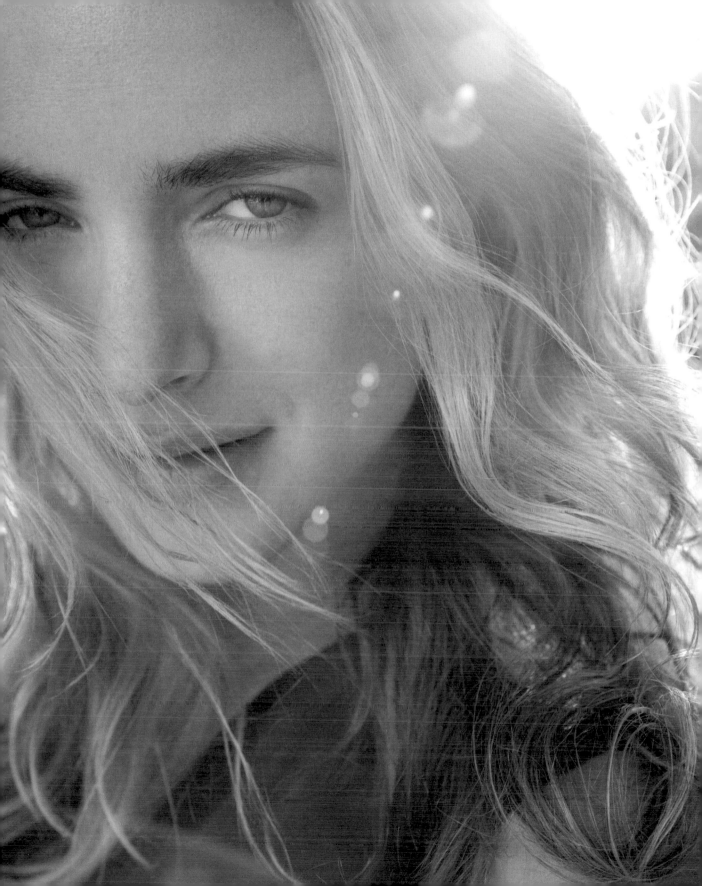

Hair Color: From Bleach to Black

Hair color contains some of the most toxic chemicals in the beauty business: Bleaches irritate and damage hair and skin, sometimes even burning it. Much worse, though, elements in the pigmenting process, particularly with brown shades, are carcinogenic. That said, there aren't great clean options at this point, which means that this is one of those toxic hits that so many women (including most GOOP staffers) take—making it all the more important that the rest of your routine is clean.

Just as a brilliant chef takes the same ingredients you might cook with and turns out something truly incredible, there is no substitute for the work of a brilliant colorist. By the same token, you do have access to the same or similar ingredients, so depending on how complicated your particular color is, you may be able to color it yourself some or all of the time.

A great colorist is incredibly useful in arriving at the perfect color for your face, hair, and skin tone. All the apps, charts, and tips in the world can't replace the intuition of someone experienced in hair color. If you're lucky enough to have access to a colorist you trust, definitely go for a consultation before you do anything. Single-process dirty-blonde, brown, or black hair is often so straightforward that you may not need to return to your colorist every time you need your roots done; once- or twice-a-year visits to refresh your whole head might be all you need, or you may be able to find an out-of-the-box, allover color you can do at home, period. Everyone's comfort level is different. For double-process color—where you're changing the allover color, then further altering it with highlights and/or lowlights—more skills are definitely required. There are people who successfully do their own highlights on a regular basis, but they are rare.

YOUR COLOR OPTIONS

- **Permanent vs. semi-permanent:** Permanent color is precisely what it sounds like: While it may fade over time, it permanently alters the shade of whatever hair it touches. As your hair grows, there'll be a line of demarcation between the colored hair and the new roots.

  Semi-permanent is a temporary dye that washes out over the course of twenty to thirty washes. It fades completely over time, so there are no roots, no long-term commitment. You can't go lighter with semi-permanent color, however: It deposits pigment, rather than taking it away (permanent color takes away pigment in hair, then chemically alters its color, rather than depositing pigment). Semi-permanent is less damaging, in general.

- **Double process:** Colored hair that has highlights on top of the color involves two separate coloring processes, layered over one another. The most extreme double process is full-on Edie Sedgwick/Marilyn Monroe platinum, which looks amazing but can absolutely trash hair. While you can do it yourself, a shade this intense is much better done with a colorist, to minimize damage and to attain the perfect shade.

- **Highlights:** Whether done all over, or just a few judicious pieces around the face, highlights can make your hair look naturally lit by the sun, not to mention more dimensional, which is how natural, uncolored hair looks. Highlights are less intense, in general, but they require more skill than the average non-hair-colorist has—for most people, it's best to get them done in a salon. Lemon juice and sunlight, or chlorine and sunlight, can often create some natural highlights on virgin hair; on over-colored hair, they tend to look brassy.

- **Crazy colors:** From pastel green to full-on fuchsia, out-there colors go in and out of style. If you use bleach to achieve a color, rather than the less-dramatic temporary options, you've got the same damage and roots problems that you get with any colored hair.

- **Gloss:** Applied in a salon or at home, a gloss refreshes your color and shine, so you can go longer between coloring. Similar to semi-permanent color, a gloss deposits temporary pigment and shine ingredients; colorists use glosses to correct and tone fading color. You can get clear glosses that just enhance shine, too—upping only the shine actually makes the color look better just on its own. But a colored gloss will definitely help fix fading that looks like the color has gone off.

- **Roots:** There are people who color their hair once a week to cover any trace of roots, and there are people who grow out their roots on purpose for the cool look of it. Most people fall somewhere in the middle of that spectrum. Touching up your roots is vastly preferable to re-coloring your whole head: It minimizes damage to hair so it looks and feels better, saves time, and limits your exposure to hair color in general. At a salon, a root-touch-up service is often combined with a gloss for an overall refresh. You can create the same effect at home: Do a root touch-up one week, and a gloss (colored or clear) the next. DIY root-touch-up products have become pretty sophisticated and are worth trying.

There are also pens, mascaras, foams, and powders formulated to temporarily (until the next shampoo) color roots. While most of these are made with conventional beauty formulas and chemicals, those chemicals pale in toxicity to that of permanent hair color, so they represent a much healthier, if imperfect and less permanent, option. Some of them are pretty amazing and well worth having around, if only for emergencies. For people who don't wash their hair often, the powders (we like Color Wow), especially, can be a brilliant, relatively nonchemical solution for roots, period.

FIXING FADING/BRASSINESS/GREENISH TINGE

The more you wash your hair, particularly with detergent (sulfate-containing) shampoo, the quicker your color fades, making it look dull and/or orange-tinged (what colorists refer to as *brassy*). The reason for the orange color is that even dark-brown hair color uses a small amount of bleach to help the dye penetrate the hair, so when the color fades, it ends up lighter than your original hair color, and bleach plus brown adds up to something that's reddish.

Red hair color, on the other hand, fades the fastest, no matter what brand/colorist/shampoo you use. It too can look peachy/orangey, or it can simply look dull after time and repeated washing.

Blonde color can turn brassy just like brown hair; its tone is best countered with purple shampoos or glosses, which restore the proper coolness. The other blonde-fading issue is a green tinge, caused by the water in swimming pools (there is copper in chlorinating chemicals, which causes the green color) and is definitely best fixed by a colorist.

Lastly (and very importantly): Most colors are categorized as either "golden" or "ash." Golden or warm fades to red, so if you hate brassiness, err on the side of ash or cool.

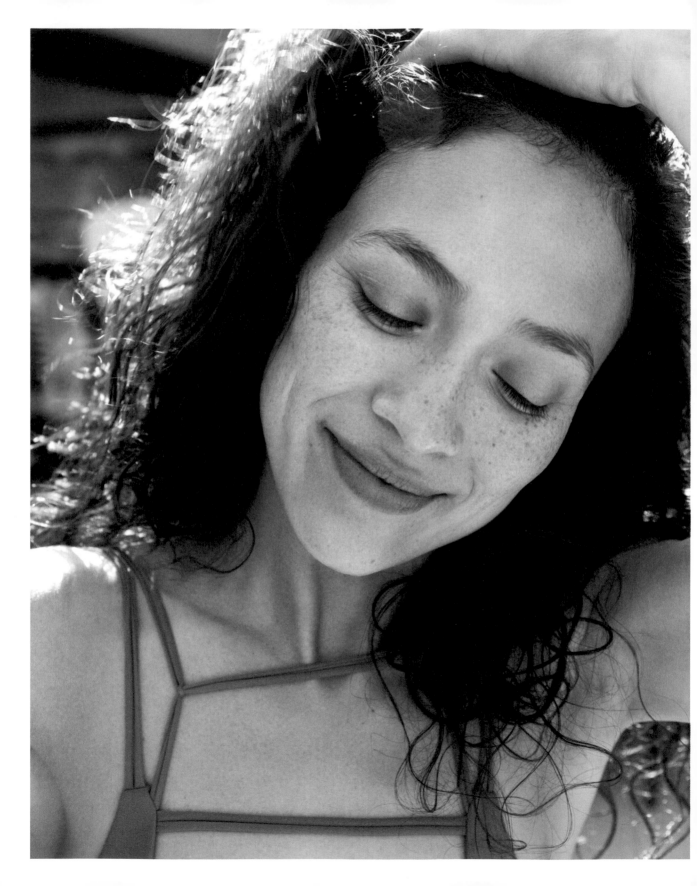

Relaxers, Straightening Treatments, and Perms

Even more powerful than most hair coloring ingredients, the chemicals in hair straighteners can be seriously damaging to hair, not to mention overall health. Chris Rock's brilliant 2009 documentary *Good Hair* points to some of the dangers of hair straightening technology, not to mention the dangers of a culture that insists on a single standard for beauty. Relaxers, Japanese straightening, and keratin treatments can straighten hair completely, or simply calm curlier hair into waves, or merely treat it so frizz is tamped down. Be extremely careful about combining hair color with any sort of straightening technology, as the combined damage can literally break your hair.

That said, the amount of time and money straightening processes save on styling makes them worth it to many women, despite the health concerns; consult with your most trusted hair expert (your stylist or colorist) about which straightening technology is going to work best on your particular hair.

Hair Crises

There are a few common problems that plague our hair. A really ubiquitous one, product buildup, is a no-brainer to fix. Frizz and flyaways take more effort to control. Thinning hair, which can be devastating emotionally, is unfortunately harder to treat, but there are a few solutions that can make a difference.

PRODUCT BUILDUP

Styling products can build up in hair; so can shampoo and conditioner if they're not rinsed out properly. Hair guru Philip Kingsley points out that many people don't get their hair wet enough in the shower before shampooing to begin with—so it doesn't get a chance to wash out existing product. This leaves hair dull and hard to style. Always spend a little extra time getting hair—especially at the scalp—wet. It sounds so obvious as to be silly, but doing it right will make a huge difference in your hair immediately. Likewise, make sure you thoroughly rinse everything off your hair before getting out.

You don't need special products to fight buildup; if you really feel it's a problem, rinse wet hair with a few capfuls of apple cider vinegar before shampooing.

FRIZZ

Frizz and poufiness can strike even the smoothest-haired among us from time to time. Caused sometimes by the hair texture you're born with and in other cases by humidity filling the hair shaft with moisture, the key is sealing out moisture with ultra-conditioning oils and creams, and smoothing hair texture. Sulfate (detergent)-free shampoos with lots of moisture, conditioners, stylers like hair oils and balms, and heat from blow-dryers and flatirons—all of these can tamp down hair temporarily; keratin treatments can be full of serious toxins like formaldehyde (see page 158), but they do work, often for months on end.

THINNING HAIR

It's estimated that some 30 million American women deal with thinning hair at some point in their lives. Sometimes the condition is temporary—often brought on by shifting hormones that later stabilize, and the hair grows back, as in pregnancy—and sometimes it is not. Perimenopausal and menopausal changes can cause hair loss similar to that of pregnancy—most people regain most of what they've lost after these major hormonal shifts. Thinning hair can indicate underlying health problems, from vitamin deficiencies to cancer, so definitely see a doctor if you feel that you're losing hair for no reason. (And keep reading for answers from one here.)

BREAKAGE

Strengthening the hair that you do have is key for people with thinning hair; follow the dietary guidelines (to come) in this chapter, and seriously consider taking biotin—it's one of the few supplements that even the medical community agrees has some impact. Protein treatments (along with dietary changes) can help further strengthen hair—remember that hair is mostly protein to begin with. The caveat with protein treatments is that too much will cause hair to become brittle—it is critical to maintain the balance between strength and flexibility. So create a regimen that combines protein hair treatments with ones designed purely for moisture and conditioning.

Hair color (particularly extreme bleaching, as in a double-process blonde) and straightening (from relaxer to keratin treatments) can take a serious toll on the health of your hair, sometimes causing so much breakage that it looks like your hair is thinning. The combination of coloring and straightening treatments is especially damaging; it can all but dissolve your hair.

Heat styling—blow-dryers, curling irons, straightening irons, hot rollers—can also weaken hair, and too much heat burns it into oblivion. If your hair is colored or chemically straightened, know that it's going to have less natural resistance to extreme heat. Heat-protective styling products

can help, but they can't compensate fully for already-compromised hair.

Tight ponytails held with even tighter elastics or barrettes can also cause breakage. The newer, wider, fabric hair ties are the gentlest on your hair; even tying a ponytail a bit looser can make a huge difference. Excessive brushing can cause the same problem, as can brushing your hair when it's wet—keep a comb by your shower, and comb through only after you put a little leave-in conditioner on the ends.

For more on hair damage and thinning, we turn to board-certified dermatologic surgeon Dr. Dendy Engelman, an associate at Manhattan Dermatology and Cosmetic Surgery, and Director of Dermatologic Surgery at New York Medical College. Dr. Engelman is an expert in Mohs surgery, dermatologic surgery, lasers, and cosmetic dermatology. She treats both men and women suffering from hair loss in her practice.

Dr. Dendy Engelman
ON HAIR LOSS

Is female hair loss mostly age-related? What age do you see it striking?
Thinning begins for women in the forties or fifties, though it can occur as early as the twenties. The good news is total baldness is rare in women; women's hair thins diffusely throughout the scalp. Genetics play a big role as well in female hair loss. If your mom or sister has thinning hair, you are much more likely to experience it as well.

Is the treatment of thinning hair the same for men and women?
There are only two FDA-approved medications for hair thinning: minoxidil for men and women, and Propecia

(brand name for finasteride) for men. Minoxidil's mechanism of action is believed to be due to an effect on the calcium channels in the hair cells. Minoxidil increases the capillary blood flow to the dermis of the skin where the follicles reside (promotes oxygen, blood, and nutrients to the hair follicles) to make them stronger and help regrow hair.

Are there any topical treatments you feel make a difference?
In addition to minoxidil used topically, I see great results with topical stem-cell treatment.

Do you think supplements and/or dietary changes can help at all?
They absolutely help with hair loss if it is the result of deficiency. Low levels of iron can lead to hair loss, and the fix may be as simple as adding an iron or vitamin supplement. Also, hair thrives on protein, iron, zinc, and vitamin B12, so consume lean meats, leafy greens, nuts, beans, and fish.

Three supplements I like are: Viviscal (fish protein) and Reserveage Keratin Booster with biotin, and a new one called Nutrafol that has been showing great clinical results as well.

Can hormones make a difference?
Some women are genetically predisposed to female-pattern hair loss, and birth control pills can suppress overproduction of male hormones that contribute to it. At menopause, thinning increases; if you're on hormone therapy, it may minimize hair loss.

Is it important to start treating hair loss as soon as you notice it?
Yes, extremely important! Studies show that once thinning is appreciable, the subject has already lost about 50 percent of her hair density. Regrowth that occurs is most often not to original density prior to hair loss or thinning, so the more you start with, the better results you get.

What are the best technological developments you've seen in thinning-hair treatments?

- Stem cells, also called pluripotent cells, are like a skeleton key that can open any lock—they have the potential to become any type of cell in the body, be it hair, skin, or muscle. One treatment, NuGene Anti-Hair-Loss Serum, contains culture medium from human adipose–derived stem cells, which has been shown to improve blood flow to the scalp and revitalize follicles. (After the fat stem cells are cultured and strained away, beneficial growth factors and cytokines are left.)

- Injecting cortisone directly into the scalp blocks the inflammatory activity that induces hair thinning. This works especially well in patients with inflammatory or autoimmune scalp disease.

- Low-level light treatment (LLLT) has been used for those suffering from male- and female-pattern hair loss. Laser red light has been shown to be effective in stimulating energy within the cells of the hair follicle. Many studies—including those performed by members of the foremost industry organization for hair transplant surgery—have shown that patients that use this type of treatment will stop hair loss and incite new regrowth, restoring perhaps 15 to 20 percent of their hair volume. It was first approved by the FDA in 2007 in the form of a laser-comb device for the treatment of mild to moderate male pattern hair loss. The problem: It wasn't practical in application, as the instructions were hard to follow correctly—so it had less-than-optimal results in non clinical use. But done correctly, LLLT for hair loss using red light lasers has been reported to increase cell metabolism and the health of blood vessels in the scalp for thicker, supple, and more durable hair shafts; stimulate the sebaceous glands for silkier-looking hair; and even increase melanin production in the hair follicles, darkening gray hairs.

• Platelet-rich plasma treatments are still being perfected, but they are reported to stimulate dormant hair follicles, thus increasing hair growth. The procedure involves drawing blood, spinning it in a centrifuge to extract the plasma, adding various nutrients (like more protein), then injecting the resulting mixture in one-inch intervals in a grid on the top of the scalp, which has been numbed with a local anesthetic.

Can you get back hair that's fallen out?
Hair follicles cycle on and cycle off, and repeat that process over the course of their life span. Each day, 100 to 200 hairs are shed, and these hair follicles are replaced by other hair follicles entering the growth phase. To maintain healthy hair follicles, it is important to have a healthy scalp. If the hair follicle is no longer viable or is surrounded/replaced with fibrosis (scarring), you cannot revive it—and the only option at that point is a hair transplant.

The Good-Hair Diet

As Dr. Engelman pointed out, our diet (as well as supplements) affects how hair looks. Extremely low-calorie diets can cause thinning hair, as can extremely low-protein diets; even when such diets don't cause hair loss, they often result in dull, brittle hair. Eating the right food supports great-looking and greet-feeling hair in powerful ways.

OUR TOP TEN LIST FOR HEALTHIER HAIR

1. **Protein:** Your hair is made primarily of protein, so get plenty of it, from beans and nuts to fish, lean meat, eggs, and yogurt.
2. **Fat:** Oily fish, raw nuts and seeds, avocado, flax—and the oils from all of these—help keep your hair soft and touchable. It's important to note that without fat, many of the nutrients in food (and supplements) don't get absorbed.
3. **Omegas:** Particularly helpful fats are omega-3s, -6s, and -7s. Oily fish and cold-pressed flaxseed oil are excellent sources.
4. **Iron:** Iron supports circulation—critical for healthy skin and hair. Beans, eggs, meat, broccoli, and spinach are ways to get more.
5. **Vitamin A:** Found in carrots, sweet potatoes, spinach, peaches, cod liver oil, and krill oil, vitamin A encourages the healthy growth of sebum, which keeps your hair soft and healthy—not to mention preventing breakage.
6. **Vitamin C:** This antioxidant—in citrus, bell peppers, guavas, kale, kiwis, and cantaloupe—helps you absorb minerals like iron (for circulation) and magnesium.
7. **Vitamin E:** The same reason vitamin E is good for your heart—it encourages capillary growth and is anti-inflammatory, among other things—is why it's so good for your hair. Find it in dark leafy greens, almonds, avocados, sunflower seeds, shellfish, fish, and eggs. (You can also apply vitamin E oil directly onto hair.)
8. **Zinc:** Low levels of zinc in the body can directly cause hair loss. Oysters have the most zinc of any food; beans, crab, lobster, chicken, and nuts all have zinc in them, too.
9. **Biotin:** This B vitamin—found in yeast, liver, egg yolks, soy, and walnuts, plus hair-growth supplements—supports healthy hair growth like few other compounds.
10. **Vitamin B5:** Helps prevent hair loss and encourages healthy hair growth. Greek yogurt, also packed with protein, is a great way to get it.

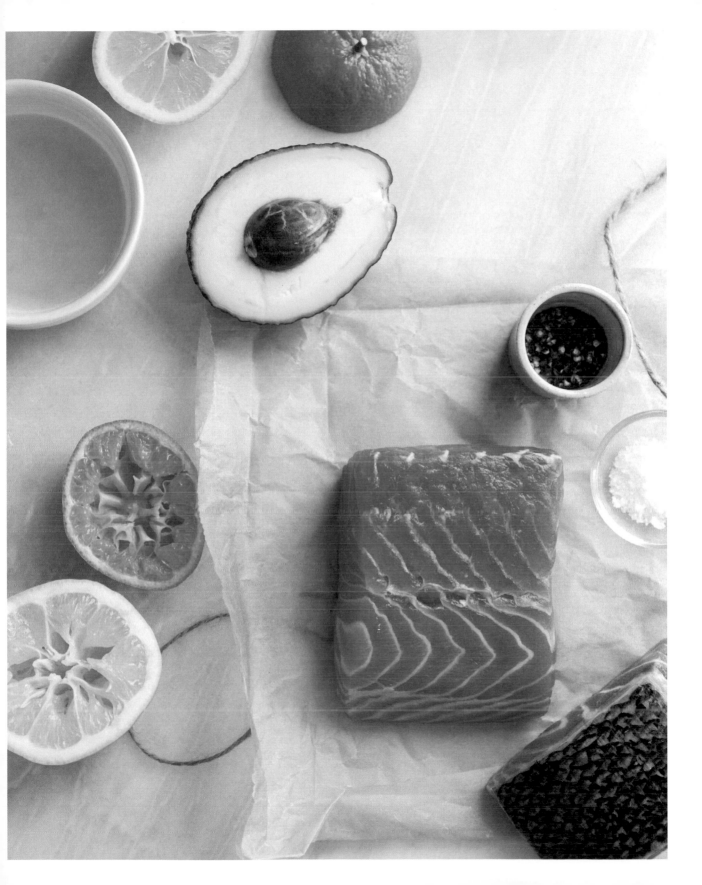

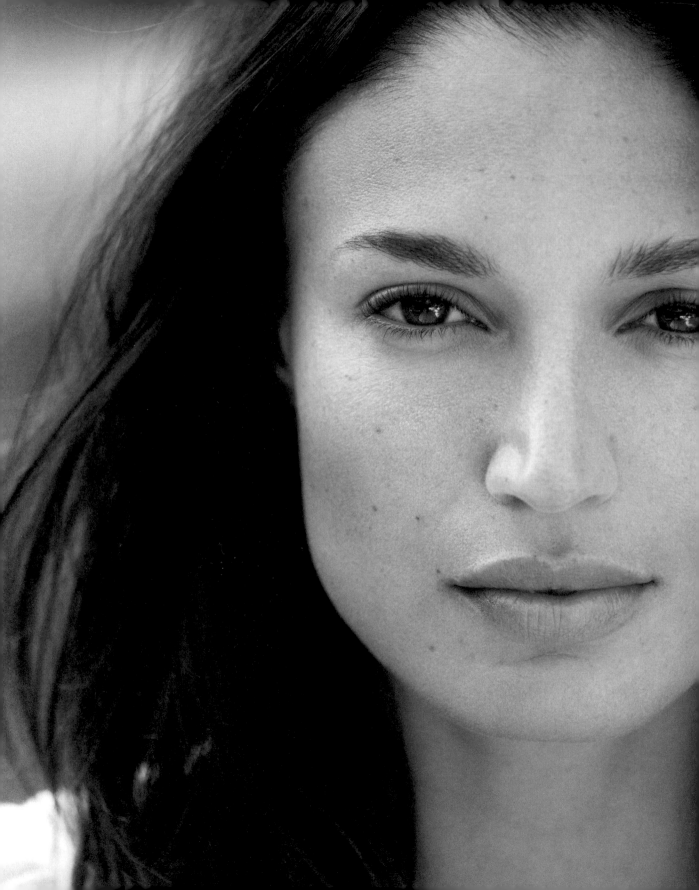

8.

Your Skin As You Age

Take Care of Your Face

Everybody—even a newborn—is aging. It's neither bad nor good, it just is. The specific signs of aging skin, however, are unloved by most. It's common in our culture to overemphasize the *awfulness* of the visible markers of aging. Trying to erase all evidence of aging from your face is both futile and a fool's errand—with some of the solutions ending up looking much worse than the original "problems" did. Attempting to look your best, for whatever age you actually are, is for sure the most happiness-inducing strategy, not to mention the most realistic.

Taking care of your skin at all stages of your life makes an enormous difference. Chapter 4, on sun, smoking, and pollution, is worth reading and re-reading: Wearing sunblock regularly and not smoking are the anti-aging measures that pay off the biggest, by far. Moisturizers, peels, and even injections pale in comparison to not smoking and consistent sunblock use.

That said, there is a great deal you can do beyond those two critical measures. Inflammation is now believed to cause most of what we consider

to be visible aging, so look at your overall lifestyle and try to curb as much inflammation-causing behavior as you can—from glycation (caused by consuming sugar, alcohol, and barbecued meat, to name a few) and exposure to pollutants, to making sure your teeth and gums are well taken care of (unhealthy gums are thought to raise inflammation levels throughout the body). A clean diet and regular exercise make an enormous difference in the way you look and the way you feel (and thus act); what makes a person seem old or young depends a lot on these factors. Energy, enthusiasm, and glowing skin do take you pretty far, actually.

To understand more about aging, it's helpful to look at children's skin. It's incredibly beautiful—and it all but takes care of itself. Cell turnover is quick, collagen and elastin are being produced at maximum rates, circulation is at its top efficiency (increased circulation is also why pregnant women seem to glow). The color and texture of a child's skin is something to behold, and to treat aging skin most effectively, use products and techniques designed to mimic the way children's skin takes care of itself. As we age, cell turnover slows, for instance. Exfoliating agents—from face scrubs to dermatologist peels—speed the process back up. Similarly, compounds that recharge collagen production or encourage circulation give skin the firmness and glow of youth. Below, the GOOP team has put together a (partial, as it is constantly expanding) list of anti-aging approaches and what to expect from them.

The Basics

First up, the fundamental components of your regular routine and the product choices for moisturizing skin from the common moisturizer to GOOP–favorite face oils:

MOISTURIZERS AND CREAMS

Moisturizer…moisturizes. It doesn't smooth wrinkles (though it plumps them up so they look smoother temporarily, which is why it's always great to moisturize before putting on makeup, for instance). On its own, it also doesn't firm skin or fade dark spots. It doesn't fight signs of aging except in the moment: It makes our skin look and feel better for as long as the moisturizer lasts. It does strengthen the skin's barrier function, so it's less vulnerable to inflammation and irritation, so it is anti-aging in that sense, though those sorts of benefits depend on the moisturizer being applied.

Eye Cream

The skin around your eyes produces very little oil, and it's the thinnest skin you have—that's why you see aging around your eyes first. Eye cream is moisturizer designed not to irritate your eyes or the eye area; most do not have special powers. In fact, because of the need to be non-irritating, most are milder than regular anti-agers. Some have peptides or other ingredients to stimulate collagen—any bit of which helps, especially if you have dark circles (the darkness is mostly blood, showing through the thin skin). If you can tolerate it, a bit of a retinoid (see page 187) around the eyes is something dermatologists often (privately, as it's not prescribed for the eye area) recommend. Other eye creams focus on soothing, to calm redness and puffiness.

Ask any makeup artist what his or her no-fail first step is and they will tell you eye cream. Like regular moisturizer, it plumps and smoothes lines, so makeup doesn't catch in them. Eye creams can also contain de-puffing ingredients like caffeine; these work to some degree, though don't expect miracles. Cold helps in the de-puffing department—some people keep eye cream in the fridge, but something that stays cold, like a gel pack, or a cucumber, is more effective.

DOES ANTI-AGING MAKEUP WORK?

The short answer: It works so marginally as to be statistically insignificant. Makeup has to do so many other things—smooth, even, tint, feel nice, look nice, spread perfectly—that the amount of active ingredient in any formula is going to be super-small. The most anti-aging makeup formula is the most moisturizing, least harsh one. Look for a product that feels wonderful, leaves your skin dewy and fresh, and never dries it out—that is your best choice.

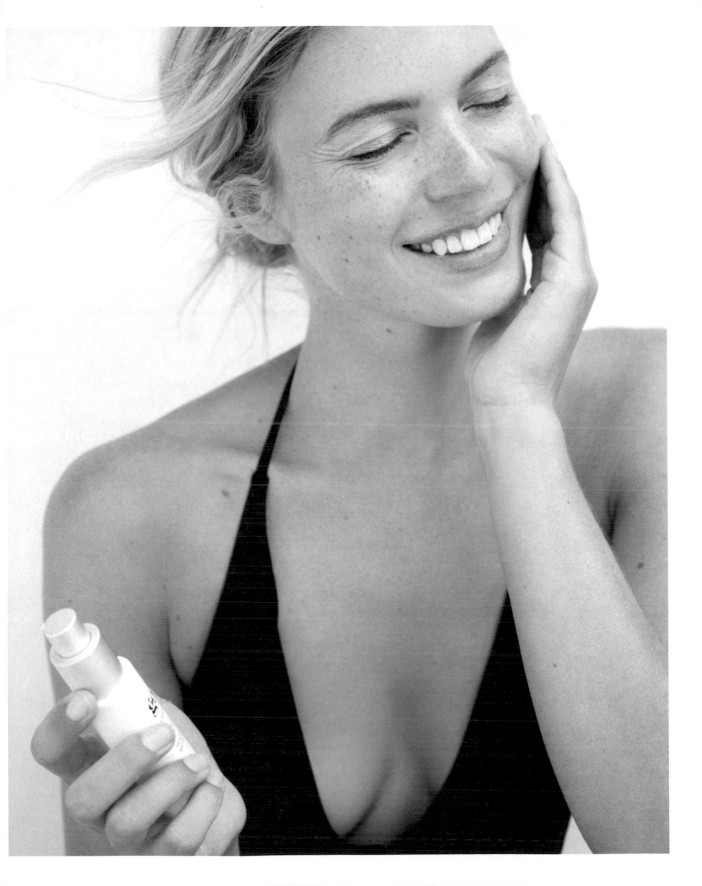

Oils

When you talk about oils, there aren't stacks of impressive clinicals, or convincing before-and-afters, but there is most of human history: Women have been pressing and smoothing oils into their skin for centuries. Moisturizers and creams are relatively new inventions, and they aren't more moisturizing than oils—they simply have a different texture. Conventional moisturizers are often made with so many fillers and stabilizers to affect texture and shelf life that they are actually considerably less moisturizing than straight-up oils. Oils feel incredible, and they can leave your skin glowy and ultra-hydrated. Like moisturizers, they don't get rid of wrinkles, but plump them up, smoothing them temporarily.

goop PICKS

We're face-oil obsessives at GOOP. We made a face oil that we love in the GOOP by Juice Beauty line, though our face-oil fixation goes even further: For ultimate anti-aging, we love Vintner's Daughter; for custom-made-for-each-season exquisite luxury, de Mamiel; for ultimate anti-inflammatory action and healing, May Lindstrom.

Serums

The idea behind most serums is that instead of suspending active ingredients in a moisturizer formula—which changes the pH and can render the active ingredients much less active, or dilutes the actives so you get less of them on your skin—

you can create a formula that's mostly just the actives, for more powerful results. Of course, some conventional brands add fillers and stabilizers and the rest to serums, too, but in general, a serum is a more direct route to treatment ingredients than regular moisturizer. A good serum infuses your skin with actives (say, an antioxidant like vitamin C) and is best used on bare skin, before moisturizer. If it's summer or you're not particularly dry, serums can sometimes be used as moisturizers, as many are mildly hydrating.

TONERS/WATERS

If they feel nice, or help get your makeup off without drying or irritating, these are fine to use. Some can leave treatment ingredients behind, or prep skin to better absorb more active treatments to come. Toners and waters are probably the least crucial part of a skincare regimen, but many people absolutely swear by them.

DOES YOUR CLEANSER MAKE A DIFFERENCE?

There are cleansers designed to treat everything from dullness to acne to wrinkles, but because the ingredients mostly wash off, cleanser is probably not going to affect the way your skin ages too much—unless it's too harsh. Avoid foams and gels for the most part, concentrating on cleansing oils, balms, or creams. The ideal cleanser leaves your skin clean but soft and supple as opposed to tight.

THE ANTI-AGERS

To get serious anti-aging benefits, you need to go beyond plain old (but perfectly good and entirely useful for other reasons) moisturizing products, into targeted anti-aging treatments:

Retinoids

Ask any dermatologist for the gold standard in anti-aging and the answer will be the same: retinoic acid. It's a vitamin-A derivative that does all sorts of things, from building collagen in the skin and increasing cell turnover to discouraging precancerous growths in skin (a related compound is even aspirated into lungs to discourage cancer). Available only by prescription, retinoids treat acne as well as the signs of aging (wrinkles, age spots, lack of firmness, enlarged pores, and more). Retinoic acid does increase sun sensitivity, so if you use it, apply it only at night, never in the morning, and you've got to use sunblock religiously. It can also cause irritation for many people; if you find it causes you to peel, start by washing it off 5 minutes after applying it, and use it only every other night. Gradually, your skin will acclimate to the retinoid and you'll be able to leave it on overnight, and may even be able to use it every night. Some women find they're more prone to irritation from retinoids around their periods; the easy fix is to tone it down during that time.

Cosmetic companies—both conventional and nontoxic/clean ones—market retinol, a related but less-powerful compound, in skincare. Retinol can absolutely make a big difference in your skin, but if you love the results, you might consider prescription retinoids for a more intensive dose. But an over-the-counter retinol may be perfect for your skin if you find the full-strength versions too irritating.

On the flip side, there are plenty of aestheticians who will tell you too much retinoic acid damages your skin. (It does not, as some will tell you, thin the skin.) In any case, if retinoids or retinols cause sensitivity or long-term irritation in your skin, there are plenty of anti-aging alternatives to choose from.

AHAs, BHAs, and Fruit Enzymes

Alpha (AHA) and beta (BHA) hydroxy acids speed cell turnover in much the same way retinoids do, and they have a milder collagen-stimulating effect. Fruit enzymes like papaya have a similar effect. All sweep away dead skin cells chemically—an advantage over physical scrubs, which can scratch and create microscopic tears in skin. (The plastic microbeads so toxic to the environment are thankfully now banned, but they did have an advantage over the less uniform particles in many natural physical scrubs, which create the microscopic tears.) AHAs and BHAs can be incredibly mild or incredibly strong, depending on their concentration in a formula and/or pH level. The primary BHA, salicylic acid—otherwise known as willow bark, or aspirin—has anti-inflammatory and antibacterial properties that make it brilliant for acne, but can also be used for anti-aging. Treatment with these acids brightens, softens, and smoothes skin, as well as moisturizes. Counterintuitively, AHAs were actually developed as a treatment for ichthyosis, a disease that causes extremely dry skin. Overuse will irritate skin, but AHAs can be incredibly useful in treating the signs of aging. You can find AHAs and BHAs in all manner of creams, serums, toners, and wipes, not to mention serious peels, from daily exfoliants to major, in-office dermatological peels.

Collagen

Collagen is the protein that is your skin's structural support; as we age, it breaks down, so we lose firmness and volume within the skin. Cosmetic creams with collagen as an ingredient have been around for a long time, but it's unclear that simply smoothing collagen on the top layer of dead skin will in any way help replace what's been lost below, where it counts. Creams that spur the body to start making more collagen on its own—from retinoids to peptides—do seem to have a more significant effect.

Back in the day, dermatologists used collagen injections to fill depressed areas of the skin like acne scars or hollows under the eyes; they worked, but the effects didn't last long. Today, fillers (more on page 191) perform a similar but longer lasting and more predictable role; some of them may even help stimulate collagen production to some degree.

Ingesting collagen—through bone broths, gelatin, or, now, supplements specifically designed for skin—can also have an effect, though it's not well tested. Some ingestible collagen supplements have had pretty impressive clinical trials in terms of their effect on skin; the caveat is the collagen generally comes from ground-up cow and/or rooster parts from Germany and China. Industry experts often give the tip that the collagen from Germany is higher quality, but for many of us, the specter of mad cow disease makes the whole enterprise decidedly less appealing. There are plant collagen supplements emerging as well, but their effect is not as clear yet.

Peptides

Peptides are short chains of amino acids that signal cells in the skin that collagen has been lost—prompting it to generate more collagen. In general, they're a pretty fantastic addition to an anti-aging product or regimen: They don't usually cause irritation, and their clinical results are hard to argue with. They build collagen, smooth wrinkles, and improve skin texture—and you can find them in conventional and nontoxic products.

Vitamin C and Other Antioxidants

Again, antioxidants like vitamin C and idebenone are wonderful for skin, as they are for the rest of your body. (Antioxidant molecules scavenge free

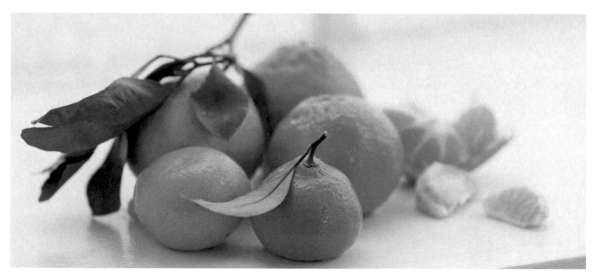

radicals and neutralize them.) You can and should eat them—vegetables, fruits, and fish oils are some prime sources—and you can and should slather them on your skin. Vitamin C is perhaps the best-known topical antioxidant: It has a clarifying, brightening, mildly exfoliating, mildly tightening effect on skin. It's an easy compound to love, because the results are relatively perceptible and immediate, and it works with practically any treatment regimen. Vitamin C is especially great to apply in the morning, because it's been shown (both topically and internally) to a have a sun-protective effect—though you'd still want to wear sunblock. Sunblock can't block every free radical that hits you, so adding antioxidants into the mix creates something of a safety net—every bit makes a difference.

Vitamin E is another well-known antioxidant—it's brilliant for healing and moisturizing. You can simply burst an oral vitamin E capsule and smooth it on skin, or you can get it in any number of products, conventional or nontoxic.

Vitamin D is an antioxidant your body makes for itself, with the aid of sunlight or supplements; it's generally not applied topically, unless you count the sun as a topical. (More on vitamin D on page 118.)

Vitamin A and its many derivatives (the aforementioned retinoids and retinols) are amazing for skin, as are resveratrol (the antioxidant that makes grapes and blueberries so healthy) and green tea. All are wonderful taken internally and topically.

New antioxidants and antioxidant sources are being discovered all the time; it's well worth experimenting with topical products to find one you like—applying one every morning is essential for staving off the signs of aging.

Anti-Inflammatories

Consuming anti-inflammatory compounds in food or supplements can make a serious difference in the way you age and topical versions can, too. Inflammation (from internal, body-wide inflammation that isn't immediately visible to something obvious like a rash or a puffy face), now considered to be the cause of most of the aging that goes on in our bodies, builds on itself, so intervening where there is any bit of inflammation makes an enormous amount of sense. Many already-anti-aging substances are also anti-inflammatory, from salicylic acid to most antioxidants. Certain types of mushrooms and mushroom extracts are great anti-inflammatories, so are some topical probiotics (even plain old yogurt on the face works), aloe, and omega oils, to name a few. If the anti-ager you're already using has anti-inflammatory properties—say, something made with green tea extract, or vitamin E—brilliant. If not, incorporate anti-inflammatories into your regimen. Either way, keep seriously soothing treatments (aloe, vitamin E, or orally taken aspirin) on hand for inflammatory emergencies like a sunburn or a hangover.

Peels

Peels are another (usually fairly instant) way of exfoliating skin, clearing pores so that they're minimized, and potentially stimulating collagen. They can be anything from a DIY pad that gives you a little extra glow and smoother skin, to a dermatologist-office procedure with recovery times and more potent and long-lasting results. The most common ingredient in peels are AHAs of varying strengths and pHs; some are also made with fruit enzymes that are similar in action to AHAs, and others with different types of synthetic acids. Peels can definitely improve the look of your skin, but the key is to not do too much. Over-exfoliation—with peels or with product or a combination of the two—creates irritation and inflammation, both of which are decidedly aging, defeating the original purpose.

Mild peels done at home on a regular basis are probably your best bet for keeping your skin fresh and smooth; as you experiment with products, err on the side of less powerful until you really feel you know your skin. If you do end up irritated, pour on the anti-inflammatories.

Light Exposure
Dermatologists use both red- and blue-light therapy to fight aging as well as acne (red is most common for anti-aging). They stimulate collagen to some degree and also have great anti-inflammatory benefits—for that reason, they're often used after peels or other mildly invasive dermatological procedures to reduce irritation and redness, and even speed healing time. There are at-home versions of dermatologists' light-therapy machines that do show some clinical results in terms of anti-aging; the key with them is that they're weaker, so they require much longer exposure, repeated over a long period of time, which can get tedious.

SERIOUS (DERMATOLOGICAL) WORK
At the other end of the spectrum from basic skin-care steps are dermatological procedures. Following is a list of available treatments, and what you should consider before committing to any:

Botox
Derived from what is literally the most lethal substance on earth, botulinum toxin, Botox weakens muscle tissue, usually for between three and four months. It got its start around fifty years ago as a treatment for muscle spasms and twitches, and is used today to treat everything from migraines and muscle pain to crossed eyes (strabismus) and, most famously, wrinkles. It works: No wrinkle cream on earth is going to give you the results you'll get from Botox. It's expensive and it carries some (relatively minimal) risk, but, unlike practically every other "wrinkle fix" available, it does precisely what it promises.

Botox has become something of a shorthand in our culture for "bad plastic surgery" and/or "female vanity run amok." When someone says, "Oh, she's had too much Botox," the work they're referring to is probably actually plastic surgery or too much filler. In the early days of Botox, there were people who overdid it a bit and ended up with a frozen, faintly waxy look, but that's an uncommon mistake today.

Dermatologists most typically inject the forehead just between the eyebrows; Botox also can help with crow's-feet, and can be injected above the outer brows for a lifting effect on the upper eyelids (overdone, that technique can result in too-high eyebrows). It also can be used in the neck, both to smooth the look of the neck, but also to decrease sagging in the face overall—your neck muscles pull your facial muscles downward, as it turns out. While "neck Botox" sounds extreme, the results are natural looking. Harder to make look natural is Botox around the mouth area; only try it if your dermatologist is extremely experienced in that particular application.

This last point is the most important: Any facial intervention risks an unnatural-looking outcome, and the best cosmetic dermatologists are artists as much as they are scientists and technicians. If you're going to spend the (serious) money that anti-aging dermatology costs, don't try to save a little by going with anyone less than the best. Look at before-and-afters, and if at all possible, at actual people who've undergone treatment from the doctor you're considering. It's not Botox that's going to make you look younger, or look overdone; it's the person injecting it.

HOW TO PICK A DERMATOLOGIST

The tough thing about figuring out who might be the best dermatologist for you is that the best ones do work that's invisible; this applies to plastic surgeons as well. Of course you're going to choose someone accredited by the American Academy of Dermatology, someone who's gone to schools you've heard of and has privileges at hospitals you're familiar with. But beyond the basic, legitimate doctor screen, you've got to look further. People you know who look fantastic but unworked upon and rave about their dermatologist are definitely worth listening to. In the absence of a raving, trusted friend, set up an appointment to see before-and-afters and to talk about what treatments the dermatologist thinks might be best for you. If the dermatologist immediately launches into all sorts of fixes for "problems" you don't consider problems, find another one. A gifted dermatologist—just like a gifted hairstylist or makeup artist—will really look at you, and ask you questions about what bothers you, rather than projecting a one-size-fits-all vision of anti-aging onto you. Take your time with treatments, too: Don't go in for the full, do-everything-all-at-once procedures. Start small—a laser treatment, a small amount of Botox—and see if that does it.

Fillers

The advice regarding Botox goes double time for injectable fillers (Restylane, Juvéderm, Sculptra). Fillers—sometimes made with hyaluronic acid, the compound used for moisture within your skin—can seriously rejuvenate your face, or they can make you look like a crazy person. The overblown lips and cheekbones often attributed to "too much Botox" are actually too much filler. And filler is easy to overdo: Find a dermatologist whose work is imperceptible, but gorgeous.

We lose volume in our skin as we age—the collagen loss is the primary cause, but there are other factors, up to and including bone loss—and filler, done right, can restore the volume of youth. Much of what people think of as sagging skin is actually skin that's lost its support system. Fillers can be pretty long lasting, depending on the product, from 8 months to 2 years, and most of them can be reversed if you don't like the results.

Subtle filler around the cheekbones and jawline can restore structural support for the skin; lips are much trickier, so proceed at your own risk. Avoid getting filler in the nasolabial folds (worst name for a body part ever) around your mouth leading up to your nose: Extra volume there leaves people looking decidedly chimp-ish. Avoid obsessing over nasolabial folds in general, because people also tend to overdo cheek filler in an attempt to get rid of them. Filler sadly doesn't work well around the eyes, so also pay attention (and have your dermatologist pay attention) to the point where your cheekbone and your under-eye meet: Too much cheekbone filler will cause an unnatural dent where your under-eye begins. The right amount of cheekbone filler, however, can lift your entire lower face—again, imperceptibly but beautifully.

Threading

Somewhere between dermatology and plastic surgery, threading is another technique for supporting aging skin that's lost collagen and its firmness and structure. Typically, a natural or synthetic thread that dissolves over three weeks to a month is inserted under the skin by a dermatologist or plastic surgeon; the thread itself promotes the growth of new skin tissue, fibers, and collagen around it. The effects can last up to two years. Downtime is minimal; bruising and swelling is a possibility, as with fillers and even Botox. Used with modalities like fillers and Botox, the effects can be pretty amazing—and, in skilled hands, incredibly natural-looking.

ANTI-INFLAMMATORIES AND DERMATOLOGICAL PROCEDURES

Fish oil is great for skin—except if you're about to have an injection. The same goes for arnica, aspirin, and anything else that thins your blood: If you take them during the week before you see the dermatologist, they seriously up your chances of developing a bruise. Skip it and you're much less likely to look as if you've had something done.

Lasers, Heat, and Radiofrequency Treatments

A good dermatologist has an arsenal of machine treatments that fight aging. They fall into a number of categories, so we'll discuss them according to the issues they treat.

- **Wrinkles, crepiness, and rough skin:** Resurfacing lasers work by remodeling existing collagen and stimulating new collagen production, as wrinkles, texture, and crepiness are caused by thinning collagen in the dermis layer of the skin. They do not, as old-fashioned lasers once did (and as deep chemical peels and deep dermabrasion still do), thin the skin or take away its top layers. Most resurfacing lasers now are fractional—meaning that the laser targets the skin in dots, each separated by an expanse of untreated skin, speeding healing time and reducing the chance of side effects like abnormal pigmentation.

  Resurfacing lasers make a serious difference in the look of your skin (and they're being shown in studies to treat precancerous lesions in skin as well), but they do involve downtime. Depending on your lifestyle, your dermatologist's advice, the state of your skin, and your tolerance for downtime, you can try non-ablative (non-wounding) lasers like Clear + Brilliant or Fraxel Restore, or go with a stronger, ablative (superficially wounding) laser like Fraxel Repair—the latter option will leave you with serious redness and scabs for about a week, then about a month's worth of your skin being pinker than usual.

  A new, less known and less downtime-intensive option called a *picosecond laser*, originally developed to treat pigment (especially tattoos), is now being shown to promote the same sort of collagen response produced by fractional lasers, but with much less downtime—usually only a few hours of pinkness.

- **Redness:** Lasers can also get rid of redness from sun damage, genetics, hormones, and rosacea. They work by zapping (medically unnecessary) blood vessels while leaving the surrounding skin untouched. A pulsed-dye laser like the Vbeam is the ultimate in redness removal—it can even remove port-wine-stain birthmarks. Newer lasers like the Excel V work with different wavelengths of light than pulsed-dye lasers do, so they can target larger blood vessels that look like red lines/squiggles or blue paths on the face. Redness-reduction lasers don't hurt much and leave skin pink for a few hours, so downtime is minimal.

- **Sagging/loss of firmness:** Radiofrequency and ultrasound technologies can both be used to tighten and firm skin. Both procedures used to hurt a lot, though they have minimal downtime; technology has improved so that they now hurt a great deal less. The results don't show up right away, and they depend on the individual, but they can be dramatic in terms of firming and tightening. Dermatologists disagree across the board over the two technologies' relative effectiveness; whichever machine a given dermatologist has, that's the one thought to be superior. Talk to people who've had both procedures and research results...but both do, in general, have a pretty significant effect and little to no downtime.

    Radiofrequency treatment—for example, Thermage—heats underlying collagen fibers and stimulates remodeling of collagen and the production of new collagen. Downtime depends on the depth of the procedure; it ranges from none at all to several weeks of redness.

    Ultrasound—the most popular is Ultherapy—uses focused sound waves to heat the underlying collagen, stimulating collagen remodeling and collagen production. It hurts (less than it once did), but there's no downtime whatsoever.

- **Dark spots:** As soon as a spot appears, treat it with a laser. The topical "dark spot" treatments from both conventional and nontoxic beauty brands are never going to completely erase a spot. The exception to that rule is a prescription compound called hydroquinone that is so toxic it's banned in most other developed countries besides the U.S.

    Pigment-specific lasers—ruby, YAG, or Alexandrite, to name a few—target a particular spot, from freckles to larger dark spots, and zap them. The procedure is relatively painless but leaves a small scab wherever the spot was, which usually flakes off after a few days. Fractional resurfacing lasers can also treat dark spots and pigmentation through exfoliation.

    It should be noted that without constant sunscreen use, whatever you have spent time and money zapping away will quickly reappear.

For Good Measure

Again, because it can't be overstated: Choosing to have a procedure done, and settling on a doctor, should be a carefully thought out series of decisions. Pick the best dermatologist you can find, one who can show you before-and-afters, or, best of all, one whose work you were surprised to learn was work. The best procedures have subtle, natural results—and there are numerous ways to achieve them. Talk with your dermatologist about cost before having anything done—and factor how long the effects of a given treatment last into the cost. And in general, do less at first. You can always do more, but take it slow.

Why Hormones Are Always a Thing

Whether or not you're considering any of the procedures mentioned, it's worth understanding one of the major factors in the body's aging process that we haven't thoroughly covered yet—hormones. Although we commonly associate hormones with young/teenage skin, they affect our skin (and bodies) throughout our entire lives.

As hormone expert Dr. Laura Lefkowitz notes, "Hormones become especially confusing as we start to age. The information on hormones, hormone replacement therapy, and perimenopause is often conflicting. And it is hard to get anyone to address the issues." Which is, of course, what Dr. Lefkowitz does for us here. Her thorough descriptions of the roles hormones play in our latter decades will inform everything from diet and exercise routine to the treatment options that you consider potentially viable and appealing.

Dr. Laura Lefkowitz
ON HORMONES THROUGH THE DECADES

How much of skin aging is related to hormone levels?
Hormone levels are an important factor in skin aging. The natural process of skin aging depends on both *extrinsic* and *intrinsic* factors.

Extrinsic aging is more variable and occurs as a result of sun exposure and environmental damage (e.g., tobacco use, alcohol use, diet, exposure to pollution, surgery, and injections).

Intrinsic aging is the natural aging process that takes place over the years due to genetic predetermination and hormonal influences. Estrogen (a sex hormone) is the number one player in beautiful-looking skin. Estrogen modulates

skin physiology (how a cell functions) by influencing all the cells that our skin is made of: *keratinocytes* (produce keratin, making skin water-resistant), *fibroblasts* (produce collagen and elastin, which provide plumpness and elasticity to the skin), *melanocytes* (produce skin pigment), *hair follicles,* and *sebaceous glands* (produce oil to lubricate skin). Also, estrogen improves angiogenesis (small blood vessel growth) in the skin so that nutrients and oxygen can be effectively delivered to skin cells for proper functioning, vibrancy, elasticity, wound healing, and immune responses.

As we age and our ovarian function decreases, estrogen levels drop until we reach menopause. This progressive estrogen insufficiency decreases skin's defense against oxidative stress (extrinsic factors) and intrinsically skin becomes drier and thinner with less collagen. The elastin fibers become thicker, more clumped, and looser, resulting in decreased elasticity, brittle skin, and increased wrinkling. With all these hormonal changes, the skin's protective function becomes compromised with impaired wound healing, hair loss, pigmentary changes (skin discoloration), and skin cancer.

Hormone replacement therapy clearly does something to maintain the look of healthy skin (and hair): elasticity, moisture retention, firmness. Health practitioners are often reluctant to discuss this, lest they encourage a potentially cancer-causing agent to treat a cosmetic problem. What is your stance?
Supplementing with sex hormones like estrogen, progesterone, and testosterone can return a more youthful appearance to the skin and vaginal mucosa. But at a certain age we are not naturally supposed to have these hormones circulating throughout our bloodstream, so there are risks as far as blood clotting leading to strokes, weight gain leading to diabetes, or hormone-sensitive cancer cells growing rapidly in response to exogenous hormones that genetically would not be circulating post-menopause. The medical community takes an oath to "do no harm," so

traditionally we don't recommend adding something that has potential harm for a cosmetic benefit.

I believe supplementing with sex hormones is a personal decision. All cosmetic medical interventions have risks and side effects. Having a facelift, breast augmentation, Botox, fillers, laser, etc., all have potential risks, such as anesthesia complications, infection, nerve damage, and scarring. But many people feel they are willing to take the risk to look better.

If you have no family history of hormone-related cancers, have good medical care, and are really suffering emotionally and physically from the drop in hormones, are willing to take the risks with the benefit, and go for regular screenings (mammogram, Pap smear, ultrasounds, etc.) then hormone replacement may be the right decision for you after a thoughtful consultation with your physician.

Does it make a difference—looks-wise or health-wise—whether a woman uses regular commercial hormones or bio-identical ones from a compounding pharmacy?
It does not make a difference looks-wise if you use commercial or bio-identical hormones. They are structurally the same thing. From a health perspective, there is a difference, though, because dosing is more variable with bio-identical hormones, which are not currently approved by the FDA. They therefore have a higher risk of side effects—e.g., blood clots, heart attack, stroke, breast cancer, or gall bladder disease. Let me explain...

The term *bio-identical* is a misnomer—it should really be *bio-similar* or *bio-mimetic*. Real bio-identical hormones would be using hormones from another woman or human being. Both commercial and bio-identical hormones are plant-based, and neither are chemically identical to hormones made by human beings.

All hormones dock in receptor sites on cells and cause a reaction within the cells that results in the desired effect, i.e., increased production of collagen and elastin. Both conventional and bio-identical hormones dock on the same receptor sites and create the same downstream effect and desired outcome whether or not they are "natural" or "synthetic." And all plant-derived hormones (whether they come from a compounding pharmacy or a large FDA-regulated commercial pharmacy) require a chemical process to synthesize the final product, the active hormone, which is then put in a pill, cream, spray, or patch.

So both hormones work the same; the difference is in the dosing and delivery system. To make bio-identical hormones, a pharmacy purchases the active ingredients from the same manufacturer that sells to a commercial pharmaceutical company, and then "compounds" it into a usable form. Compounding is the creation of a particular pharmaceutical to "fit the individual" by custom-mixing these products according to a health care professional's order. The mix contains not only the active hormone, but other inactive ingredients that help hold a pill together, or give a cream, lotion, or gel its form and thickness so that it can be applied to the body.

Bio-identical hormones do not go through FDA testing, standards, and quality assurance. It is unknown whether these mixtures provide the appropriate levels of hormones needed in the body. It is also unknown whether the amount of drug delivered is consistent from pill to pill or each time a cream or gel is applied. And the hormones can be mixed with other ingredients that can increase or decrease absorption through the gut or skin. So you really don't know, day-to-day, batch-to-batch, what dose you are getting.

On the other hand, FDA-approved commercially available hormones must undergo a rigorous evaluation process, which scrutinizes everything about the drug to ensure its safety and effectiveness. From early testing, to the design and results of large clinical trials, to the severity of side effects, to the conditions under which the drug is manufactured, FDA-approved "commercial hormones" have met all federal standards for approval.

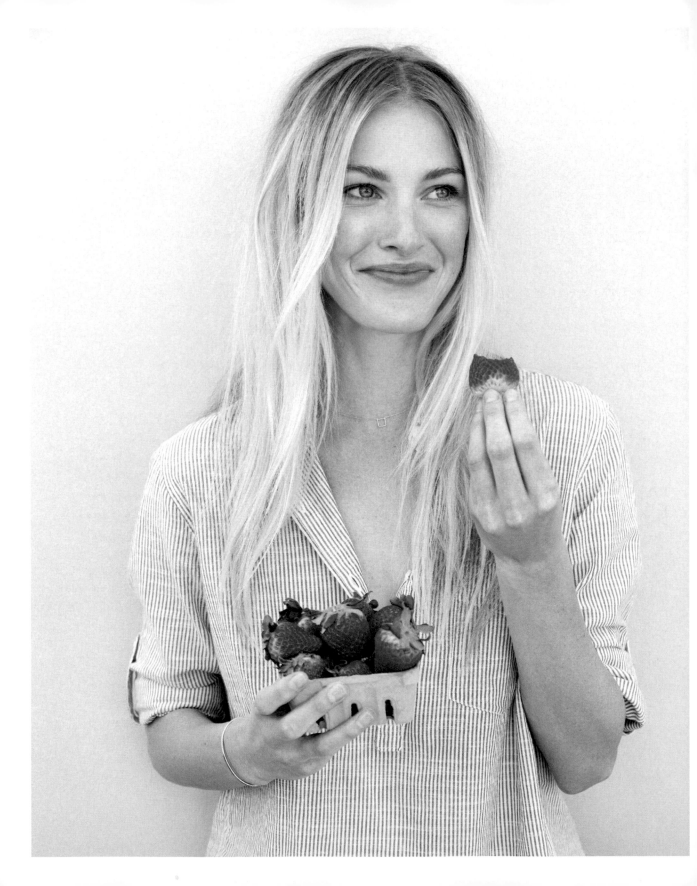

FDA-approved commercial drugs are sold by prescription only, and usually for effective relief of menopause symptoms, such as hot flashes and vaginal dryness. Whereas the end goal of bio-identical hormones is usually to reverse signs of aging, the FDA-approved use is not for "anti-aging" benefits, even though you may see skin or hair benefits with its use.

So, bottom line...commercial and "bio-identical" hormones work exactly the same. With commercial hormones we know the exact dose you are getting. With bio-identical hormones, we do not know the exact dose you are receiving. You may look better because of higher hormone levels, but you may also be at higher risk for side effects.

Can diet or exercise make a difference in how your hormones behave/affect the look of your skin and hair?
The old saying, "You are what you eat," still rings true. Diet, exercise, and toxin exposure all have a significant impact on how your hormones are produced and how they function.

To produce sex hormones (estrogen, progesterone, etc.) you need to ingest healthy fats and have some basic fat stores. Women who restrict the fat in their diet or have a too-low body fat percentage will stop menstruating because they literally don't have enough fat in their diets to produce hormones needed to menstruate.

To make good-quality hair cells you need adequate protein, zinc, biotin, and other vitamins and minerals. To produce nice plump skin cells you need vitamins like vitamin A, C, and E, and fatty acids.

Hormones and healthy functioning cells cannot be produced from a diet of diet soda and protein bars/shakes. Diets high in processed foods, sugar, flour, artificial sweeteners, and trans fats cause inflammation in the body by raising insulin levels and producing cytokines, which directly affect the production of other hormones and the body's ability to produce high-quality, functioning cells.

To look and feel radiant you must provide your body with the raw materials (essential nutrients) to make the best cells and hormones. Eating a colorful diet, specifically a variety of colorful vegetables, lean proteins, healthy fats, with small amounts of whole grains and fruit, and staying well hydrated with water are essential to looking younger than your age.

Exercise is very important for hormone production. Cortisol, our fight-or-flight hormone and the hormone that enables us to stay up when we need to pull an all-nighter, is an inflammatory, abdominal fat-storing, blood sugar-elevating hormone. Cortisol affects many other hormones in the body, specifically insulin, another fat-storing, inflammatory hormone. Moderate exercise for 30 to 90 minutes per day has been shown to lower cortisol levels. Lack of exercise or excessive exercise has been shown to increase cortisol levels. So in order to maintain proper hormone balance, moderate daily exercise is essential.

Exercise is also important for skin and hair appearance, growth, and cell turnover. Many people don't realize it, but our skin is our largest organ. It is capable of many duties: protection from the environment, thermoregulation (temperature control), and detoxification, to name a few. When you exercise and sweat, toxins are eliminated from your pores and dead cells are shed, which is great for maintaining cell health and improving skin appearance. Exercise increases blood flow to the skin. As the body heats up during exercise, our smallest vessels, called capillaries, dilate in an attempt to dissipate heat from the body surface so we don't overheat. These dilated capillaries not only let off heat, but can more adequately deliver oxygen and nutrients to the skin for cell growth and repair. These dilated vessels can also reabsorb toxins and shuttle them back through the bloodstream to the liver and kidneys to be removed from the system. So exercise really makes a difference in delivering nutrients and removing waste from the skin and hair follicles, improving their overall health and appearance.

What can a woman do at age forty, fifty, sixty, seventy to keep her hormones at optimum levels for health/ happiness/appearance?

The best way to have optimal hormone levels over forty is to start taking care of yourself in your twenties and thirties. But it is never too late to fix things. Most women blame their thyroid for the changes in weight, skin, and hair they see around menopause, but the thyroid gland usually is not the main problem. It is true that as we age there can be a decline in thyroid function, which affects its ability to produce hormones that regulate metabolism and other systems. By eating a diet rich in colorful vegetables, lean protein, and healthy fats you provide your thyroid with the essential nutrients—specifically minerals like iodine, selenium, iron, copper, and zinc—that are essential for proper thyroid function. Supporting your thyroid health is definitely important as you move through the decades. I recommend thyroid function screening with appropriate blood chemistry to make sure your thyroid levels are adequate.

But let's talk about the real players responsible for the hormonal shift and changes in weight and appearance that we see with menopause. Estrogen (the hormone that makes us look beautiful and youthful) is produced in the ovaries, adrenal glands, and adipose (fat) tissue. The high levels of sex hormones we see prior to menopause are essential for fertility. As you age, your ovaries make progressively less and less sex hormones until you reach menopause, when ovarian hormone production completely shuts down. Adrenal gland hormone production also goes through changes during menopause to further complicate the situation.

Once you reach menopause, although no longer capable of reproducing, the body still needs a baseline level of sex hormones for other bodily functions such as bone health, blood vessel health, etc. So if the ovaries, the main producer of sex hormones, are no longer producing estrogen, and the adrenal glands are going through

changes, too, where can the body produce baseline levels of circulating sex hormones?

Adipose tissue to the RESCUE! By increasing fat stores of course!

As the levels of sex hormones decline toward menopause, changes happen on cell surface receptors, causing cell membranes to become less sensitive to insulin, the hormone responsible for shuttling glucose (sugar) into our cells to be used for energy. This phenomenon is called *insulin resistance*, and causes sugar to be diverted into the liver, where it is converted into cholesterol, as well as adipose (fat) tissue, which is usually deposited in the abdomen. This is the cause of the "thickening of the waistline" commonly seen in menopausal women.

This shift in insulin sensitivity and fat deposition can get out of control and set off a vicious cycle: The more weight you gain, the worse the insulin resistance becomes, and the quicker you store more fat. This is why we see woman gain ten, twenty, thirty or more pounds when they reach menopause, even though they may be eating and exercising the same way as they did prior. Their behaviors haven't changed, but the system has changed, and it is now primed to store fat. Insulin is a very inflammatory hormone, so the increased levels not only cause weight gain, but the inflammation becomes visible in the skin and hair.

Although the body is happy with its new menopausal fat stores and its improved ability to make enough estrogen for cellular function, when you look in the mirror you are very unhappy with your new thick waist that puts you at risk for diabetes, high blood pressure, and cardiovascular disease. Furthermore, the excess circulating estrogen and sex hormones that we see from gaining too much weight after menopause (BMI above normal) puts you at higher risk for certain cancers, specifically hormone-sensitive cancers like breast cancer.

In all actuality, you don't need to gain any weight around menopause to make baseline levels of estrogen. At a normal BMI you have enough fat supply to adequately produce estrogen for bodily functions.

The key to looking well through the menopause transition and thereafter is to be proactive beforehand by maintaining a normal BMI and controlling your hormones through diet, exercise, and sleep. Once the sex hormone levels start dropping in perimenopause, you need to change your diet and limit the ingestion of foods that your body perceives as sugar and utilizes insulin to process. For example, a diet rich in fruit may have served you well prior to menopause, but fruit contains a lot of fructose (sugar) that needs insulin to be processed. With the drop in sex hormones and rise in insulin resistance, your ability to metabolize fruit has changed, and it will be more easily converted to fat.

Exercise may have the biggest effect of any measure you could take to improve your insulin sensitivity. Any type of physical activity has the potential to make your insulin work better, and combining aerobic activities with resistance/weight training appears to have the greatest effect. Aerobic activities burn more calories (and glucose) per session, but resistance training builds muscle, which is what burns glucose during exercise, so having more muscle is better long-term. The more muscle you have, the more calories you burn, increasing your resting metabolic rate. More intense and longer-duration activities can improve insulin sensitivity for up to 1 to 2 days, as muscle glycogen that was used during the exercise is being restored. To improve insulin sensitivity on a continuing basis, you should plan on exercising at least every other day, with daily workouts having an even more beneficial effect.

Controlling the insulin resistance we see around menopause is the key to maintaining a normal BMI well into your seventies and eighties, decreasing inflammation, and supporting healthy cell function, which makes you appear and feel younger and healthier. So, as you move through the decades, eat a low-glycemic, nutrient-dense diet, and commit to regular daily exercise and consistent restorative sleep.

Big Picture

How your skin looks and feels as it ages depends on many factors, including genetics. But somewhere on the spectrum between the occasional dab of cream here or there and a trip to the dermatologist, it's important to find your comfort zone. Nurturing and loving your skin—as opposed to fighting every change tooth and nail—will leave you looking and feeling most yourself, and most beautiful.

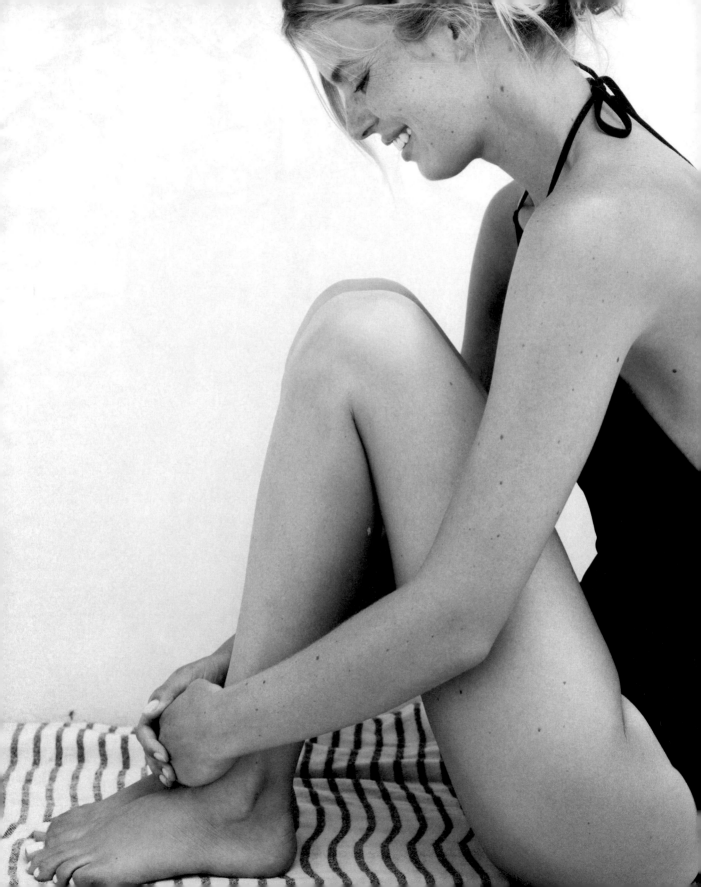

9.

Breakout-Prone Skin

Dealing with Acne

Having acne in high school is not fun. Having acne as an adult…still no fun. If you've struggled with acne at any point in your life, you'll already know that there is a huge number of approaches to treating it. The approach that works for you depends entirely on your specific skin and body type. And it's important to remember that there really is no do-this-and-you're-done cure for acne. Like any chronic condition, you have to keep treating it, even when you see absolutely no evidence that it's still an issue.

Acne is caused by bacteria that most people have on their skin; when skin is oily and/or irritated, bacteria have an easier time taking hold. Whether you're forty and suddenly breaking out after a lifetime of clear skin, or a teenager with prom dress anxiety, hormones are often a big part of the problem. Hormones help power an increase in oil production and a decreased resistance to infection and inflammation. The combination isn't pretty. The skin condition rosacea can also be a contributor to or cause of breakouts.

Keeping your skin as healthy and balanced as possible makes a serious difference; conventional treatments have long focused on fighting acne—note the violent word—with harsh chemicals and alcohol to dry it out. But since the main problem with acne is the inflammation it causes—and inflammation within the body feeds on itself, with a bit of inflammation causing a cascade of ever-larger flare-ups—a gentler, steadier approach is generally far more effective.

CREATE A CLEAN ROUTINE (AND STICK TO IT RELIGIOUSLY)

Your routine—day in, day out, no matter whether your skin is broken out or clear—is everything. We'll outline a plan if you don't have one in place already, but we can't stress enough the power of a routine that remains a constant. Gently cleansing and treating the entire face, both morning and evening, is the most critical step you can take. Problem skin can motivate people to constantly try new products—this is a mistake when dealing with acne, and can definitely exacerbate it. Any given product can take up to 6 weeks to work properly, so select what you want to try with care, then give it a real chance. When starting a new regimen, your skin can definitely go through a period of getting worse before it clears up; sometimes it's a question of breakouts just beneath the surface being drawn out more quickly, sometimes it's the skin simply reacting to change, sometimes it just *is*. Be as patient as you can. Also try adding only one new product at a time, so you'll be able to see which product is making what sort of difference.

If rosacea turns out to be the problem (you need to see a dermatologist to diagnose it, but breakouts combined with a tendency for the skin to flush after exercise, alcohol, etc., can be symptoms), an even gentler routine is required, with as few products as possible (see page 229 for suggestions). For anything but the mildest rosacea, it's a good idea to see a dermatologist.

DON'T FEAR OIL

"Oil free" is the cornerstone of conventional acne-treatment formulas, because people with oily skin naturally think that putting oil on their skin can compound their troubles. Mineral oil, to be sure, causes acne and should never be in any sort of oily-skin formula. But many natural oils have the opposite effect than you'd expect—they cleanse skin without the use of irritating detergents. (You know how oil and water don't mix? You need either detergent or oil to break up the extra sebum produced by acne-prone skin.) Harsh detergents can actually cause excessive oiliness—the skin reacts to being stripped of all its oil by producing more. In addition, a number of natural essential oils actually help to treat acne and oiliness. So "oil free" isn't the useful filter it appears to be in treating acne.

Ingredients That Help

Among those of us at GOOP who are more familiar with breakouts than we'd like to be, we've personally tried (in addition to researched) a lot of potential ingredient heroes. Here's what actually works:

- **Salicylic acid:** Otherwise known as aspirin, otherwise known as willow bark, salicylic acid is the gold standard in acne treatment: It's a powerful anti-inflammatory, a gentle but extremely thorough exfoliant, and antibacterial as well. (The percentage of salicylic acid in a given product doesn't really indicate how strong it is, because how the pH is balanced affects the strength much more than percentages, so higher is not necessarily stronger, and lower is not necessarily gentler.)

- **Retinols:** Derivatives of vitamin A, retinols and retinoic acid are both anti-acne and anti-aging. Retinols help the skin function better in many ways, from rebuilding collagen to increasing cell turnover. The degree of intensity in retinols varies dramatically: There's retinol as it appears in cosmetic products, then the retinoic acid of prescription products like Retin-A and Tazorac, all the way up to a related form of the compound that's the active ingredient in the drug Accutane, which is often used as a last resort for acne sufferers (more on page 213). (Again, keep in mind that retinols and retinoic acid increase sun sensitivity, so apply at night, and/or use sunblock along with treatment.)

- **Tea tree oil:** Grown in Australia, tea tree, or melaleuca, oil is antibacterial and antimicrobial, and has been shown to help treat acne and other skin infections. Infused into washes and treatments, or used pure as a spot treatment, it can be incredibly effective.

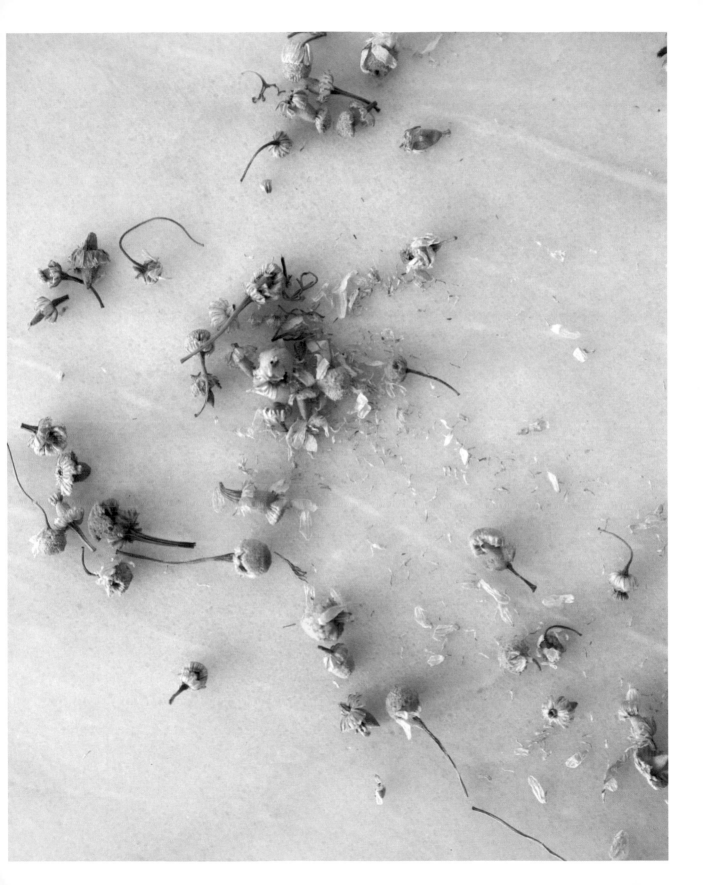

- **Lavender oil:** Antibacterial, antiviral, and antifungal, lavender oil is controversial as a treatment for acne because it can increase redness in the skin, and, depending on the concentration, can cause irritation. That said, many people use it against breakouts with great success. If your skin is sensitive, lavender is probably not the best treatment for acne; if your skin rarely reacts, it might be worth a try.
- **Clay:** Natural clays can be amazing as washes, masks, exfoliants, or spot treatments, drawing out infection without irritating skin. Clay can also give foundation and moisturizer formulas a more matte finish. Some clays are more drying than others; finding your skin's ideal formula/ideal clay definitely involves a little trial and error, but if you find a clay too drying, the easy and obvious solution does really work: Leave it on for less time.

goop PICKS

May Lindstrom's The Problem Solver mask is life changing. An anti-inflammatory miracle worker, it soothes and treats acne…like nothing else.

Drunk Elephant's Vitamin C serum is made with skin-loving vitamin C, E, and ferulic acid, and is less drying and more potent than conventional versions of the same thing.

- **Benzoyl peroxide:** A powerful antibacterial agent that gets into your pores and kills the acne bacteria there, benzoyl peroxide is also surprisingly relatively clean, with a 3 hazard rating from EWG. (A low hazard is 1, a high hazard is 10.) Its downside: It can cause dryness and irritation. Always start with the

goop PICKS

Herbivore's Blue Tansy line is full of azulene—in the oil, mask, and toner—as gentle as it is effective as it is beautiful to look at.

lowest concentration of benzoyl peroxide to avoid those side effects as much as possible; stay with a particular concentration for at least 3 weeks before you decide it's not working for your skin. Using too much, too soon is a common mistake.

- **Azulene:** A gorgeously blue anti-inflammatory compound derived from chamomile, azulene helps take down redness and irritation from acne (or from harsh acne treatments), so skin stays in balance and is less likely to break out.
- **Vitamin C:** Vitamin C's powerful free-radical-scavenging effects work well to treat acne. It can be used topically as well as taken orally, with the best strategy being a combination of both forms. Oral vitamin C is especially effective, as it bolsters the immune response in general and soothes irritation from free radical formation, as well as preventing it. Take it daily as part of your acne regimen. Topical vitamin C is one of those products practically every skin type should use—for acne, it helps bring down inflammation, kills some of the bacteria, loosens clogged pores, evens skin tone, and helps eradicate the red spots left after acne has cleared. You can use it any time, but it's best applied in the morning, as it also has a sun-protective effect.

Diet Changes That Make a Difference

As it does with any infection, sugar feeds acne bacteria. It also increases inflammation, exacerbating breakouts. Low glycemic diets have been shown in studies to help treat acne (although treating acne with only diet changes is rarely completely successful). Other studies have shown a weak link between dairy (specifically skim milk, which has the highest sugar content) and acne. Chocolate, long considered to cause acne, has never been proven to be a factor. Greasy food, also long blamed for causing breakouts, also appears to have little effect on skin. Obviously, if you notice a particular food exacerbates your breakouts, avoid it. Doing the beauty detox in Chapter 1 can help you figure out which foods are causing you problems; anyone with acne problems (or worried about aging, for that matter) should cut down on sugar and high-glycemic carbs.

Elements of an Ideal Routine

Here's how to put your skin steps together:

- **Cleanse:** A gentle, non-drying cream, oil, foam, gel, or bar (whatever formula appeals/works for you) used every evening to take everything off and prepare the skin for treatment is essential. Many people like to cleanse in the morning as well; it isn't absolutely necessary, as your skin isn't dirty at that point, but since oil/bacteria/dead skin cells may have accumulated overnight, it's a good idea. The same holds true post-workout.
- **Exfoliate:** Exfoliation is key for preventing breakouts. You can exfoliate at different points in your

routine, depending on personal preference, and at different intensities, depending on your skin's sensitivity. In any case, the goal is to sweep away grime, dead skin cells, makeup, and anything else clinging to your skin so that (a) the gunk won't get stuck in pores, and (b) treatment products are allowed to penetrate more easily. Balance and perspective is important, however. Exfoliate too much and you cause irritation, which can trigger more breakouts. Just like you wouldn't want to use retinols, alpha hydroxy acids, and a daily face scrub together all at once, and you wouldn't want to use a weekly-use product daily, be aware of how much exfoliation you're doing, and how often. Too much of a good thing can really wreak havoc, so go easy.

Exfoliation comes in two basic forms: physical (a washcloth, a brush, grains, seeds, beads), or chemical (alpha or beta hydroxy acids, or enzymes derived from plants like papaya). Both are great, and you can even use them (carefully) in combination.

A sonic brush is one of the gentlest and most effective ways to exfoliate. A good one is an investment (they're around $100, depending on the model—we like Clarisonic), but one that quickly pays for itself: Use it daily with your favorite cleanser and your pores will be clean and your treatment products will really sink in. In short, sonic brushes make a huge difference for many acne sufferers (they're also good for anti-aging). Non-sonic brushes tend to be less gentle on skin, or, if they're gentle enough, not terribly effective. If you're doing a brush, make it a sonic one.

Scrubs like sugar, apricot kernel, or even crushed marble can work well, too. Super-intense scrubs can be harsh and micro-tear skin, though so use the gentlest version you can.

Chemical exfoliants are present in cleansers, masks, toners, and treatments to varying degrees and can be mild or extremely powerful, depending on the concentrations of acids or enzymes within a given formula, and depending on how long you leave the product on. Salicylic acid is particularly useful for breakouts, as it disinfects and soothes inflammation as it gets rid of dead skin cells.

- **Tone** (if you love it): Some people like to add a toner in between cleansing and treatment; a mild one can layer in additional breakout-discouraging ingredients, along with an extra bit of exfoliation. They're definitely not necessary for everyone; it depends on your skin. (If you have rosacea, see page 230 for an expert esthetician's recommendation on toner.)

- **Treat** (all over): To truly fight acne, you need an all-over-the-face product that kills bacteria, tones down inflammation, and de-gunks pores. The best are made with salicylic acid, which does all of the above. It's important to continue treating the entire face even once your skin has cleared. This is probably the hardest step to follow, but killing bacteria, mild exfoliation, and free radical defense is a constant if invisible necessity. Many products have moisturizers built into the formula; properly hydrated skin is more resilient and less vulnerable to acne.

- **Spot-treat** (only when you need it): Exfoliating/soothing/antibacterial treatments can reduce the severity of and the length of time you have to suffer with a breakout. Confine spot treatments to the area in question—as a general rule, spot treatments are more drying and irritating than any other category, so you should limit where you apply product. We always hear that myth that toothpaste is a great spot treatment, and while it has slight drying and anti-inflammatory properties, it's an

okay spot treatment at best. Clay, salicylic acid, or benzoyl peroxide are far superior solutions.

- **Sun protection:** The breakout-prone are understandably wary of sunscreens—conventional formulas are among the most skin-irritating in the entire beauty space. Physical sunblock, made solely of minerals, has the opposite effect on acne skin: It soothes. Physical sunblock is harder to rub in (see why in Chapter 4), but it is a small price to pay for seriously reduced breakouts. That said, a given sunblock might be better or worse for your individual skin, so experiment with formulas.

- **Masks:** Masks can kick-start a new acne treatment routine, and they can supercharge your efforts when you need it most. Look for exfoliating masks to sweep away dead skin cells and leave your skin refreshed and glowing, soothing ones to tone down redness and overreaction, antioxidant masks to stem and prevent free radical damage, or clays to disinfect, soothe, and detox.

- **At-home extractions:** Most dermatologists and aestheticians will tell you not to attempt at-home extractions. Careful extraction with a metal extraction tool (you can get them at beauty supply stores) can work, but it usually takes practice. Less invasive, over-the-counter pore strips can clear some blackheads and general congestion.

goop PICKS

Coola Mineral Face SPF 30 blends into skin as if it were chemical or nano, which it is not, and it soothes and protects skin, never causing breakouts.

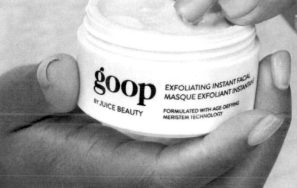

GOOP PICKS

The GOOP by Juice Beauty Instant Facial is made with papaya and other enzymes to gently but super-effectively sweep away dead skin cells and dirt. As we designed the product, GP's directive was always: "It needs to just take everything off." The result is a product that leaves your skin perfectly and evenly exfoliated for maximum glow.

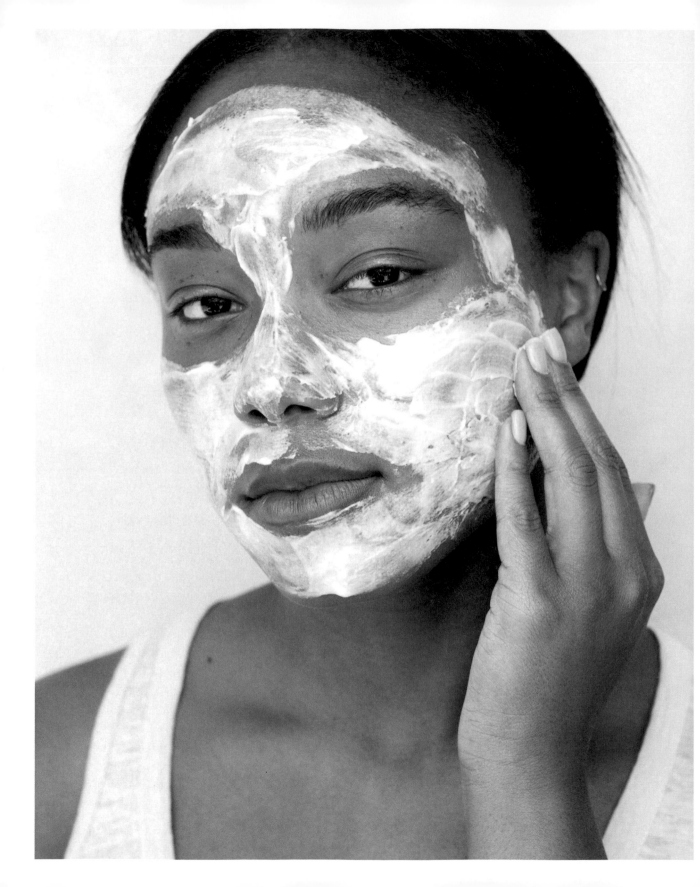

Beyond DIY

If over-the-counter regimens and diet changes aren't working, don't put off seeking expert help for potentially more powerful interventions. Living with serious breakouts can really damage your self-esteem, and treating the problem can be easier than you think.

Cystic acne—large, red, and painful breakouts that are deep in your skin—should never be ignored; it can leave lifelong scars on your face, not to mention your psyche. Cystic acne can be complex to treat, but most people do find the right solution eventually, whether it's Ayurveda or Accutane.

SEE AN AYURVEDIC DOCTOR

The Ayurvedic approach to treating acne (and any other disease) seeks to balance the *doshas*. There are three—Vata, Pitta, and Kapha—each an aspect of human mind/body tendencies. In the case of acne, imbalances in all three doshas affecting digestion, toxin load within the body, and sebum (oil) production cause there to be more acne bacteria on the skin than there would be otherwise. If you only treat acne as a surface issue, even with the help of oral antibiotics, you never really cure the underlying problem, which is why it continues. Ayurvedic medicine treats the imbalances with diet, along with teas made with particular herbs; it can take months, but the benefits do appear, and extend beyond your skin to better health overall. As with any other acne treatment, once your skin is clear, continue with the regimen—the diet and tea, along with good basic skincare—to maintain it. (For more from an Ayurvedic doctor, see page 227.)

SEE A DERMATOLOGIST

People spend serious money on product after product, thinking the dermatologist is going to be expensive; the reality is, a lot of medical acne treatment is covered by insurance, and they have an awful lot of super-effective solutions that work for many people:

- **Blue and red light treatments:** Light therapy can be extremely effective at killing bacteria, helping control oil, and decreasing inflammation; for some patients, it completely resolves their breakouts. There are over-the-counter blue and red light treatments as well. As with other at-home light devices, you can often achieve similar results if you're incredibly dedicated—they require many more treatments because they're much less powerful.

- **Prescription retinoic acid:** Retinoic acid—a.k.a. Retin-A, Differin, and Tazorac—is a prescription-strength form of vitamin A, and it's one of the best acne treatments there is (it's also an incredible anti-aging topical treatment). Retinols in over-the-counter products work in a similar way, but are generally less powerful. Retinoic acid increases cell turnover, helps the skin better resist infection, decreases inflammation, stimulates collagen production, and essentially gets your skin all-over functioning better. Beyond acne and aging, it's even used to treat certain kinds of skin cancer. All retinoids cause sun sensitivity, so you definitely need to wear sunblock in conjunction with treatment, and retinoids should be applied only at night. Most cause some degree of dryness and/or peeling; the best way to deal with it is to ramp up slowly. Put the cream on for only 5 minutes before washing it off the first few times you use it, build up to using it every other day, and when it's finally not causing any peeling, try once a day. Prescription retinoids are definitely not clean, it should be noted. Some clean cosmetics companies make products with retinol in them; retinol has some, but not all, of the benefits of actual retinoids.

- **Accutane:** Accutane is a controversial, powerful drug with major side effects that nonetheless changes the lives of severe cystic acne sufferers. It can cause birth defects, so patients are required to sign documents indicating they won't become pregnant during the course of treatment. It's not an option to be considered lightly, but for some people, it's truly life changing. (More on page 213.)

- **Cortisone injections:** If you've got the biggest interview of your life/you're getting married/going on TV/something major that just won't work with a breakout, make an emergency appointment with the dermatologist for a cortisone injection: While it's not cost- or health-effective to do on a regular basis, it solves your problem—usually within 24 to 48 hours—when you really need it solved.

- **Hormone-balancing prescriptions:** Because your hormones power much of the overproduction of oil that occurs in your skin, not to mention some of the vulnerability to infection, various forms of the contraceptive pill are often prescribed to help clear acne—and the treatment works for many people. The drug spironolactone is also used off-label to tamp down testosterone in the blood, treating acne in some patients.

- **Topical and oral antibiotics:** Given the amount of antibiotic resistance in this country and the damaging effects, especially to your gut, that antibiotics can have, long-term antibiotic use for acne—and some dermatologists readily prescribe it—is rarely the best course of action.

SEE AN AESTHETICIAN

A talented aesthetician can transform your skin. A bad one can make things worse, emotionally and otherwise. If you leave a facial feeling ashamed of your skin, never go back. A great aesthetician will treat your skin *and* leave you feeling attractive and hopeful.

- **Facials:** A facial here or there is unlikely to make a difference in any sort of acne, but a regular routine of them—depending on the aesthetician—can make a huge one. Every aesthetician's process is different; get recommendations from friends and even consider asking for before-and-after photos of clients with acne. Definitely choose facials designed to treat acne: You need products and processes focused on healing your particular complexion.

- **Extractions:** A good aesthetician can perform extractions in a way that minimizes potential damage to the skin and eases a breakout. Too much or a poorly performed extraction can seriously irritate skin, causing more problems.

- **Microdermabrasion and peels:** Microdermabrasion and in-salon peels exfoliate skin, usually to a more dramatic degree than over-the-counter peels or scrubs—but not always. If you're regularly using retinols or alpha hydroxy acid preparations, along with a sonic skin brush or other consistent exfoliation, the cost of microdermabrasion or salon-administered peels may not be worth the benefit. That said, if you're not a big at-home exfoliator, regular microdermabrasion or a series of peels can have a big impact on your skin. As with all exfoliation, too much can cause irritation and thus more breakouts, so balance is key.

Ask a Dermatologist

Dr. Karyn Grossman is an internationally renowned, board-certified cosmetic dermatologist with offices in New York and Beverly Hills. Trained at Harvard Medical School, she's a leader in the field, helping to develop new techniques and technologies. She's known for a cautious, careful, innovative approach to everything from aging to acne.

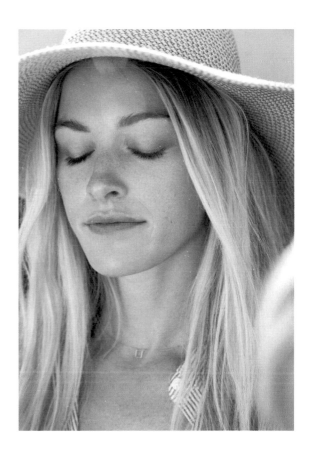

Dr. Karyn Grossman
ON GETTING CLEAR SKIN

What are the best tools at the dermatologist's disposal to treat acne?

Prescription medications, facials, extractions, peels, and lasers. Depending upon the extent and type of the acne, the amount of scarring someone is getting, and many other things, we use some or a combination of these tools to most effectively treat a patient. Unfortunately, one product does not work for everyone. So, while dermatologists make educated decisions regarding a patient's particular regimen, it may need to be adjusted. What works for a while may wane in its response, and medications may need to be changed.

Topical medications fall into several categories:

- Topical antibiotics like erythromycin, clindamycin, and metronidazole are most effective on red or inflammatory acne. These work to reduce the bacteria on the skin to decrease acne.
- A new "anti-mite" medication, topical ivermectin, has also been recently shown to improve some forms of acne.
- Retinoids—Retin-A, Differin, Tazorac—also help with acne (and aging for adults). They work by normalizing the superficial layer of the skin and decrease clogging of the pores, blackheads, whiteheads, and cysts.
- Alpha and beta hydroxy acids also work by normalizing the growth of the surface of the skin and help with comedones and pores, but are less effective with inflammatory acne.
- Benzoyl peroxide helps to decrease the bacteria on the skin, as well as to unclog pores, but can be quite drying and can "bleach" patients' clothes, towels, and bed linens.
- Azelex/Finacea works as an antibacterial, helps with clogging, and may also help to decrease pigmentation in the skin from acne.
- Aczone works predominately as an anti-inflammatory.

- Sulfur-based medications work somewhat as an anti-inflammatory, but also tend to significantly dry out the skin, so are used these days more as spot treatments.

The most common **oral medications** prescribed for acne are antibiotics with tetracyclines—tetracycline, doxycy-cline, and minocycline—as the main agents prescribed. These work on reducing the amount of bacteria in the skin, but are also anti-inflammatory. Often for back/chest acne, patients will need oral antibiotics to get the acne under control. Oral antibiotics tend to be very effective with even severe acne, but they should always be prescribed with topical medications, so that a patient can get off the oral medications sooner, then maintain the skin with topi-cal medications. This helps to prevent the development of antibiotic resistance and other possible side effects from long-term antibiotic usage.

Extractions are an important part of treatment, since acne medications work best on preventing acne from coming—and less well on treating the acne that is there. To get someone's existing breakouts to clear more quickly, extractions are very important. Also, leaving blackheads and hard cysts under the skin encourages inflammatory acne to start in that spot in the future, so extractions are useful in fighting that tendency.

Different lasers can be used to help acne as well: IPL (intense pulse light) helps treat red inflammatory lesions, as well as the red and brown spots that can remain after a pimple resolves. The heat may also help to destroy some of the bacteria in the skin. IPL with a suction device is called Isolaz: The suction can help to draw out some of the acne lesions, then the IPL light helps with the red and brown spots. IPL can also be combined with extractions for signifi-cant improvement in the skin. Levulan, a topical medication, can also be used with IPL or blue or red light: The Levulan-

and-light combo helps to decrease the oil gland production and can dramatically improve acne. Blue light alone, without Levulan, can also be helpful in reducing bacteria.

Heat-generating lasers can be helpful for some patients, but generally are less effective and reliable compared to other treatments. The mechanism of action in these is also not well understood.

How severe a breakout problem warrants a trip to the dermatologist?
Any breakout that is not going away with over-the-counter topicals after 2 months, is leaving red or indented scars, or is getting worse over time should send you quickly to your dermatologist. While acne is, for many, temporary (but can also last for many years), scars last a lifetime and can only be partially treated to decrease their appearance later on. Also, occasionally acne that was well controlled suddenly gets worse. This can often be a sign of a staph infection that has developed in the acne. Any acne that is painful, tender, or deep under the skin also warrants a trip to the dermatologist. Also, back acne and chest acne are often very difficult to treat and are more likely to need prescription medications.

How long should a person try an OTC regimen in order to determine whether it works for his/her skin?
Topical medications, whether over-the-counter or prescription, take longer than oral medications to work. Many patients come in after trying a regimen for only 1 to 2 weeks, complaining their skin has not improved. In reality, it takes 4 to 6 weeks to really start to see a change in the skin from topicals. In order to truly evaluate these products, you must use them consistently to begin to see improvement in the skin. (One or 2 times a week is not consistent; they need to be used daily, over time.) It can take closer to 3 months to see the total benefit from a new regimen.

Very important: When using any topical medications—use them daily, on all the areas prone to acne. Do not just spot-treat the pimples you see. Topical skincare is designed to help prevent acne from developing, so you need to treat all of your skin. If you wait until you already have the acne and spot treat, you are doing yourself a disservice.

What are the differences between teen acne and adult acne? Should they be treated differently?

Teen acne is almost always hormone modulated. During puberty, hormone levels skyrocket and cause changes in the skin that lead to the development of acne. In girls, typically, the beginning of acne correlates roughly to their menstrual cycle starting in a year or so. This hormonally influenced acne can continue into the early twenties for many individuals.

Adult acne can also be hormonally driven. Women will often notice a correlation between their menstrual cycle and acne flares. Acne can develop with their period, with ovulation, just after their period, etc. Women who suffer from polycystic ovarian syndrome can get hard-to-control acne, also due to persistent elevated levels of hormones. And, just as during puberty, skin tends to act up for women as they head through the long perimenopausal stage. Typically this acne tends to be located away from the more traditional T-zone area and affects the lower face, jawline, and neck.

Bacteria on the skin and in follicles can also aggravate acne in both teenage years and adult years. So adding a topical medication that decreases bacteria on the skin for both of these ages can be helpful. However, we often choose a different vehicle, or delivery system, for people in different age groups. Since younger patients tend to be more oily, I like to prescribe solutions and some types of gels that contain alcohol, which is helpful for those with more oily skin. For adults suffering with acne, I tend to prescribe lotions and creams that are often alcohol-free, causing less dryness.

Inflammation is a key factor in both adolescent and adult acne. People with just blackheads and whiteheads have less inflammation in their skin, but this is relatively unusual. Certain types of "acne"—rosacea and perioral dermatitis—have significant amounts of inflammation. Topical products with anti-inflammatory properties can have a significant benefit. Interestingly, low-dose antibiotics have also been shown to have more anti-inflammatory properties than antibacterial properties. It's important to note that certain oral medications should not be used in children under age 12—such as tetracyclines—as they affect tooth development.

How do you feel about Accutane?

Accutane is an entire discussion in and of itself—it's highly effective and something I have taken twice myself. However, it is controversial because of some of the legal issues surrounding its usage. There are some definite known significant side effects of Accutane—elevation of cholesterol, dryness, and photosensitivity. These can and do happen to many patients and I consider them to be part of the process of the treatment. Dryness and photosensitivity can usually be moderated by topicals and SPF. Some patients have some elevation of cholesterol, which reverses when stopping the meds. These side effects are also dose-related—so lower-dose therapy will cause less of them than higher-dose therapy. Occasionally, people have issues with their other liver enzymes, especially if they drink alcohol. This can prove to be more serious, and usually will resolve if the patient moderates the behavior. If it is not related to alcohol consumption, either the dose needs to be adjusted lower, or the medication may need to be stopped.

There are a host of other rare side effects, which have been reported, documented, and are true, but highly uncommon. These include things such as liver problems and muscle issues. However, pregnancy is a big issue during Accutane use: Babies born to moms who take Accutane during pregnancy can have some very specific birth defects. The iPledge program was developed to deal with this, plus each pill has a red X over a pregnant woman on it. Women need to have pregnancy tests each month in order to receive the medication. There have also been some reports, claims, and lawsuits regarding depression, suicide, and irritable bowel syndrome. I give all patients the American Academy of Dermatology position paper on this, so they can make up their own minds on what to do.

With all that said, Accutane is still a great drug for decreasing acne and giving patients a long-term remission from it. There is nothing else out there that can decrease acne for 8 to 10 years. So in my office, it definitely has its place—as long as we have a lot of paperwork to go with it.

What treatments are available for people who break out severely while pregnant?
Acne during pregnancy can be difficult and frustrating for many patients. Obviously, topicals are going to be the mainstay of treatment—there are really no drugs for acne that have been studied in pregnant woman and carry no risk. Again, I balance risk with benefit. The most commonly prescribed medications during pregnancy are topical clindamycin and erythromycin. These can be helpful for many women. Occasionally I will add light peels. I tend to use short-contact, low-strength TCA peels, as these have minimal risk of absorption. Extractions can also be very helpful during this time. Occasionally, patients will even need large acne cysts injected. When prescribing any medications during pregnancy, though, I always have patients check with their OBs first—as they have the final say.

What's the single most effective at-home step a mild acne sufferer can take to treat the problem?
Good skincare every day is definitely the most effective and best way to handle acne. Using topical treatments daily—even OTC—is the best mechanism we have to prevent your skin from breaking out. Also, don't pick the acne you have—

it can increase the problem and cause scarring. In addition, pay attention to behaviors like leaning your face on your hands, the hair care products you're using, and anything else that you may be doing that touches/leans on your face. Even your cellphone can contribute to acne flares.

Are there any alternative therapies that you've seen work for people?
Alternative therapies for acne are always difficult to evaluate, usually because most patients are using traditional therapies as well. However, anything that seems to be working and doesn't cause harm is something that in my mind may be reasonable. I have seen patients happy with acupuncture, special diets, and meditation. However, I often see a flare in acne from "cleanses" and "juicing"—I suspect from the stress that it puts on the body.

Ask a Hormone Expert

Deciding whether or not a hormonal treatment—which comes with its own set of advantages and disadvantages—is right for you can be tough. We went back to Dr. Laura Lefkowitz to help make the decision a bit easier. (And while we had her on hand, we asked her another skin question we've always wondered about.)

Dr. Laura Lefkowitz
ON HORMONES AND YOUR SKIN

Do you have opinions on the use of the pill or topical, off-label hormone-affecting treatments like spironolactone for hormonal acne?
I am a huge proponent of using both oral contraceptives and spironolactone for treating hormonal acne. In my late teens I suffered from painful cystic acne. I tried

everything—topical and oral antibiotics, topical ointments, steroid injections, topical retinoids—and nothing worked. When I finally started oral contraceptives, after 3 months my skin cleared up and I was forever converted.

Androgens, defined as "male sex hormones," e.g., testosterone and DHEA, are present in both men and women. They cause hormonal acne flare-ups by over-stimulating the sebaceous glands (oil-producing glands), and alter skin cells that shed on the surface to become abnormally sticky, accumulate, and clog up the hair follicles in the skin. In conjunction with an overgrowth of acne-causing bacterium, *Propionibacterium acnes*, you get skin inflammation and the appearance of acne.

Androgens are also responsible for thinning or balding hair. Many women with polycystic ovarian syndrome (PCOS) have an androgen imbalance and present with hair growth on the face, chest, back, and stomach. Hormonal testing is recommended for females who have acne accompanied by excess facial or body hair, deepening voice, or irregular or infrequent menstrual periods to rule out PCOS. The majority of women with hormonal acne who do not have PCOS have normal androgen levels, but their androgen receptors are more sensitive than normal, so acne develops.

The FDA has approved the use of combination oral contraceptives, which contain estrogen and progesterone, to effectively clear acne in women either when used alone or in conjunction with an anti-androgen medication, such as spironolactone.

The active hormones in oral contraceptives work together to alter the levels and activity of the androgen hormones that trigger the acne. In some cases, the addition of estrogen and progesterone is not enough and you must augment treatment with anti-androgen medications, such as spironolactone.

Spironolactone works by lowering the overall level of androgen production and the conversion of testosterone into DHEA, the hormone responsible for male-pattern scalp hair thinning, body hair growth, and acne. Spironolactone is very effective in reducing body hair growth and improving acne for young women, especially in conjunction with oral contraceptive pills. Most women taking spironolactone will see positive results; however, it can take up to 6 months to see an improvement in symptoms (scalp hair regrowth, decrease in facial hair, improvements in acne, etc.).

Why is skin more sensitive (not just to pain, but more reactive) during your period?
After you ovulate (mid-cycle, around day 12 to 16 in a typical 28- to 30-day cycle), if you do not become pregnant, estrogen hormone levels start to drop in preparation for menstruation (we steadily lose the beautiful-skin hormone during the second half of our menstrual cycle). Progesterone levels briefly increase after ovulation, which can make skin oilier and more spot-prone. Progesterone stimulates the production of sebum (oil). As progesterone levels rise, the skin swells and squeezes pores shut, leading to clogged pores and breakouts. After the brief increase in progesterone after ovulation, its levels dramatically fall right before your period begins. So by the time you are menstruating, you have very little female hormone (estrogen and progesterone) production that is responsible for making your skin calm and beautiful.

On the other hand, the androgens levels (testosterone and DHEA) build up toward menstruation, which also create sebum and acne and further aggravate the problem.

On the first day of your period, the body produces a hormone called prostaglandin that causes contractions in the uterus to shed the lining of your uterus, which causes the actual "bleeding." Prostaglandins increase pain sensitivity, so your skin will be more tender and spots will feel more painful than usual. Prostaglandin also makes blood vessels constrict, so you may flush more easily and have a mottled appearance. With less soothing estrogen in your blood, skin will feel drier and blotchier, and lines or wrinkles will appear more obvious.

Makeup for Clear-Looking Skin

Lots of makeup layered on top of a breakout usually looks like…lots of makeup layered on top of a breakout. It's a catch-22; in trying to minimize a problem area, you can end up highlighting it. The trick is to do as little as possible: Many people with oily skin will swathe the whole face in foundation, even though the breakout covers only a small portion of the face. Instead, leave the clear spots on your skin as makeup-free as you can—there's nothing prettier than bare skin, and it'll distract the eye from the less alluring area. If you prefer some kind of coverage, keep it light: tinted moisturizer, a sheer foundation, or BB cream applied sparingly.

Conceal the breakout with concealer. This sounds obvious, but many people attempt concealing with layers of foundation—concealer is 100 percent more effective, it stays where you put it, and you need much less of it. Just the way foundation is not much use in concealing acne, neither is sheer, liquid concealer. A super-thick, drier formula, applied with a small brush, is so much better at concealing that it'll actually save time, along with making you look better. Dab the concealer on with the brush, covering *only* the area you want to conceal—not on the perfectly fine skin surrounding the breakout (the brush gives you the precision). Gently pat to blend—if you rub to blend, you'll move the concealer off of what you're trying to conceal and onto skin that doesn't need it, and then you'll have to reapply, and you'll end up with too much concealer on your face. Instead, pat softly: It will seem like it isn't going to blend, and then suddenly, it'll be blended perfectly.

Oil control: Some people love powder, some people love under-makeup mattifiers; both are fine unless they irritate your particular skin. Oil-absorbing sheets easily fix shininess if you're not a powder or mattifier person; keep them in your makeup bag and use as needed. Powder users should choose loose translucent powder applied with a big fluffy brush whenever possible—dust it on when you're finished with your makeup—and a compact powder with a brush (not a sponge, which can leave too much product on skin) for on the go.

Powder blush is definitely preferable to creams or gels if the skin on your cheeks is at all oily or broken out. The powder, just like translucent face powder, reduces shine, not to mention the color lasts significantly longer throughout the day.

Beyond concealer and shine control, makeup for acne-prone skin is like makeup for any other skin. To be sure, a dramatic eye or lip can distract a bit, so your breakout stands out less (remember, though, it stands out to you about a billion times more than it does to anyone else).

Don't Obsess (Because No One Else Is)

Regardless of whether or not you're too damn old for acne: Once you do whatever makeup you're going to do, as you go through the day, think often about the unblemished parts of your skin and how they are shining through. And think about how what you say, the way you smile, and your overall energy is what makes an impression on people. Feeling bad about a breakout can deeply impact your interactions with people if you let that feeling take over. A temporary detail on the surface of your skin in no way defines you; at the same time, treating that temporary detail is absolutely worth it.

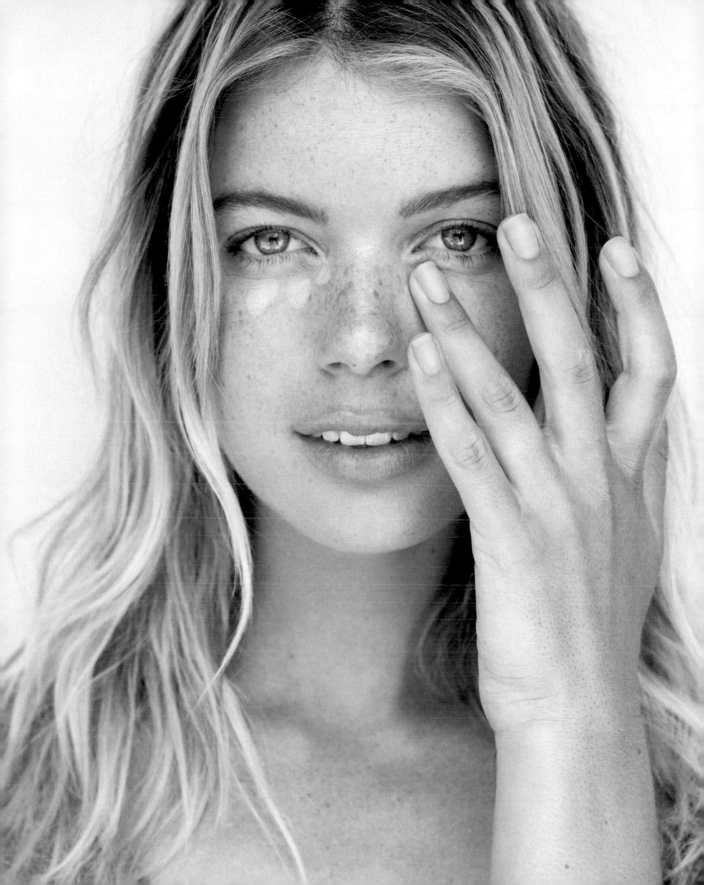

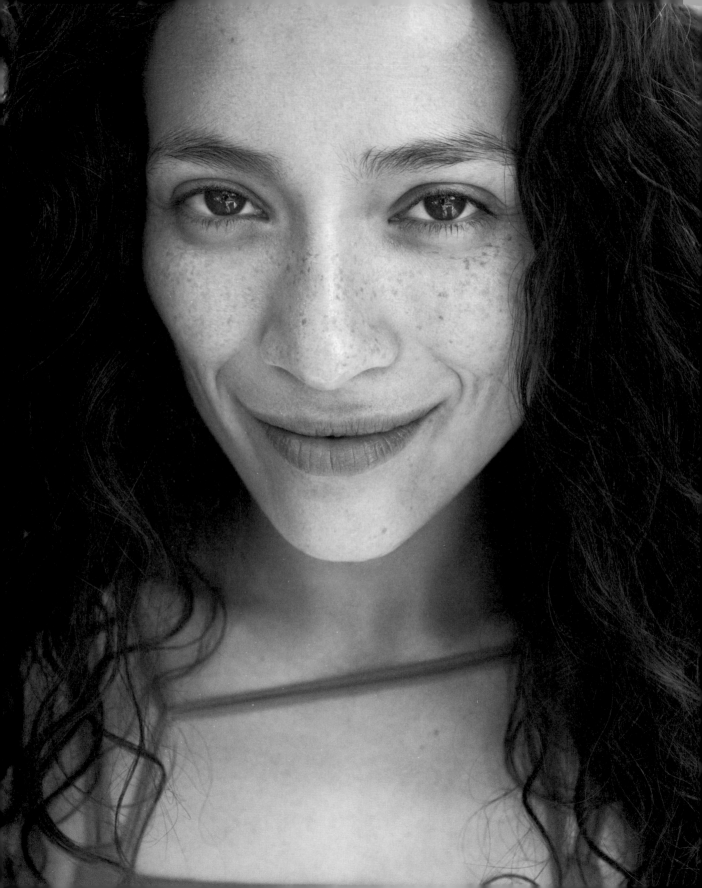

10.

Dry and Sensitive Skin

Keeping Moisture In

A major component of feeling beautiful is feeling comfortable in your skin. Treating dry or reactive skin so it just feels...*normal* can make a world of difference in terms of your entire outlook. Dry or irritated skin can be caused by a laundry list of potential factors—extreme weather, contact allergens, airborne allergens, diabetes, psoriasis, eczema, rosacea, thyroid malfunction, drug interactions, vitamin deficiencies... you name it. Zeroing in on the causes is critical in returning your skin to a happy, healthy state.

Your skin is full of moisture—we're more than 70 percent water, after all. The challenge is retaining that moisture. The skin is also full of oils and lipids designed to keep moisture within, but sun exposure, aging, temperature extremes, and outside aggressors (alcohol, detergents, or other chemicals) can dry out your skin. Moisturizers of all types—from oils to serums to gel-creams—form a barrier that keeps moisture from escaping, in different degrees. Irritation also interferes with the skin's barrier function, which is why dryness and skin sensitivity can be so intertwined; one can definitely lead to the other. Inflammation naturally builds on itself, so ignoring the problem or leaving your skin alone is not the solution.

Whether you suffer seasonally or constantly, and whether the problem is severe or mild, arriving at the ultimate regimen that keeps your skin supple, dewy, and comfortable is an achievable goal for most people. It does involve experimentation and tinkering with your routine, however; no one solution works for everyone, especially because the causes of dryness and irritation are so varied.

Behavioral changes can absolutely make a difference—for instance, limiting the time you spend in the shower or bath can help since water, especially hot water, is counterintuitively drying. Dietary changes like consuming more healthy oils can also work wonders. Exercise is amazing for increasing circulation, which can help with skin hydration. The detergents you wash your clothes and bedding in can cause sensitivity and inflammation, and they can contribute to dryness; ditto dishwashing liquids and other cleaners. A switch to clean detergents and cleaning products formulated for sensitive skin might make a difference.

Your Hydration Routine

You can tailor your routine to your particular preferences and sensitivities to a certain degree, but the core elements of your routine should include: cleansing, moisturizing, layering, exfoliating, and taking internal supplements. Here, how to put it all together:

CLEANSE

How you cleanse your skin—both face and body—is an essential factor to look at if you are struggling with dry or sensitive skin. Pretty much anything that foams or lathers is your enemy. Lather = detergent, in most cases. Conventional "moisturizing" body washes, for example, combine moisturizing ingredients with detergents (not to mention perfumes, which can further irritate and dehydrate)—which can spell serious trouble for dry skin. Consider oil, cream, or balm cleansers (nontoxic, clean ones are much more likely to include only moisturizing ingredients as opposed to fillers and texturizers), and consider cleansing less. Your skin isn't dirty when you wake up in the morning—so don't bother disrupting it with cleansing. If you must cleanse in the morning, finish immediately with an oil or moisturizer. In the shower, cleansing oils or creams are ideal, and a super-gentle (the gentle is important), very oily scrub can lightly exfoliate and moisturize all at once.

MOISTURIZE

How thick a cream or lotion is often indicates how moisturizing it is. But what you see isn't always what you get. Conventional moisturizers can appear thick, but much of that richness can be added fillers and texturizers. Silicones are particularly deceptive; they add nothing to the actual hydrating power of a moisturizer, but are used to make products *feel* more moisturizing, blendable, and comforting. Another extremely common texture-enhancer, propylene glycol (a.k.a. antifreeze), makes products feel softer and gentler, but does nothing to actually nourish or help skin. Conversely, there are ultra-hydrating serums that feel like practically nothing on the skin. Still, in general and especially when you're working with

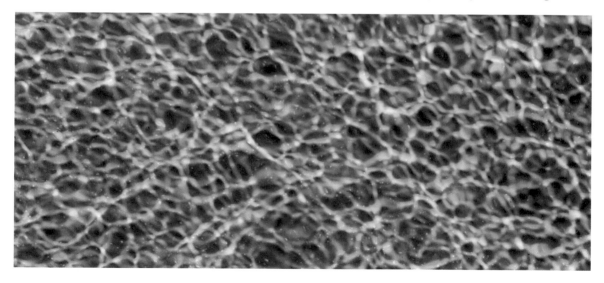

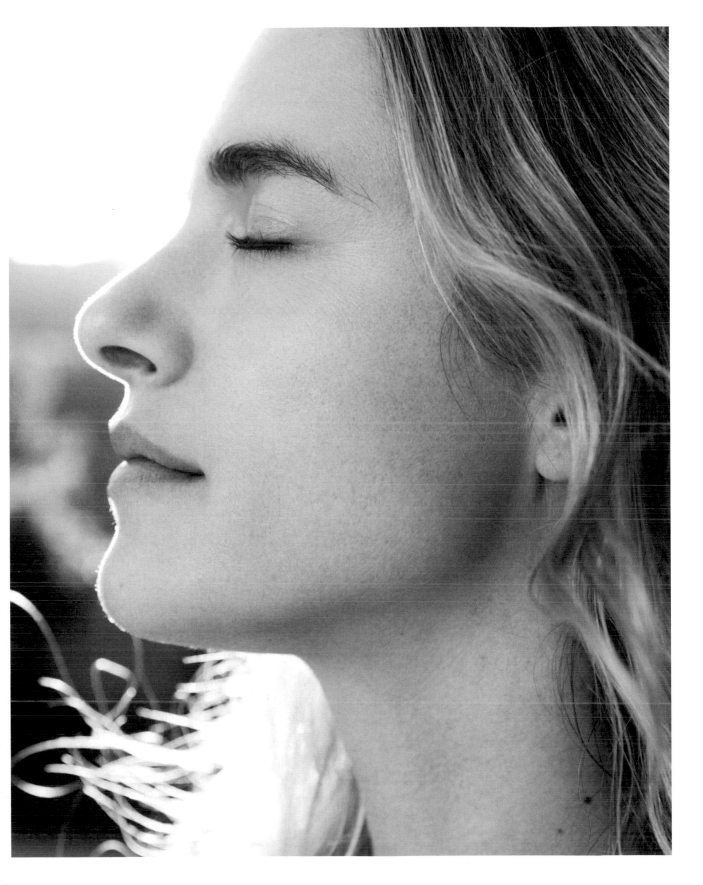

clean, nontoxic products, thicker is a fairly reliable indication of more moisturizing power.

Applying moisturizers—or any nontoxic products, really—when your skin is wet is a good idea for two reasons, the obvious being that it seals in the water that's on your skin. But the more important aspect is that wet skin is more porous, so treatment ingredients—in this case, hydrators—can penetrate into deeper layers of the skin, where they can do the most good.

In addition to moisturizers, there is a handful of other classes of products that deliver the same results. Below we outline the philosophy behind using balms, oils, creams, lotions, and serums:

- **Why use a balm?** The thickest, most skin-coddling, nourishing option in moisturizing, your average balm is not something you're going to want to put on under makeup: A good one is thick, occlusive, and super-healing. Most balms are nicely multipurpose and great on skin, but also on lips, and on dry or rough spots all over the body. You can also use them over sunblock in extreme weather situations like skiing.

- **Why use an oil?** Oils are the original moisturizer; women have been using them for centuries. They vary in texture, depending on the type of oil, so definitely experiment with a few before deciding yea or nay. You can use an oil just like a regular moisturizer, though they generally take a few minutes to sink in enough to apply makeup over. Apply face and/or body oils as often as your skin seems to like. You can use body oil in your bath instead of products labeled "bath oil," which, especially in the world of conventional beauty products, mix oil with detergents to make the oil disperse evenly. (Yes, this is as drying as it sounds.) The general rule of thumb: If it foams, it's seriously no good for dry skin. Body oil—100 percent oil—will leave your tub a little slippery (and be careful, as the number one place household accidents occur is the bathroom), but will also leave itself on your skin, gloriously if unevenly. Because hot baths (*who, except someone in an extremely hot climate, wants to take the oft-recommended tepid bath?*) are drying, using body oil in the tub can help you retain moisture.

  The other thing oils are amazing for is, oddly, refreshing makeup. You know that 4 p.m. slump when your skin looks faded and tired and you feel like you should redo your makeup? Smooth a little face oil onto your fingertips and pat onto your skin over makeup—it will enliven your face and freshen your whole look without requiring more layers of makeup.

- **Why use a cream?** One of the serious advantages of a nice, rich face or body cream is the texture. A cream distributes moisture more evenly than other products and it lasts longer on the skin than your average oil or even balm. Creams are also fantastic for sealing in an oil or a serum.

- **Why use a lotion?** Some people don't like the feeling of a heavy cream on their faces; lotions are generally lighter. They can be a little less moisturizing, but not necessarily. The key is, if you love a lighter texture, pick a lotion and use it as often as necessary. If you enjoy the experience, you'll stick to it—and consistency is key.

- **Why use a serum?** The light texture of most serums means that, for the most part, they're less moisturizing. While there are exceptions to that rule, think of most serums as the best way to deliver active ingredients (brighteners or firming or anti-wrinkle ingredients). Most people with any sort of dry-skin issue are going to want to *layer* a moisturizer or oil over a serum.

LAYER

Smoothing on product after product can leave you with irritated skin and/or product piled up on your skin in weird clumps. But done judiciously, it's a great way to (a) get more moisture into skin, and (b) treat dry skin with anti-aging or anti-acne ingredients without overdrying. Keep the number of products as minimal as possible, and leave time—a few minutes at least—between your layers, so each product has an opportunity to sink into your skin.

Dermatologists advise applying sunblock first. *Always* use a physical/mineral sunblock as opposed to chemical sunscreens, even in gentle-looking "daily moisturizers." Chemical sunscreens are some of the most irritating compounds we put on our skin; they're right up there with fragrances, and sometimes even worse. (They also quickly degrade in sunlight, rendering them useless after a few hours, but see Chapter 4 for more on that.) The added benefit of physical sunblock is that because of the minerals they're made with, they're actually soothing to reactive skin: As you're taking that extra minute to rub in the extra whiteness of a sunblock, consider that the same stuff that makes it hard to rub in also soothes severe skin irritations like diaper rash; it's also the same stuff cosmetic companies mix into foundations to "blur" and minimize skin imperfections.

After sunblock, assess whether you need more moisture (most people with dry or sensitive skin will, but know that even a dry-feeling sunblock does have a skin-barrier-reinforcing, hydrating effect). For some, an oil will feel great, others might love a cream, still others might need only a serum (and for those who prefer to apply serum or moisturizer first, wait a few minutes for it to sink in, then apply sunblock).

Remember that any tinted moisturizer/CC or BB cream/foundation is essentially another layer: It, too, has a protective, mildly hydrating effect. If you're using a product made with a physical sunblock and you like to use it all over your face, it's probably a good-enough sunblock layer on its own for a day when you're going to the office or otherwise mostly inside. For an outside day or if you're always by a big window, do both sunblock and whatever foundation-ish product you like.

INTERNAL SUPPLEMENTS

Supplementing with omega-rich oils—from salmon or cod-liver to flaxseed or evening primrose—can make a serious difference for people with dry skin. As with everything else, the only way to know is to try. Keep oils fresh in the refrigerator, and be sure to get them— particularly salmon-oil capsules—from a reputable provider: New studies have shown that rancid oils, particularly fish oils, can actually cause inflammation—the reverse of what you're trying to do. Some people have also had good results with anti-allergy compounds like quercetin.

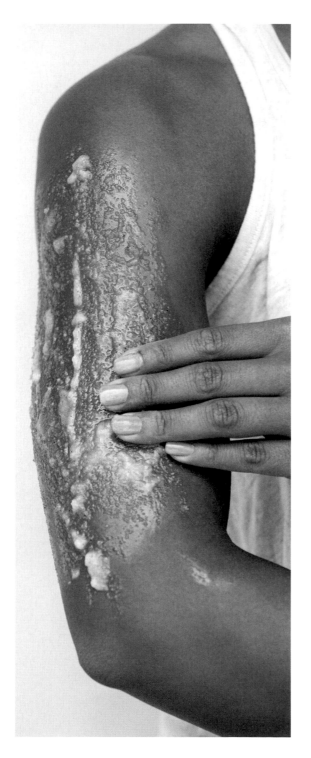

EXFOLIATE

People with irritable or dry skin often avoid exfoliating because it seems like it would worsen the problem. Exfoliating too much will absolutely dry skin, and can seriously disrupt the protective mantle of the skin and compromise its barrier function. But the right amount of exfoliation makes skin function better all over, plus it allows treatment ingredients to sink in further.

Scrubs made with lots of oils and emollients feel especially good if your skin is dry; you have to watch your step in the shower, but you'll emerge fully moisturized, without having to apply lotion or cream after. At the very least, they give you a head start in terms of layering on product, and sealing in moisture.

Chemical exfoliants—AHAs, BHAs, and plant enzymes like papaya—are often the best solution for dry or irritation-prone skin, but use them extremely cautiously, because their strength varies widely. AHAs were actually initially developed to treat an extreme dry skin condition called ichthyosis; their exfoliating qualities allow treatment to penetrate and smooth the surface in a way that can help treat irritation, too. But a too-harsh AHA on dry or irritated skin can compound the problem; so again, proceed with caution and consult a dermatologist if need be.

A Dermatologist's Perspective

One of only a small handful of physicians in the country who is board-certified in both derma-tology and psychiatry, Dr. Amy Wechsler adds another dimension to her practice. Using the latest technologies and techniques, she treats a wide range of dermatologic conditions—beginning with a careful evaluation of the patient's psychological stressors and skincare concerns. Here, she weighs in on sensitive-skin issues.

Dr. Amy Wechsler
ON TREATING SENSITIVE SKIN

How much of chronic skin sensitivity do you find is caused by purely environmental factors?
A great deal—there is a lot of over-scrubbing and cleansing that can cause skin sensitivity, in addition to dry winters, not enough humidity, not using humidifiers, and other factors. Americans tend to overly cleanse their skin—I think we're ingrained with the thought that if one's skin isn't squeaky clean, then it's not clean enough, but squeaky-clean skin means that the natural oils were stripped away. Also, unprotected sun exposure dries the skin and can cause sensitivity. Pollution is another cause of chronic skin sensitivity, and as pollution worsens, so does skin sensitivity.

We also use too many products. Fragrance often causes sensitivity; other ingredients can do it as well.

Exfoliation can help dry skin—to an extent, and then it quickly becomes a negative. How should people modulate their exfoliation use?
Anyone with dry or sensitive skin should be really careful with exfoliating. Do it infrequently, and use something gentle that doesn't sting, burn, or hurt in any way. Someone with sensitive, dry skin can exfoliate just once or twice a week. Toners or exfoliants with a low concentration of salicylic acid (0.5%) or brown sugar are typically gentle enough for sensitive skin. I like my patients to wash their faces with their clean hands instead of a washcloth or device, since the latter can often be too harsh.

How do stress and other psychological factors play a role in sensitive skin? Does stress play a role in dry skin as well?
The brain and the skin have myriad interconnections. Stress and sleep deprivation can induce temporary sensitivity in someone who is typically not sensitive, and they can also worsen sensitivity in someone who is constitutionally sensitive. Stress causes an increase in cortisol, and cortisol does many bad things: It causes inflammation, collagen breakdown, and also an increase in trans-epidermal water loss, which makes the skin's barrier function less healthy, leading to both dryness and sensitivity. A product that someone usually tolerates well can all of a sudden cause an itchy rash in someone experiencing temporarily sensitive skin.

What are the best at-home steps a person can take to control dry skin?
Take short showers only once a day, and use a mild cleanser or soap—and no washcloths. Moisturize right after showering, and at least one other time during the day. Use a humidifier during winter, and you can try whole-milk compresses if you have eczema.

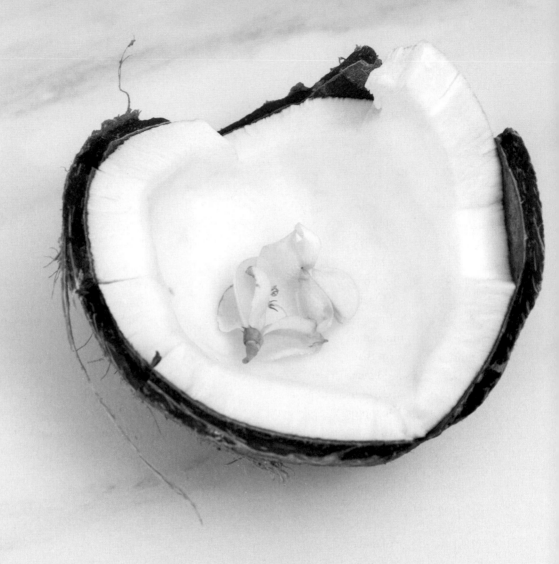

Labels Decoded: (Potentially) Soothing Ingredients for Dry or Irritated Skin

Here are some good ingredients to look for as you shop for products specifically tailored to dry or sensitive skin:

- Aloe
- Azulene
- Honey
- Vitamin E
- Omega-3, -6, and -9 oils
- Calendula
- Clay
- Feverfew
- Cucumber
- Oatmeal

- Salicylic acid (BHA, otherwise known as aspirin and willow bark)
- Zinc oxide
- Evening primrose oil
- Flaxseed oil
- Coconut oil
- Prickly pear seed oil
- Argan oil
- Chia seed oil

Beyond Sensitive

If you have eczema and rosacea, you may need to do more than the routine outlined so far in this chapter to find some comfort.

ECZEMA

Eczema is a not-terribly-well-understood auto-immune reaction. It's often a lifelong problem that flares up when the sufferer is under physical or mental stress. Standard medical treatments include topical steroids, which are problematic to use on any sort of long-term basis. Doctors also often recommend occlusive balms (most doctor-recommended options are made of mineral oil or petroleum jelly, which can do more harm than good), but moisturizing eczema does not do much to make it go away.

Some sufferers have had incredible (as in: no-more, never-again symptoms) results with homeopathy; acupuncture can also help. Natural healing agents from calendula and chamomile to clay treatments can also have an effect. Keep trying: Doctors will tell you there's little to do beyond what they offer, but the truth is, no one modality seems to have the answer for everyone.

And, if you haven't landed on a solution yet, an Ayurvedic approach is absolutely worth pursuing for multiple health benefits. Our head merchant, Blair Lawson (see her gorgeous skin on page 235), introduced us to a pioneer in Ayurvedic skincare, Dr. Pratima Raichur, a chemist, botanist, aesthetician, and Ayurvedic doctor who has developed a holistic system for skin wellness along with her own line of organic skincare products. Dr. Raichur has treated and healed thousands of patients for more than forty years in her New York City salon. We asked her to explain the causes of eczema and how best to treat it.

Dr. Pratima Raichur
ON AYURVEDIC HEALING

What is your approach to treating eczema?
My approach to treating any skin disease is rooted in the holistic science of Ayurveda. Ayurveda is a mind-body healing system that recognizes that an individual is the totality of his/her experience. So a person's condition—be it a skin ailment or otherwise—is affected by everything in his/her life, including diet, what one thinks, feels, what behaviors one inherits from parents, lifestyle patterns, and stress levels. While a person may not have imbalances within all of those arenas, my approach is to help address each area and find a state of balance where it's needed.

Some of the specific diagnostics I perform include assessing the person's nails, tongue, eyes, and skin to help identify the body's nutrient levels, patterns of toxicity or accumulation, and other markers of health. I also observe the person's energy level, emotional state, eye movements, speech pattern, and more. All of this can tell me about the person's condition and give me insight into the root causes of the eczema.

Because Ayurveda teaches us that the outer manifestation of illness and disease comes from an imbalance of either the physical body, the energetic body, the mental body, and/or the consciousness, it's important to address all four of these levels, otherwise issues will continue to return. One main component of these four levels is nutrition, so I always begin treatment with customized dietary guidelines in tandem with ionized herbal supplements. In addition I assess stress levels, offering stress management techniques and other healthful lifestyle practices. All of these steps, when used with therapeutic skincare formulations, can offer extensive healing and treatment.

Is eczema dry skin? Irritated skin? A fungal infection?
Eczema can be dry or moist, known as *oozing eczema*, but in most cases it is irritated patches of skin. Depending on

each individual's *dosha*, or mind-body type, you may see different forms of eczema manifest on the skin, which can range from dryness with itching and pain (Vata dosha type) to an oozing form of eczema that may be accompanied by redness, burning, and severe itching (Pitta dosha type), to thick and whitish or paler near the affected area, along with fluid retention and itching at the site (Kapha dosha type). So while eczema is not considered a fungal infection, it can certainly take many different forms on a person's skin.

Mainstream medicine seems to offer mostly steroids and petroleum jelly—do these things work?
These things may appear to offer some relief, but it's only temporary and superficial. Steroidal creams might clear up eczema for a little while, but eventually it will come back because the treatment only masks the symptoms. The root causes are not actually being corrected; the imbalances causing the eczema haven't been balanced. If the diet hasn't changed, allergens are still present within the blood and stressors are still unmitigated, and the system still contains the inflammatory patterns that are causing the eczema. Unfortunately, anything you simply suppress will come back, and oftentimes it will come back more aggressively. Eczema on the skin is a sign that other aspects of the mind and body need more help and support, and if those other aspects are not properly treated, eczema will continue to be present.

What do you feel is the cause of eczema?
The main causes of eczema are allergies and stress. Allergies can be a result of many things, including what Ayurveda refers to as *ama*, or "undigested food or emotion." A good example of something that causes a buildup of *ama* is genetically modified foods, which contribute to inflammation and sensitivities because they are foreign to our bodies. Allergies can also result from irritants in our environment, such as detergents and air contaminants.

Allergies, when combined with stress, increase the inflammation in our bodies, and cause imbalances that can ultimately lead to eczema, as well as to other skin conditions.

Stress is key. When combined with an allergy of some sort, it is often a strong recipe for eczema. I've seen an increase in the cases of eczema over the years, and I believe, in addition to allergy and food sensitivity, this is due in large part to an increasingly pressurized modern-day lifestyle. Ayurveda has taught for centuries (and modern-day research into neuroplasticity now confirms), that the mind can really focus on only one thing at a time. So despite our best efforts, our minds cannot actually multitask, and trying to do so may lead only to further stress. We also know that our bodies can be in only one place at any given moment. Yet our current lifestyles pull us in many different directions at once. All of this causes a tremendous amount of stress on the physical body and the mind. Stress is how our bodies respond to these pressures. This leads to compromised health, resulting in such things as eczema. You can think of stress as a self-preservation response to the pressure on, or the struggle within, the mind and body.

Are certain foods problematic for eczema?
Diet plays a huge role in the health of our bodies. It can trigger allergies and stress, but it can also be incredibly healing. Some of the most common food allergens associated with eczema are milk, cheese, fried foods, fermented foods, nightshades, peppers and hot spices, certain citrus, alcohol, overly processed foods, GMOs, and preservatives. Eliminating these potentially irritating foods can have a huge impact. Once we identify and eliminate dietary intolerances, we can then purify the body and liver, and strengthen the immune system with the appropriate anti-inflammatory, replenishing foods, along with herbal nutrition, to help the body eradicate old patterns and find a new state of balance.

What kind of skincare works best for eczema?
Generally eczema benefits from herbs, oils, and minerals that reduce inflammation, calm allergic reactions and irritations, and deliver cooling, soothing, and healing properties. Ingredients that I incorporate into my Ayurvedic herbal eczema formulas—such as neem, white or red sandalwood, white turmeric, and pure *shilajit*—are wonderful for these purposes.

I use traditional Ayurvedic methodology to harness the optimal healing power of the herbs, exploiting their medicinal and calming benefits to alleviate and ultimately heal the symptoms of eczema. All of our herbal formulations also go through an ionization process, which is important to maximize the herbs' efficiency and potency so they can truly heal and boost health, as well as help the body to better assimilate the herbs. All of these preparatory steps play just as important a role, if not more so, than the ingredients themselves.

Is there an eczema personality type?
While all of us are a combination of all three of the doshas (Vata, Pitta, and Kapha) in varying proportions, eczema is prevalent in people who are most dominant in Pitta dosha. Not surprisingly, Pitta is governed by the fire element and these types naturally have more heat in their system, which can produce "fiery" traits, such as competitiveness, being highly ambitious, passionate, driven, very intelligent, prone to anger and frustration. Physical traits for Pitta include strong digestion, combination/sensitive skin, being warm to the touch, and having the propensity for physical transformation, including weight fluctuations.

Sometimes Vata types experience eczema as well, but, as mentioned previously, it will be drier. This is due to the fact that Vata is governed by the air and space elements. Kapha types, governed by earth and water elements, yield the thicker eczema conditions with moisture retention.

Does Ayurvedic-based eczema treatment have other benefits?
Since we are not simply treating the skin, an Ayurvedic-based treatment journey brings with it an entire life balance. Skin is just a manifestation of our inner being, so a holistic healing path works to balance every aspect of our life experience. Through a dietary elimination process, you can identify root allergens. Therapeutic herbs help detoxify the blood and liver, while proper nutrition and lifestyle strengthen the immune system, address mental stresses, and establish a new state of health and vitality. In treating your eczema, you treat everything else. An Ayurvedic approach to healing affects the entire human being—body, mind, and spirit.

ROSACEA
Rosacea, a chronic skin condition with symptoms including redness and small bumps, is particularly intractable and often takes serious experimenting to find products and/or a regimen your skin responds to. Rosacea patients often think what's bothering them is acne (it can cause inflammation that can look like pimples), dry skin, or allergies (a very common symptom is flushing of the skin after exercise, drinking alcohol, or eating certain foods). Untreated, it can build on itself and eventually lead to broken capillaries. If your budget allows (and rosacea treatments are usually at least partly covered by insurance), consider seeing a dermatologist—at the very least to confirm a diagnosis. For some patients, topical prescription drugs like Metrogel help; for others, they don't at all.

Whether or not you choose prescription treatments, when buying any sort of skincare go for the gentlest products you can find. Conventional beauty products are made with all kinds of skin irritants and toxins that are terrible for rosacea patients—often even in products that claim to be for sensitive skin. And even natural or clean products can still irritate your skin. Take it slow, read labels, and choose carefully.

Also, although you may have been told that facials are too risky for sensitive skin, we've found that specialized facials (and the really talented aestheticians behind them) can go a long way to clearing up rosacea. Christine Chin has been transforming the skin of in-the-know New Yorkers for decades—eradicating acne, shrinking pores, and beating back the signs of aging—into dewy, poreless loveliness. And she's incredible with rosacea: Her atypical approach has changed the lives and skin of many sufferers, including several now-perfect-skinned GOOP staffers. Her hour-and-a-half facials are not easy (she's been nicknamed Mean Christine after her no-pain-no-gain philosophy), but they are unbelievably thorough—and the results are pretty much impossible to argue with.

Christine Chin
ON SAYING GOOD-BYE TO ROSACEA

How do you know a client has rosacea, rather than just sensitive skin?
It's pretty obvious—people don't come to me for mild problems, generally. I get a little disappointed when they do! I like to really help a person, change their skin. People come to me with their whole faces disfigured, often using thick camouflage makeup. I see very bad acne—cystic acne, bad scarring—and often those conditions are caused by rosacea.

Is it possible to get rid of rosacea so it doesn't come back?
I believe it is, but you have to address the plaque that forms on the skin as a result of rosacea first—you can put all the treatments you want on top of that plaque but it won't get through to the skin; it's like thick sandpaper. The reverse is also true: Whatever the body wants to get rid of won't get through that thick layer of residue on the skin. The plaque on your skin is like the plaque on your teeth—you have to clear it away before you do anything else. I believe in professional microdermabrasion. For bad cases, it may take a few times.

A month or so after we've done the microdermabrasion, if there's been some improvement I like to go in with a laser light: a healing laser that treats redness and broken capillaries.

What are some of the mistakes people make in trying to treat their rosacea?
People who think they have sensitive skin will use oily products and will avoid toner. Toner is the key to maintaining your skin if you have rosacea, and people are afraid to use it. If your skin is blotchy, most often it's because you're not using toner.

On the other hand, regular scrubbing at home is a disaster for rosacea; people end up scrubbing too hard and disturbing the skin.

Many people will use benzoyl peroxide, regular soap, and heavy moisturizer—all mistakes for someone with rosacea. Instead you want to gently cleanse, tone, and very lightly moisturize. Sometimes you can also add retinol, but it's not for everybody's skin; it can be too much.

Also, I think if you have rosacea with severe acne, it's very hard to get rid of at home. Those bumps and acne have to be taken out—you have to remove it all.

How is your approach different from that of a dermatologist?
Dermatologists give you Metrogel and antibiotics, and for some people that works, but not for many.

Once rosacea clears, how do you maintain your results?
At home you need to be on the right regimen to keep it away once it's cleared: No perfume, no alcohol, spicy food, garlic, or fast food. Life is short, so you can cheat a bit, but not too much!

Maintenance is very important, cleansing gently, using toner. Toner is like a toothbrush for your skin. The right products are important. When skin is very sensitive, you want to give it calming, beautiful ingredients like hyaluronic acid and green tea.

Again, always cleanse the skin. People wear a lot of foundation—you can't leave that stuff on at night. If your immune system's a little low, and you're not removing your foundation, the rosacea can start back up again.

And facials are key—sometimes with microdermabrasion or laser. People will say, *I don't want a facial, my doctor says it's too irritating*, but my clients' results show the exact opposite.

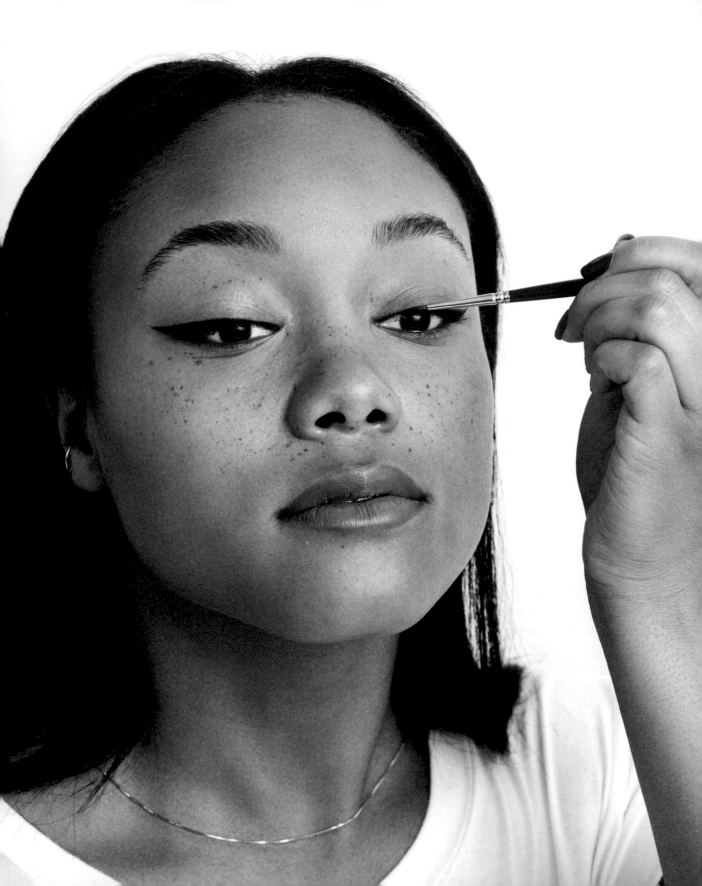

11.

Easy Makeup—
Made Easier

The Fresh Face

Clean, healthy, beautiful skin is the primary makeup look we all want here at GOOP. Chanel celebrity makeup artist Kate Lee is famous for making her clients look as if they're wearing nothing on their faces—save a gorgeous flick of eyeliner or a stunning lip color. She's responsible for many of GP's all-time greatest looks, both on and off the red carpet. Lee says her clean, real-skin aesthetic works because her clients take such good care of their complexions. "People that look really great on say, a red carpet? Part of the reason they look so good is they take care of themselves—it's not something you can necessarily apply from a bottle." That said, her step-by-step tips make just about anyone look about 1,000 times more (naturally) beautiful.

Look #1
EVERYDAY NO-MAKEUP MAKEUP

1. Skincare is everything, says Lee. "Start with very, very clean skin—the ideal client as far as I'm concerned has just come straight out of the shower." Lee smoothes the skin with moisturizer to add hydration, then waits a minute to let it settle into the skin.

2. Primer, depending on your skin, is the ultimate invisible, your-skin-but-better product. "It can help make the skin appear very fresh, particularly if the primer has a radiance to it."

3. Highlighter, if it works on your skin, is most natural-looking when it is applied before foundation: "You can use a slightly shimmery primer or cream highlighter, depending on what you prefer, just focus on the areas you want to draw attention to—such as cheekbones and the jawline. Highlighting makes the skin look more taut."

4. Put foundation only where you feel your skin needs the coverage. "I never just blanket the whole face in makeup," says Lee. "You want your skin to shine through." She prefers a light foundation to tinted moisturizer in most cases: "It just lasts better."

5. Which kind of concealer(s) you choose depends on what you're trying to conceal. Lee says she often uses three or four different types of concealer on a single client. "For blemishes, dark spots, or a freckle you don't want, I tend to use a very pigmented concealer, but I prefer a lighter, more reflective brush-type concealer under the eyes. Avoid the moving parts of the eye area—as the movement will cause the concealer to migrate and collect in creases."

6. Curl your lashes: "It makes a huge difference."

7. Groom your brows if they need it: Use pencil to fill in, or a brow powder to define the shape, and then use gel to keep the brows in place.

8. For a natural, no-makeup look, you don't necessarily need eye shadow. If your lids are too red or too dark, try a primer specifically for eyelids. "Lids can tend to be oilier so they can cause regular concealer to crease," says Lee. "Or you could blot your lids with an oil-absorbent sheet, then use a very small amount of matte concealer."

9. Use fingers or a brush to smooth cream blush on the apples of the cheeks. "Cream blushes create the most natural flush," says Lee.

10. If you've got especially oily or shiny skin, you might want a dusting of loose translucent powder. "Sometimes primer will do the job of the powder," says Lee, "but it really depends on your individual skin type. If you're oily and you do need powder, I prefer to blot and then use loose powder on a puff. I rarely use a colored compact powder—it builds up and is not as natural."

11. Apply dark, glossy, un-clumpy black mascara with a light touch.

12. Smooth on tinted lip balm to finish the look.

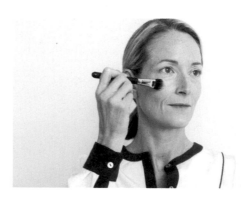

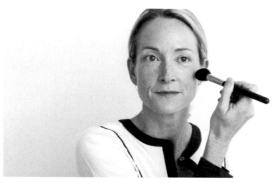

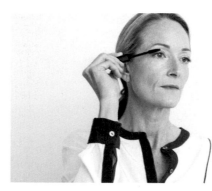

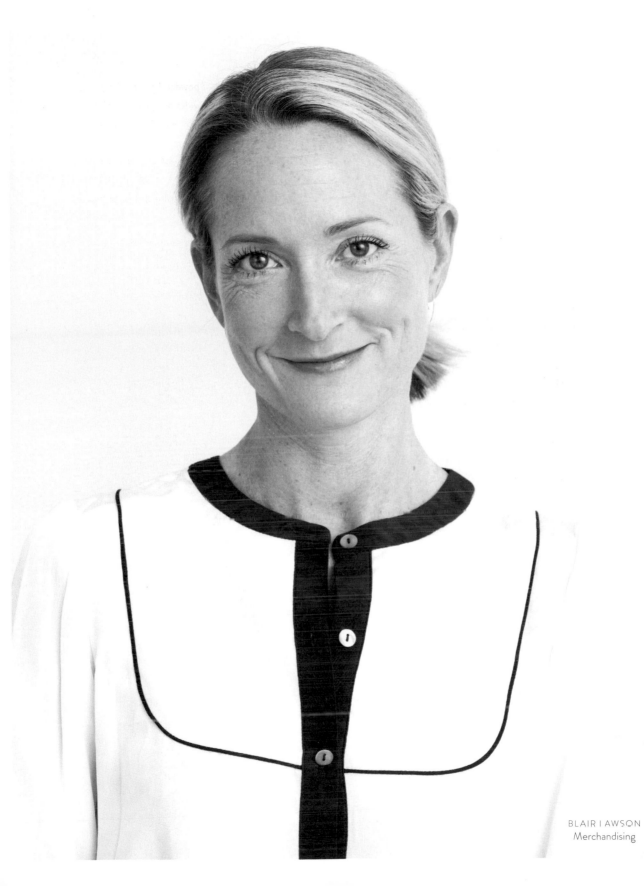

BLAIR LAWSON
Merchandising

Look #2
SOPHIA LOREN CAT-EYE

1. There are all kinds of liner: cake, gel, pencil, pen, liquid, and kohl pencil. The trick is finding the one you feel most comfortable with—whichever version speaks to you, and sounds easiest, that's the one to experiment with first. Ease of use is critical, but so is staying power. "For a cat-eye, you need something that's really going to set and won't budge," says Lee.

2. Have Q-tips with oil-free makeup remover on hand. "It's a sharp, crisp look," says Lee. "A Q-tip makes doing fixes quick and easy."

3. As you start to draw your line—starting from the middle of your upper lash line and moving outward—get the color as close to the very base of your lashes as possible. "If you don't really get it in there, it will look messy. Getting the roots of the lashes is especially important for blondes and pale redheads," says Lee.

4. How far out you wing the line depends on your eye shape, says Lee. "A very hooded eye creases over the liner if you draw it out too far, so it requires a shorter cat-eye overall. Look in the mirror and decide whether your eye socket is high enough to draw the line out. It looks good either way, you just have to be clear about your eye shape and what's going to work for you."

5. Mascara—especially on the outer corners of the lashes—heightens the effect and helps blend the liner with your lashes. "It also can help compensate if you need to do a shorter line—using mascara at the outer corners can lengthen the lash line a bit," says Lee.

6. Finish the Sophia Loren vibe with a sheer, nude lip—so sexy.

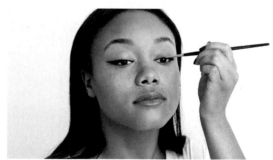

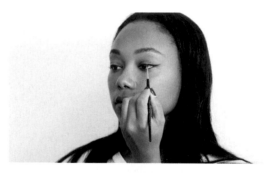

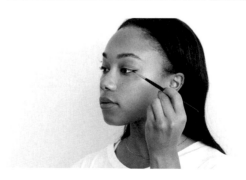

HEAVEN SAUNDERS
Operations

Look #3
RED LIP

1. Go easy on everything else. "You really want to strip the rest of your makeup back to just glowy, healthy skin if you're doing a bold red lip," says Lee.

2. If you know lipstick tends to bleed on you, trace on a neutral lip liner; if you don't need it, Lee sees no reason to use it. If you do, she advises powdering over the liner before you put on lipstick for even more staying power. Also look into formula: "A liquid lipstick sets much better, so is less likely to bleed in the first place," says Lee.

3. Highlight the Cupid's bow before putting on lipstick. "Something with a touch of shimmer generally looks prettiest," Lee notes.

4. Smooth on lipstick from the bullet or with a brush; to make it last longer, blot it off with a tissue and reapply.

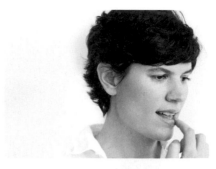
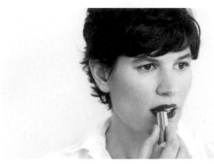
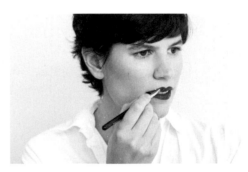
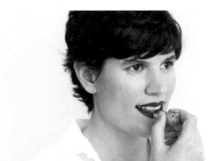

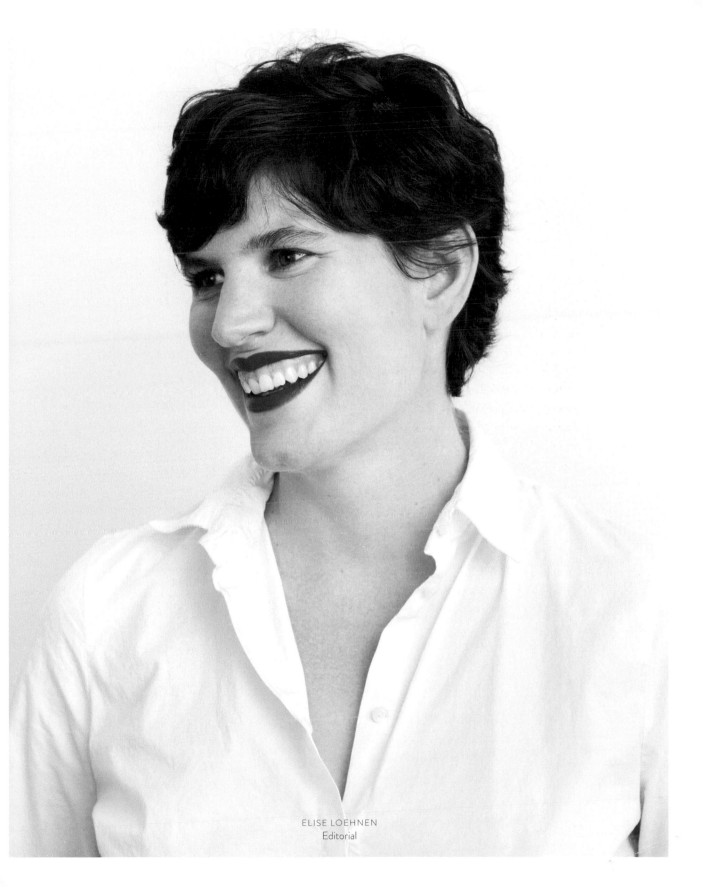

ELISE LOEHNEN
Editorial

Look #4
FRENCH-GIRL SMOKY EYE

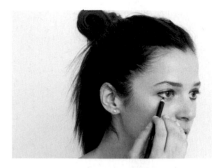

1. Pick a color, any color. "A great smoky eye doesn't have to be black," says Lee. "It could be black, it could be beautiful mid-tone brown, a deep jewel tone, a pale gray—any color you want can work."

2. Start with liner, preferably a kohl pencil in your chosen shade. "Kohl works with the moisture inside your eye, and it has a beautiful consistency."

3. Start at the outside corner of the upper lashes, and draw the initial line inward, staying as close to the lash line as possible.

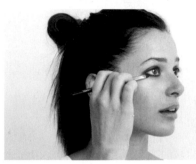

4. You can start smudging that initial line with a brush. To add more intensity, you can brush on eye shadow in the same shade over the initial line. "The most common mistake is using the same brush to blend as you do to apply," says Lee. "You need separate brushes—the difference is huge." Applying shadow over the initial line makes the color more intense and helps it to stay put, she notes. "The cream in the pencil grabs the shadow and locks it in. It's not quite as easy to blend, but it lasts longer."

5. Variations just involve intensity, says Lee: "Adding the shadow is the first level up," she says.

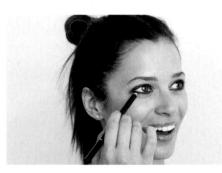

6. "Go further by doing—and smudging—a line on the lower lash line."

7. "Go further by adding kohl pencil inside the eye."

8. Go further by blending upward and inward toward the socket.

9. Lee likes a rosy, natural cheek—again, use a cream blush on the apples of the cheeks— with a smoky eye. "I think it can look dated to take all color out of lip and cheek," she says. "It can end up looking dusty and gray."

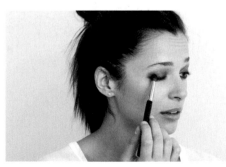

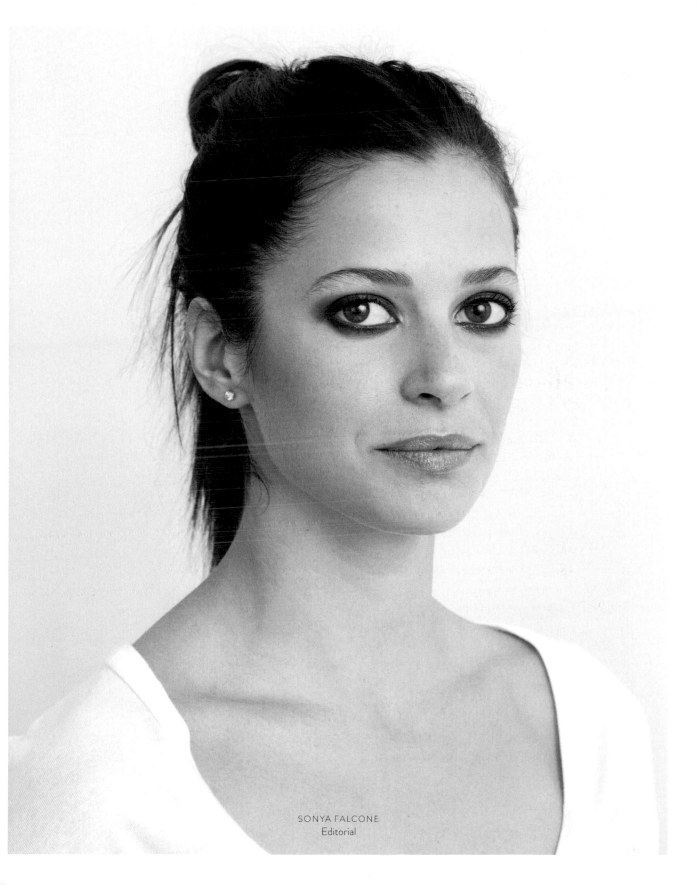

SONYA FALCONE
Editorial

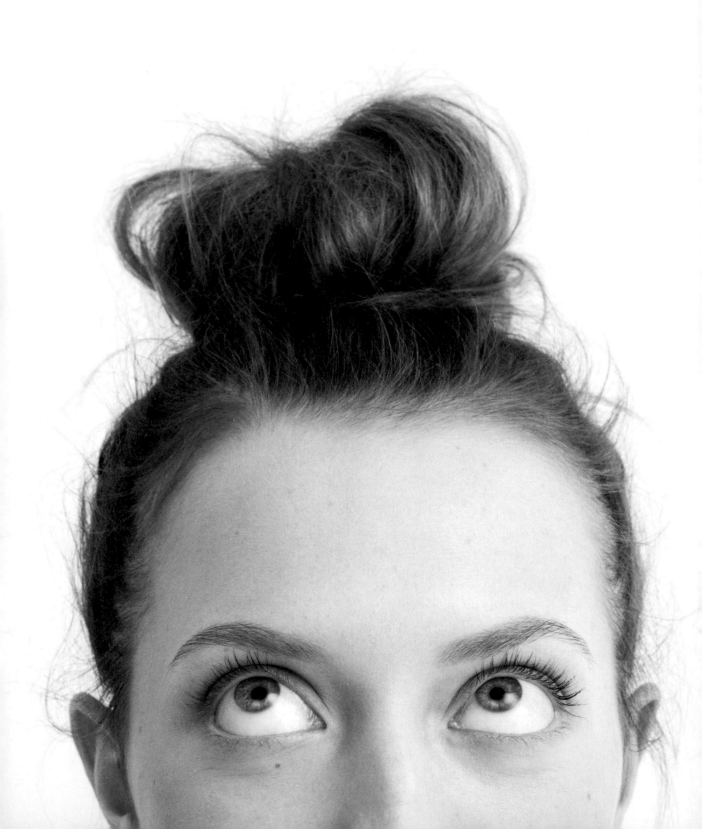

12.
Effortless Hair

Good Hair Days

If you love your hair, you feel great—and beyond a brilliant cut, beautiful color, and healthy hair maintenance, knowing how to create a few essential styles is incredibly confidence-boosting. Top hairstylist Adir Abergel, the man behind many of GP's most-loved red-carpet (and off-the red-carpet) looks, is not just amazingly talented with hair, he's also incredible at explaining how to style your hair at home. "A lot of it is just working up the confidence to feel, 'yes, I can do this,'" he says. "And really, you can." Here, he walks us through the seven styles he feels every woman should know.

Style #1
THE BLOWOUT WITH BODY

That glossy salon look—bouncy, shiny, frizz-free, totally pulled together—is worth learning to do yourself. The key is to take your time to do it right (you're already saving time by not going to the salon). One of the main reasons salon blowouts look so good is that stylists take the time. Go slow

at first, and you'll get faster as you practice—it's a skill like anything else.

1. Pre-dry your hair—not with a terry cloth towel, Abergel says, but paper towels. "If you really want that sleek, smooth look, I swear by Bounty paper towels. Scrunch them into your hair gently from your roots to your ends so you don't create friction—no back-and-forth rubbing—which creates frizz." Paper towels are also helpful for retaining your natural wave, he says: "The paper soaks up more moisture than a regular towel does, without all the friction." The other alternative is to use a towel in the same way, scrunching it from roots to tips without rubbing or moving back and forth.

2. Spritz a thickening spray generously into your roots. "You want something with both pliability and memory," says Abergel. "Not sticky, not stiff."

3. Blow-dry hair until it's about 80 percent dry, using only your fingers, on medium heat. "Too-high heat flattens your hair," says Abergel. "Medium is really important to maintain volume."

4. Finish drying with a round brush. "If your hair's above your collarbone, use a small—about two inches—brush. If it's longer, go for a medium one."

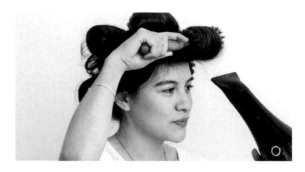

5. Section your hair into pieces no larger than the brush you're using: Start in the front (alternate sections on either side of your head), and use the brush to direct the first section away from your forehead, out in front of you.

6. Roll the end of the section around the brush, and roll up toward your scalp; heat until the section is dry.

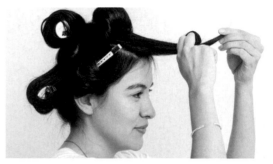

7. Don't release the hair around the brush until it has completely cooled. "Cold air locks in the shape," says Abergel. "Waiting until it cools is the secret to the perfect voluminous blowout."

8. As you remove the brush, coil the section around your fingers and clip it in place. "Let it sit while you focus on the other sections," says Abergel. Continue blow-drying sections—you should do two on the top front of your head, one on either side of your temples, and another two sections in the back.

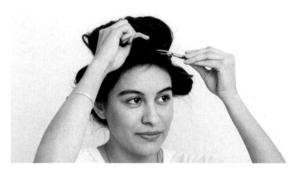

9. Wait another few minutes so all the pinned curls are completely cold, then take the clips out. If you want extra hold, mist on light hairspray while the curls are still setting.

10. To finish, you've got two options: "For a cool, deconstructed look, rake your hands through your hair and you're done," says Abergel. "For a sleek, smooth, expensive look, brush it out with a Mason Pearson brush."

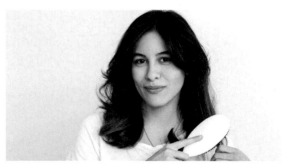

11. For extra shine, Abergel likes a light serum on the ends; if you feel like you want even more hold, mist on more light hairspray. "But nothing too heavy," he says. "It's all about leaving the integrity of the hair—let your hair shine and don't gunk it up with too many products."

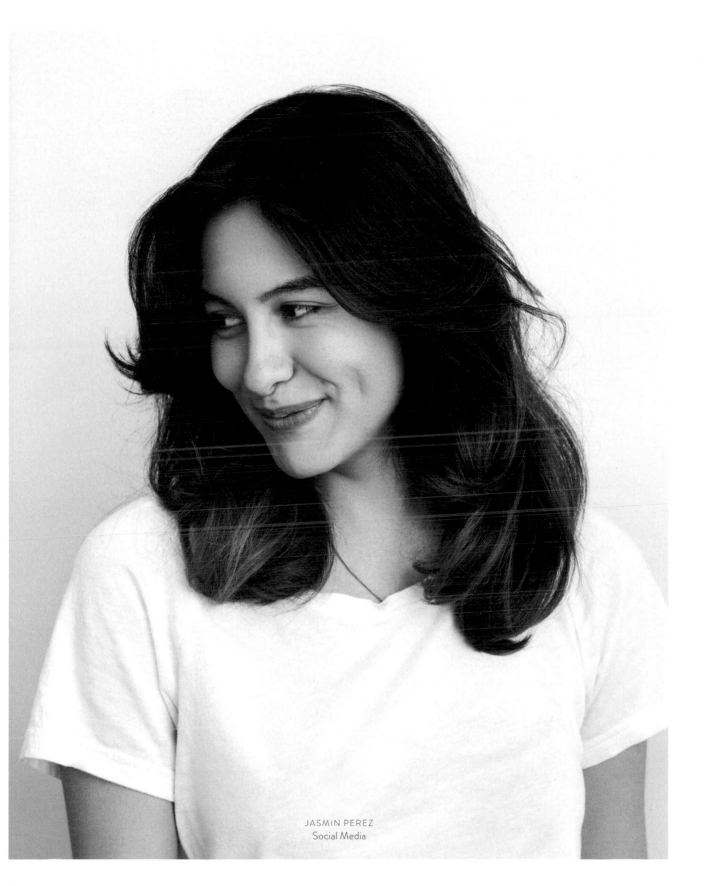

JASMIN PEREZ
Social Media

Style #2
THE SEXY BARDOT-INSPIRED TUMBLE

The '60s bombshell's look is all about volume, says Abergel. "The thing to remember is you're not re-creating her look, you're going for the spirit," he says. "You want it to be the modern version."

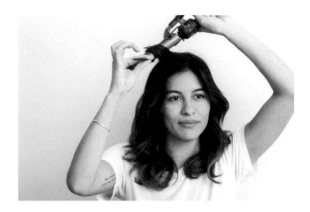

1. Do the blowout with body as in Style #1, until the point when you take the pinned curls out of the clips.

2. Heat a wand curling iron (the kind that has no clip attached) and loosely wrap large sections of hair around it. Do two sections in front and two in back; "Start the curl at the middle of the hair shaft, not by the scalp, wrap the hair around the wand but leave the ends out," says Abergel. "It'll give you a soft, deconstructed wave."

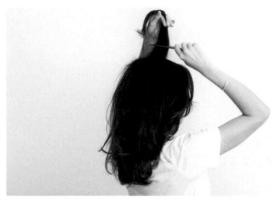

3. To create the distinctive Bardot shape, you need to create a little extra volume at the top of your head. "Make small sections at the crown area, and backcomb them with a fine-tooth comb," says Abergel. "Leave the top section alone, so it falls over the rest of the backcombing for a smooth finish. It's very '60s and Bardot-y—and it elongates your entire look and makes you look taller, which is one of the reasons it's so sexy."

4. If you want it a little deconstructed, Abergel likes to spritz in beach spray from the mid-shaft to the ends, for a bit more wave.

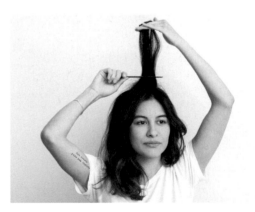

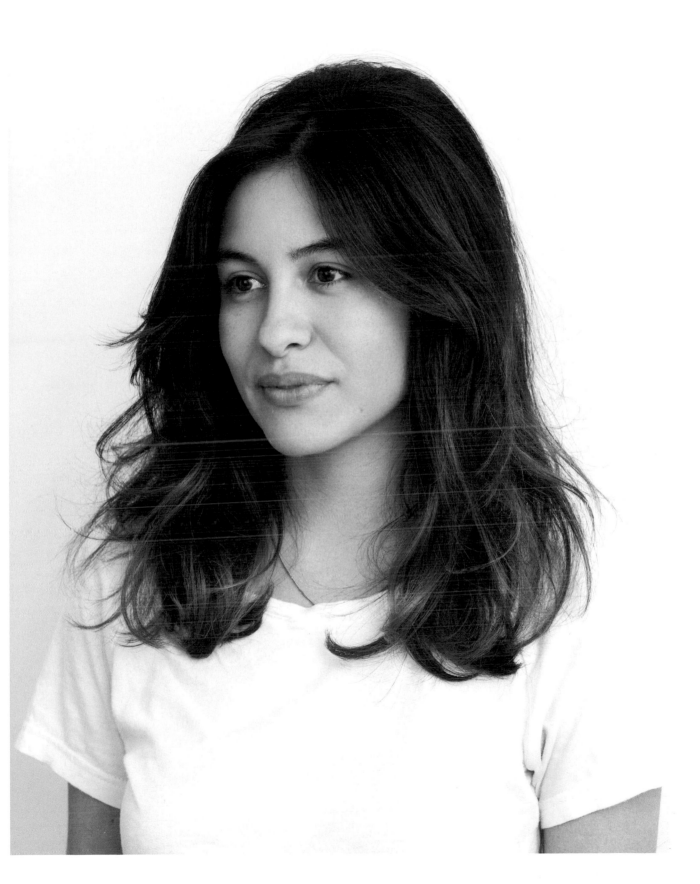

Style #3
THE SUPER-STRAIGHT BLOWOUT

Be especially methodical when you're going for flat, gleamy, stick-straight hair. "It's such a beautiful look," says Abergel. "A good flatiron is a great investment—it'll make all the difference."

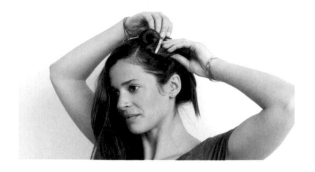

1. Use a great conditioner and conditioning shampoo—with any style, you want your hair super-moisturized, but for this one, it's especially important.

2. Starting with drying your hair with paper towels, follow the instructions for the blowout with body Style #1, but before you start your rough blow-dry, part your hair the way you want it and smooth in a light oil and a heat-protecting product. "You need both," says Abergel.

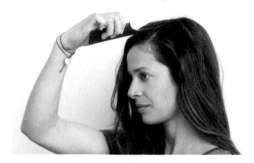

3. Once your hair is completely dry—*completely* is a key word here—begin flatironing your hair.

4. Divide your hair into four sections—two in front and two in back—and work by section, doing smaller pieces until one section is done, then move on. Start in the back. "Flatten out the cuticle as much as possible by running the iron in a downward motion," says Abergel.

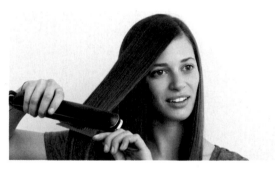

5. Once you've straightened all your hair, Abergel suggests using a toothbrush dipped in a lightweight pomade to clean up the edges: "And you can apply some shine serum or glossing cream on your ends to make it even shinier."

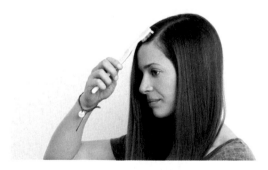

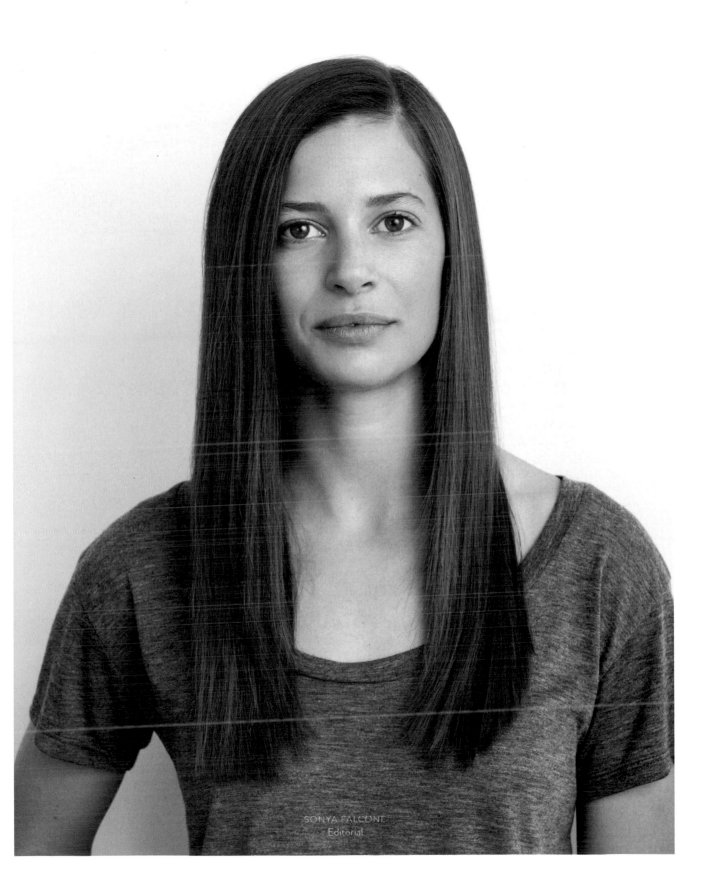

SONYA FALCONE
Editorial

Style #4
THE HIGH PONYTAIL

This simple look is super-feminine, full of energy, and it lifts your whole face up in the bargain. It requires getting the hair as beautifully smooth and shiny as possible. "You build in the sleekness and then it's easy," says Abergel. "You just concentrate on keeping it smooth and elegant."

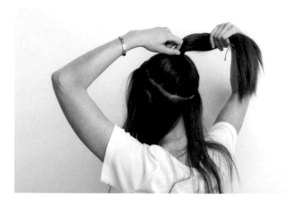

1. Start by running a light oil or serum through towel-dried (or paper-towel-dried!) hair. "It'll build in shine, reflect light, and protect your hair from the heat of the flatiron," says Abergel.

2. Roughly blow-dry hair completely, using your fingers.

3. Flatiron your entire head of hair so it's totally straight.

4. Rub a little lightweight cream or pomade thinly over your palms and smooth it through your hair, roots to end.

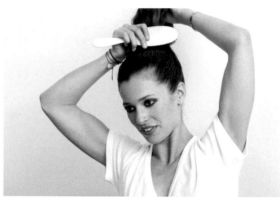

5. Make a section at the crown of your head, all the way around, and pull it into a small pony-tail at the top of your head, very slightly back.

6. Brush the remaining hair up to meet the smaller ponytail. "Keep everything super-clean and minimalist," says Abergel.

7. Secure with an elastic or bungee-cord band, then take a small section from underneath the ponytail, and wrap it around the elastic or band, so the hair covers it.

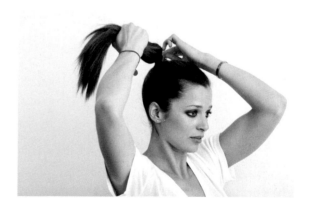

8. Tuck the ends of the section underneath the ponytail; secure it with a small bobby pin directly underneath the ponytail.

9. Tamp down any flyaways with a bit of pomade or hair cream. "It should be smooth and gleaming all over," says Abergel. "It's so chic."

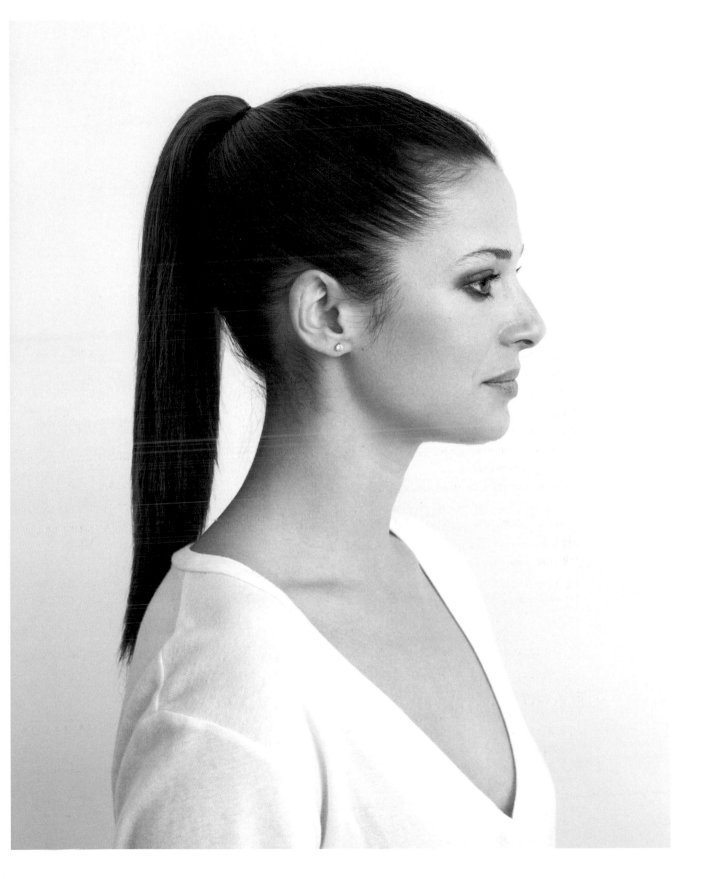

Style #5
THE TOP KNOT

It's easier than it looks, insists Abergel, and it's especially good on dirty hair, which holds the style better than freshly washed hair. "It's great for second- or third-day hair, both because it's easier and because it's a prettier, more pulled-together option at that point," he says. "It's also a great way to go from day to night, if you don't have time to redo your hair completely."

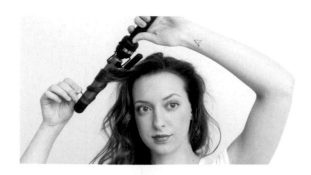

1. Spritz in volumizer at the roots, and rough-dry your hair with fingers, on medium heat.

2. With a 1-inch curling iron, randomly curl pieces of hair—in any direction. "Don't even think," says Abergel. "You're just creating texture."

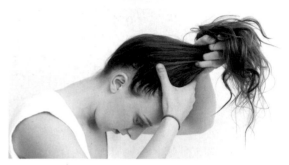

3. Pull hair into a high '80s ponytail. "A super-high ponytail will make the top knot look younger, a slightly lower one will look more classic," says Abergel.

4. Mist in texture spray—only into the ponytail.

5. With a fine-tooth comb, backcomb just at the roots of the ponytail. "You're creating a little extra bulk so the top knot will stay secure," says Abergel.

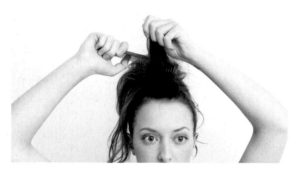

6. Twist the ponytail around your finger and coil it around itself, and pin in place with bobby pins, a hair clip, or whatever you like. "You have to not care if pieces fall out," says Abergel. "The pieces and the not-so-pristine aspect make it cool."

7. Pull out a few wispy pieces around your face, and mist with hairspray if you want more staying power.

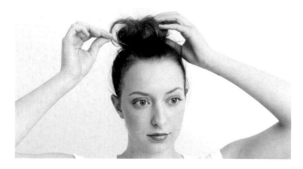

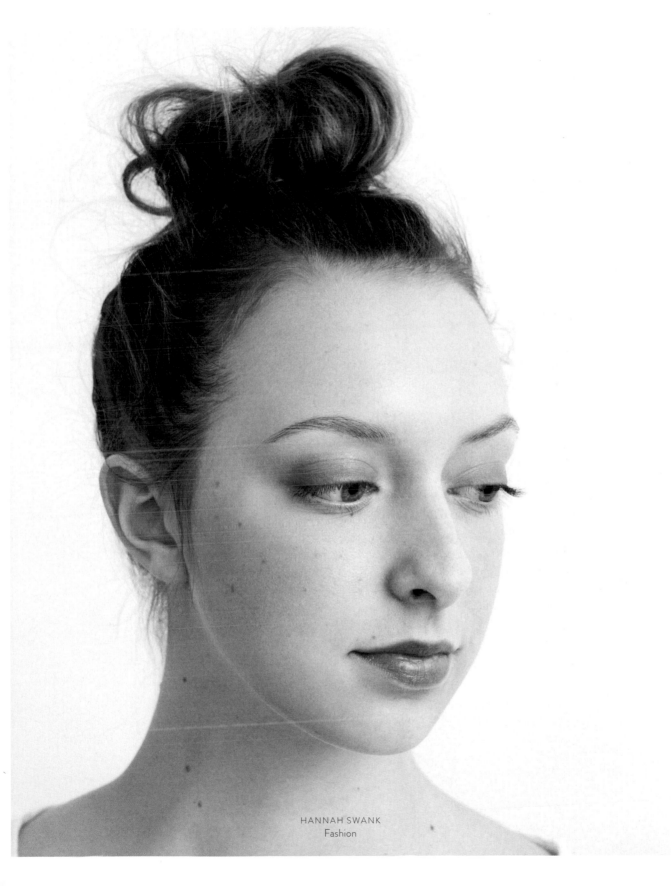

HANNAH SWANK
Fashion

Style #6
THE BEACHY WAVE

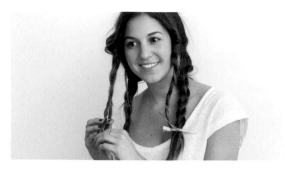

This classic tousled, salt-sprayed California look is achievable whether or not you have wavy hair. The key, says Abergel, is lack of precision. "You want a rough, undone feel," he says.

1. Towel-dry hair, then spritz in volumizing spray, directed only at your roots.
2. After the volumizer, mist in sea-salt spray, from mid-shaft to roots. "This creates that great, carefree texture," says Abergel.
3. Divide your hair into four sections; very loosely braid each section, and then dry completely—either air-drying or blow-drying.
4. Once the braids are completely dry, take them out, and with a 1¼-inch curling iron, randomly curl the hair—leaving the ends uncurled—around the outside of the curling-iron barrel. "You're trying to create an uneven texture," explains Abergel.
5. Spritz in more sea-salt spray through the mid-length and ends; scrunch your hair a little with your fingers to tousle it further.

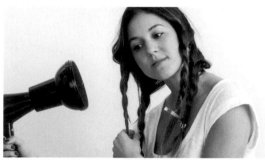

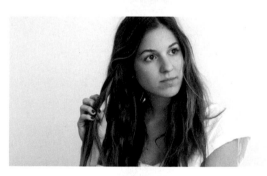

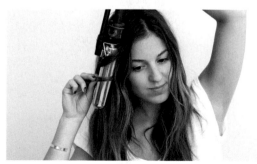

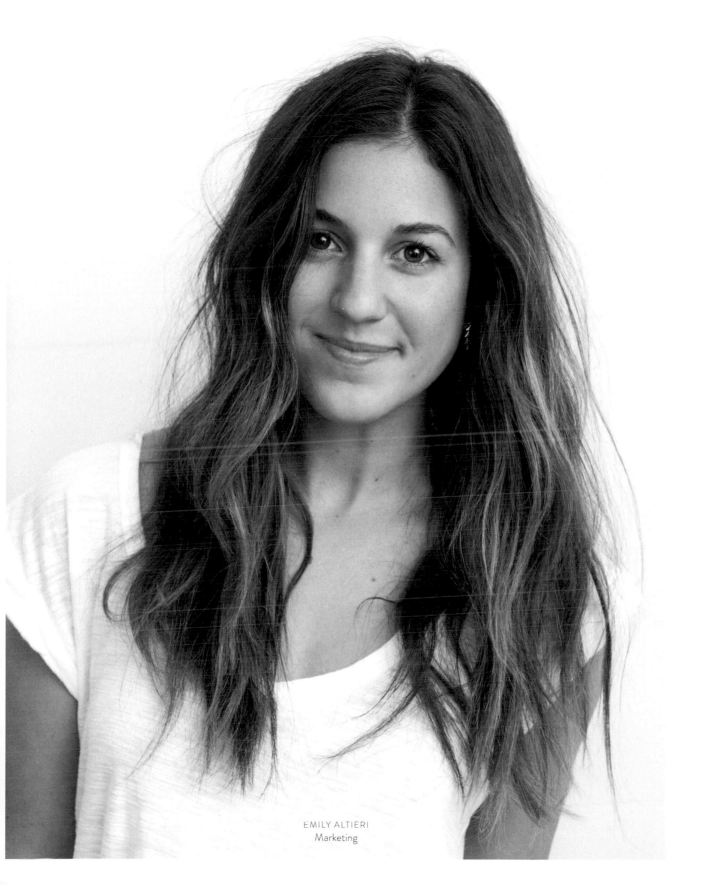

EMILY ALTIERI
Marketing

Style #7
THE PERFECT NATURAL CURL

No matter how curly your curl, the approach remains basically the same, says Abergel: "Moisture is the secret to a frizz-free curl." Start in the shower, with a sulfate-free shampoo, and an extra-moisturizing conditioner; deep conditioning treatments really help, too. "Comb your hair with a wide-tooth comb while you're still in the shower, while you still have conditioner in your hair," he says. "Treat it as gently as you can—any roughness or friction causes frizz."

1. Once out of shower, paper-towel-dry your hair, scrunching it from the ends up toward the roots. This will minimize frizz.

2. Apply leave-in conditioner or a light oil mixed with a very light gel or mousse.

3. Let your hair air-dry if you have time, or, if you need to get it dry quicker, diffuse on medium heat.

4. Define the curl with a curling iron. The size of the iron depends on the kind of curl you want, says Abergel: "If you want it tighter, use a smaller iron; if you want it looser, a bigger iron will soften your curl."

5. Mist on a bit of shine spray to finish the look. "And don't touch your hair!" adds Abergel. "Every time you touch it, you create frizz." At night, he advocates using a silk pillowcase: "Less friction, less frizz," he says.

How to Style Bangs of All Sorts

Start with a great cut so that you use as little product as possible, says Abergel: "People make the mistake of using too much product—you're trying to compensate for the wrong shape when that's happening. The secret for a universal shape for bangs is to cut straight across in the front, with a soft angle downward toward either side of your face—get the shape right, and you won't need to work so hard styling them."

1. To give just about any bangs a little life, Abergel likes to use a little volumizer at the roots. "Never use oils—they'll leave your bangs flat and lifeless," he says.

2. If you've got curly or wavy hair, use a medium-size round brush: Stretch the bangs around the brush, heat it up with a blow-dryer to get hair smooth, and remove it quickly before it cools down. "That way, the shape doesn't get too rounded but you've still got lift," he says.

3. Conversely, if you want more curve on the ends, let the brush cool down before you remove it.

4. The secret to keeping any bangs looking fresh and not oily is dry shampoo, Abergel says: "Use it whenever you need it—you can't do too much."

5. If your bangs are extra thick and you want separation, smooth in a little lightweight styling cream, just on the ends.

What to Do with Short Hair

Short hair is all about creating the right texture and movement, explains Abergel. You do this with a great cut, of course, but product also makes a serious difference. "I always have a big variety of products on hand for short hair, depending on the style I'm going for," he says. Here, what's in his bag—and what it does:

- **Pomade:** There are three types, each for different results. "Shiny is great if you're looking for a little bit more of that wet, slicked-back look," says Abergel. "Matte is fantastic if you like it textured and undone, or if you want to push your hair back into a pompadour. And cream pomades are great for creating separation on the ends, or for basic texture if your hair is on the finer side. Creams give separation without weighing hair down."

- **Dry shampoo:** Use this to prolong your style between washes, or to revive a style. "It works so well for short hair," says Abergel.

- **Texture spray:** No matter what sort of slept-in, next-day, I-just-wake-up-looking-like-this style you're going for, mist a little or a lot of this in, says Abergel. "It's great for any undone look."

- **Accessories:** Consider—and experiment with—barrettes, hairpins, and other hair accessories. "They're a great way to dress up short hair," says Abergel. "Twist little pieces, do small braids—use your imagination and have fun."

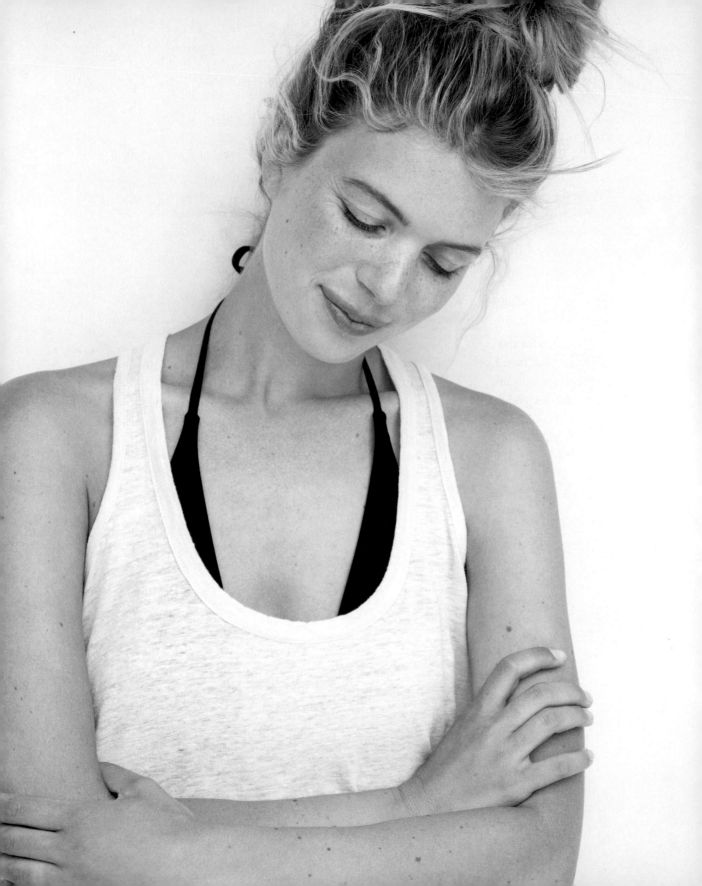

Last Gloss

Here's our two cents for staying beautiful: Be good to your body and your face: Eat clean, work out, go to bed, get sun, wear sunblock, don't smoke, seriously don't smoke, and do the extra stuff that's fun for you (yoga/mascara/meditation/face oil/sauna/foam roll/bath soak). Read labels. Or shop at places you trust that will read labels for you. Say no to toxins in the products that you put on your body and your children's bodies. Swapping out the conventional products in your medicine cabinet and makeup bag with clean beauty products feels—in two words—liberating and awesome. Share it with a friend.

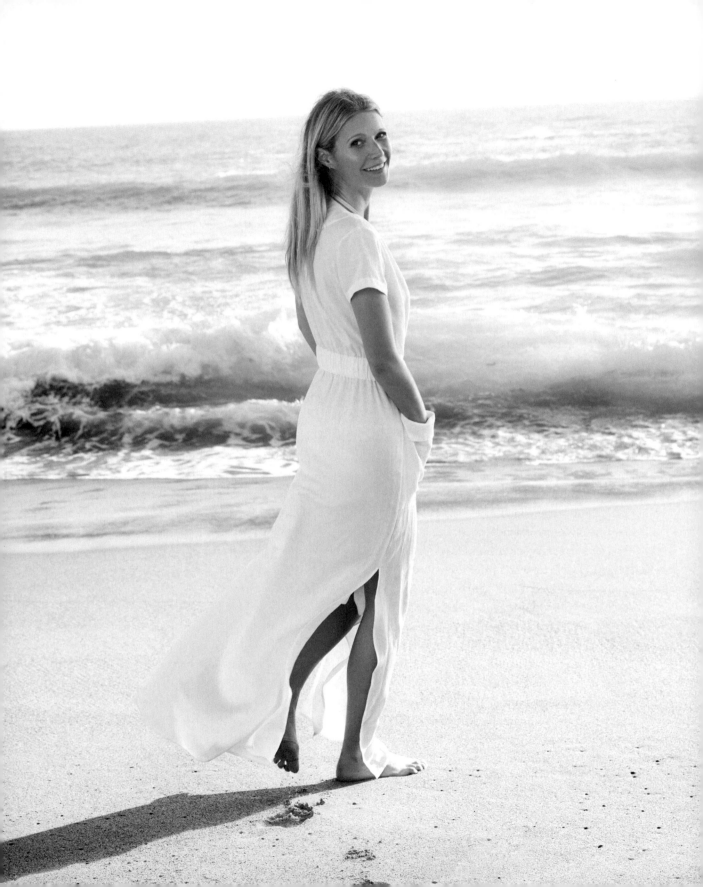

Acknowledgments

Thank you to all our experts—doctors, authors, researchers, gurus, and geniuses—who feature so prominently in this book, which exists in large part because of your wisdom and generosity: Adir Abergel, Dr. Alejandro Junger, Dr. Amy Wechsler, Christine Chin, Dr. Dendy Engelman, Eddie Stern, Dr. Frank Lipman, Karen Behnke, Dr. Karyn Grossman, Kate Lee, Dr. Laura Lefkowitz, Lauren Roxburgh, Dr. Pratima Raichur, Dr. Rafael Pelayo, Shira Lenchewski, Taryn Toomey, Tracy Anderson, and Vicky Vlachonis.

Thank you to everyone at Grand Central Life & Style and Hachette who made this a better book, and who helped it find its way to the shelf, especially: Brittany McInerney, Karen Murgolo, Morgan Hedden, Sarah Pelz, Erin Vandeveer, Siri Silleck, and Tom Whatley. Thank you to our copy editor, Deri Reed, and thanks to Shubhani Sarkar for the book's interior design.

For all the beautiful images, thank you to photographer extraordinaire Brigitte Sire. Special thanks also to Acacia, Anna Hampton, Ashlie Johnson, Barbara Schmidt, Barrie, Bethany Brill, Brentwood Farmers' Market, Caesarstone, Clare Vivier, Derek Williams, Elizabeth Saltzman, Faithfull the Brand, Frankies Bikinis, Georgie Eisdell, Ilan Dei Venice, Jeffrey Court, L'AGENCE, Natalie Shriver, Nathalie Perez, Nick Fouquet, rag & bone, Samantha Rockman, and Twig & Twine.

A big thanks to team GOOP, and particularly the *Goop Clean Beauty* crew: Kiki Koroshetz, Jean Godfrey-June, Jenny Westerhoff, Thea Baumann, Elise Loehnen, Gwyneth Paltrow, Blair Lawson, Ivy Benavente, and Julie Jen. And to the GOOP staff who modeled the hair and makeup looks in the final two chapters, thank you, too: Blair and Elise (again), Emily Altieri, Hannah Swank, Heaven Saunders, Jasmin Perez, and Sonya Falcone.

As always, thanks to our readers who made this book—and who make everything we do—possible.

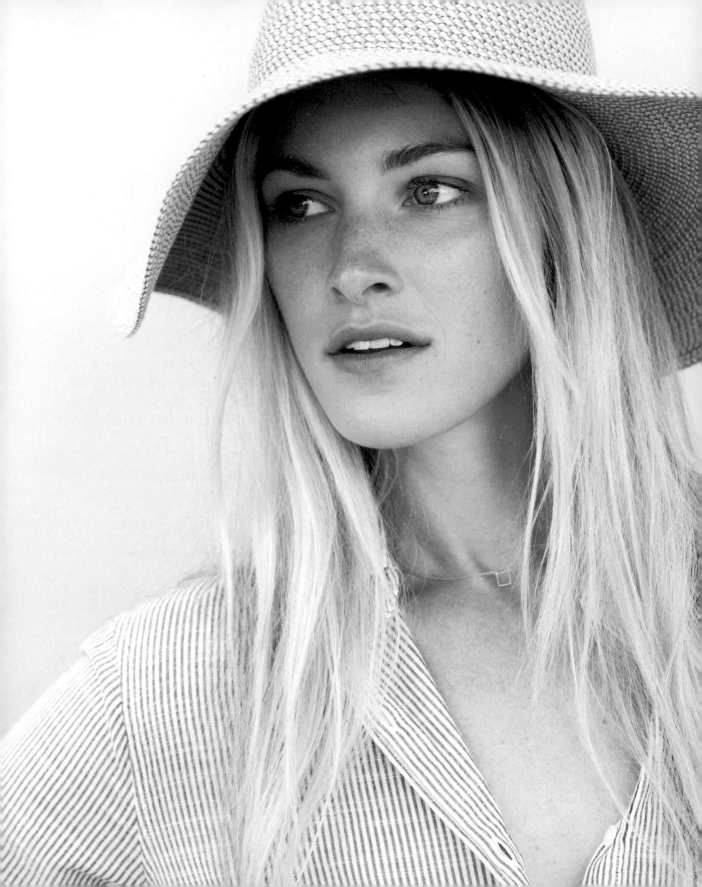

Index

NOTE: Italic page numbers
refer to illustrations.

A

Abergel, Adir, 243
acai
    Acai Bowl with Bee Pollen, *106*, 107
    antioxidants in, 91, 118
accessories, for short hair, 257
Accutane, 202, 209, 210, 213–14
acetone, 166
acne and breakout-prone skin
    aestheticians for, 210
    alternative therapies for, 214
    Ayurvedic doctors for, 209
    causes of, 201
    cleansing routine for, 201–2, 205
    dermatological procedures for,
        209–10, 211, 212
    elements of ideal routine for, 205–6
    foods for, 102, 205
    Karyn Grossman on, 211–14
    helpful ingredients, 202, 204
    and hormonal balance, 201, 210,
        213, 214–15
    Laura Lefkowitz on, 214–15
    light therapy for, 190, 209
    makeup products for, 216
    and oils, 202
    and pregnancy, 213–14
    retinoids for, 187
    supplements for, 94

acupuncture, 227
Aczone, 211
adrenal fatigue, 126–27, 137, 141
adrenal glands, 198
adrenaline, 73, 125
aestheticians, for acne and
        breakout-prone skin, 210
agave nectar, 100
AGEs (advanced glycation end
        products), 102
aging
    effect of exercising on, 68–69
    effect of meditation on, 128, 129
    effect of yoga on, 71–73
    and hormonal balance, 194–95, 197–99
    skin products for, 183–84, 186–93
AHAs (alpha hydroxy acids), 187, 211, 224
air-dry, for perfect natural curl, 256
alcohol dehydrogenase, 103, 104
alcohol use
    effect on hair, 104
    effect on intestinal wall, 59
    effect on skin, 104, 117
    and jet lag, 147
    sugar in alcohol, 103, 104, 141
allergies
    and eczema, 228
    food allergies, 5, 61
all-or-nothing thinking, 48
almond butter, Almond Butter and Sea
        Salt Cookies, 45

alpha lipoic acid, 94
American Academy of Dermatology, 191, 214
American Heart Association, 100
Ananda (Ayurvedic spa), India, 144
anchovies, Chicken Paillards with
        Radicchio and Anchovy
        Salad, 31–32
Anderson, Tracy, 67–69, 126
androgens, 215
antibiotic resistance, 62, 97
antibiotics
    for acne and breakout-prone skin,
        209, 210, 211, 212
    effect on intestinal flora, 62–63
    effect on intestinal wall, 59, 60
    for rosacea, 231
antihistamines, 148
anti-inflammatories
    and dermatological procedures, 192
    in skin products, 189
antioxidants, 91, 98, 102, 118, 188–89
appetite, 137
arctic cloudberries, 118
Aristotle, 71
aromatherapeutic scents, 142
arugula, Chicken Paillards with Fennel and
        Arugula Salad, *30*, 32–33
Asian Chopped Salad, 52–53, *53*
Asian Salmon and Avocado Salad, 108, *109*
at-home extractions, for acne, 206
autism, 96

autoimmune disorders, 59
autonomic nervous system, 130, 135
avobenzone, 123
avocados
    Asian Salmon and Avocado Salad,
        108, *109*
    benefits of, 91
    Citrus-Grilled Salmon and Avocado
        Salad, *109*, 110
    half an avocado as snack, 50
    Sweet Potato and Avocado Grain
        Bowls, 28, *29*
Ayurvedic doctors
    for acne and breakout-prone skin,
        209
    for eczema, 227–29
Azelex/Finacea, 211
azulene, 204

B

backcombing
    for sexy Bardot-inspired tumble,
        246
    for top knot, 252
bacon, 102–3
Bagna Cauda, 37
balms
    for dry and sensitive skin, 222
    for eczema, 227
    lip balm, 234, 236
bangs, 257
bath, as sleep ritual, 142
Baumann, Thea, 6
beach spray, for sexy Bardot-inspired
    tumble, 246
beachy wave, 254, *254*, *255*
beans, benefits of, 91
beauty
    concept of, ix
    detox life, 3–4, 63
    from inside out, ix–x, 1
    supplements for, 94
    See also clean beauty routine
bedding, as sleep ritual, 144
bedroom environment, 140
bee pollen, Acai Bowl with Bee Pollen,
    106, 107

Behnke, Karen, 162, 164–65, 166
Benavente, Ivy, 68
benzalkonium chloride, 161
benzoyl peroxide, 204, 211, 230
bergamot, 130
beverages, Iced Matcha Latte, 111, *111*
BHAs (beta hydroxy acids), 187,
    211, 224
bifidobacteria, 60
bioavailability, of nutrients, 95
biodegradable takeout containers, 51
bio-identical hormones, 195, 197
Blackburn, Elizabeth, 72
blow-dry hair
    for blowout with body, 243
    for high ponytail, 250
    for sexy Bardot-inspired tumble,
        246
blowout with body, 243–44, *244*, *245*
blueberries
    antioxidants in, 91
    Breakfast Porridge with Cinnamon
        and Blueberries, 10
blue light, and sleep, 140–41
blush
    for everyday no-makeup makeup,
        234
    for French-girl smokey eye, 240
body of bliss, in yoga, 71
bone structure, effect of exercising on, 69
Botox, 190–91
BPA (bisphenol A), 51, 59
braids, for beachy wave, 254
brain fog, 60, 133
brain health, and sleep, 72–73, 133, 134,
    135, 137, 138, 139
breakfasts
    Breakfast Porridge with Cinnamon
        and Blueberries, 10
    Canarino, *12*, 13
    Chocolate Milkshake Smoothie, 9
breath and breathing
    and essential oils, 130
    and meditation, 127–28
    and trigger points, 129
    and yoga, 71, 72, 73, 74
broths, Dashi, 15, *15*
brows, grooming, 234
butylated hydroxyanisole (BHA), 161
butyrate, 60

C

caffeine, 141, 148, 184
California Organic Products Act of 2003
    (COPA), 156
California State Cosmetics Program, 168
Campaign for Safe Cosmetics, 159, 168
Canarino, *12*, 13
cardio exercise, 67, 68
carrots, Ginger-Carrot Miso Dressing, 41
Cashew Crema, 24–25
cell phones, 140–41
cellulite, 78
Centers for Disease Control and
    Prevention, 62
chemical hair straightening treatments
    and perms, 162
chemicals
    effect on intestinal flora, 60
    in personal care products, 153–55
    as toxins to body, 3–4, 66
chia seeds, benefits of, 91
chicken
    Chicken Paillards with Fennel and
        Arugula Salad, *30*, 32–33
    Chicken Paillards with Radicchio
        and Anchovy Salad, 31–32
chickpeas, benefits of, 91
Chin, Christine, 230–31
chlorinated water, 60
chocolate, Chocolate Milkshake
    Smoothie, 9
Chopra, Deepak, 126
chronic diseases, leaky gut linked to, 61
cinnamon, Breakfast Porridge with
    Cinnamon and Blueberries, 10
circadian rhythm, 120, 139, 140, 146
Citrus-Grilled Salmon and Avocado Salad,
    109, 110
clay, 204
clean beauty routine
    and clean eating, 151, 259
    and personal care products, 153–62,
        164–68, 259
clean eating
    rules of, 5–6, 63
    See also foods
Clean Fifteen foods, 98, 99
Clean Fish Tacos, 24–25

clean living
    balance of, xi
    See also detox life
Clearlight Essential Nordic Spruce sauna, 67
coal tar, 161
coconut, Coconut Rice with Mango, *43*, 44
coconut nectar, 102
cod liver oil, 120
collagen, in skin products, 188
collagen peptides, 94
collagen production
    and copper pillowcases, 144
    and dry brushing, 85
    and exercise, 69
    and eye cream, 184
    and foam rolling, 78
    and peptides, 188
    promoting, 183
    and retinoids, 187, 188
    and smoking, 104
    and threading, 192
colloidal silver, 146
colonics, 85, 86–87
color, for French-girl smokey eye, 240
concealer
    for acne and breakout-prone skin, 216
    application of, 148
    for everyday no-makeup makeup, 234
conditioner, for super-straight blowout, 248
constipation, 60, 86
cookies, Almond Butter and Sea Salt
    Cookies, 45
Coola sunblock, 124
copper pillowcases, 144
cortisol
    and alcohol use, 104
    and caffeine, 141
    and exercise, 197
    and sleep, 73, 134, 137
    and stress, 127
cortisone
    for acne and breakout-prone skin, 210
    for hair loss, 179
Cosmetic Ingredient Review, 154
cravings
    for sugar, 102
    wait 15 minutes, 48
crazy colors, for hair color, 175
creams, as moisturizers, 222
Criss-Cross Back Bend, 79, *79*

cruciferous vegetables, benefits of, 91
crudités, gauging hunger with, 48
C-sections, 60
curling iron
    for beachy wave, 254
    for perfect natural curl, 256
    for sexy Bardot-inspired tumble, 246
    for top knot, 252

D

dairy foods, 60
dark, green vegetables, antioxidants in, 91
dark spots, laser treatments for, 193
Dashi
    recipe, 15, *15*
    Steamed Fish with Dashi and Soba
        Noodles, 34, *35*
Daylight Savings Time, 139
delivery food, order before leaving
    office, 50
dermatological procedures
    for acne and breakout-prone skin,
        209–10, 211, 212
    skin products, 190–93
desserts. *See* sweet treats
detergents, for dry and sensitive skin, 219
detoxification
    colonics for, 85, 86–87
    drinking water for, 66, 87
    dry brushing, 84–85
    effectiveness of, 65–66
    exercising for, 66–69, 87
    foam rolling for, 76, 78–83
    sweating for, 66, 87
    yoga for, 71–74
detox life
    beauty detox, 3–4, 63
    clean eating rules, 5–6, 63
    commitment to, 3
    GOOP Clean Beauty detox, 6
    gut system, 58–63
    recipes for, 7–47
Detox Truffles, 46, *47*
DHEA, 215
diabetes, 137
dinners. *See* lunches and dinners
1,4-dioxane contamination, 160, 161, 164

Dirty Dozen foods, 98–99
DNA, 72, 96
double process hair color, 174
dressings
    Ginger-Carrot Miso Dressing, 41
    Green Goddess Dressing, 20
driving, sun exposure from, 121
Drunk Elephant sunblock, 124
dry and sensitive skin
    cleansing, 220
    eczema, 94, 225, 227–29
    exfoliating, 224, 225
    food for, 219
    hydration routine for, 220, 222–25
    ingredients for soothing, 226
    layering, 223
    moisturizing, 220, 222
    Pratima Raichur on Ayurvedic
        healing for, 227–29
    rosacea, 94, 105, 202, 213, 229–31
    supplements for, 223
    treatment of, 219
    Amy Wechsler on, 224–25
dry brushing, 84–85
dry shampoo, for short hair, 257

E

earthing, 130
eating habits
    clean eating, 5–6, 63
    food hacks, 48, 50–51
    12-hour fasting window, 141
    See also foods; recipes
eczema, 94, 225, 227–29
Edison, Thomas, 140
EDTA, 160, 165
elimination diet, 61
emotional trauma, 75
endocrine disruptors, 154–55, 164, 165
endorphins, 66
Engelman, Dendy, 178–80
environmental impact
    and adrenal fatigue, 126–27
    on dry and sensitive skin, 225
    earthing, 130
    of essential oils, 130
    of meditation, 127–29

environmental impact (*continued*)
    minimizing free-radical damage, 117–18
    and stress, 125, 142
    sun exposure, 117, 118, 120–21, 123–24
    and vitamin D, 118, 120
Environmental Protection Agency
    (EPA), 167
Environmental Working Group
    on chemicals in umbilical cord
      blood, 153
    Clean Fifteen, 98, 99
    Dirty Dozen, 98–99
    perfumes analyzed by, 159–60
    on personal care products, 155,
      157, 164
    Skin Deep database, 158
    on sunscreen ingredients, 123–24
epigenetics, 72
Equanimity app, 126
essential oils, 130
estrogen, 138, 194, 197, 198, 215
ethanolamines, 160–61
ethoxylation, 160
everyday no-makeup makeup, 233–34,
    234, 235
exercise
    for adrenal fatigue, 127
    for aging, 68–69
    Tracy Anderson on, 67–69
    for dry and sensitive skin, 219
    effect on skin, 69, 197
    endorphins released by, 66
    frequency of, 67
    in heat, 68
    and hormonal balance, 197, 199
    for jet lag, 147
    rebounding, 68
    and sleep, 138
exfoliating agents, 184, 189–90, 205–6,
    224, 225
extractions
    for acne and breakout-prone skin,
      210, 212
    at-home extractions, 206
extrinsic aging, 194
eye care, and sleep, 148
eye creams, 184
eye liner
    for French-girl smokey eye, 240
    for Sophia Loren cat-eye, 236

F

facials, 210, 231
Falcone, Sonya, *240, 241*
farmers' markets, 98
fascia, 76, 78
fat
    and bioavailability of nutrients, 95
    for getting over sugar addiction, 102
    lipophilic toxins, 66
    omega-3 fatty acid, 91
    and sleep, 134
fat deposition, 198
Federal Fair Packaging and Labeling
    Act, 159
Fed Up (documentary), 100
fennel
    Chicken Paillards with Fennel and
      Arugula Salad, *30, 32–33*
    Roasted Fennel, 40
fermented foods, 60, 87
fiber consumption, 87
fight-or-flight reaction, 126, 127, 135
fillers
    dermatological skin care, 188, 191
    in moisturizers, 220
finish drying with round brush, for blowout
    with body, 244
fish
    Clean Fish Tacos, 24–25
    Steamed Fish with Dashi and Soba
      Noodles, 34, *35*
fish oil supplements, 94
flatiron, for high ponytail, 250
flatironing, for super-straight
    blowout, 248
foam rolling
    Criss-Cross Back Bend, 79, *79*
    Inverted Figure Four, 80, *80*
    Rolling Lunge, 81, *81*
    Rolling Swan Dive, 83, *83*
    Lauren Roxburgh on, 76, 78
    Lauren Roxburgh's sequence, 78–83
    Text-Neck Massage, 82, *82*
Food, Drug, and Cosmetic Act (1938),
    154
food allergies, 5, 61
Food and Drug Administration (FDA),
    154, 156, 162, 195, 197, 215

food-grade ingredients, 158, 162
food preservatives, 60, 96
foods
    for acne and breakout-prone skin,
      102, 205
    beauty-sapping foods, 100, 102–3
    bioavailability of nutrients, 95
    clean eating rules, 5–6, 63
    for dry and sensitive skin, 219
    for eczema, 227, 228
    food hacks, 48, 50–51
    for healthier hair, 180, 197
    for hormonal balance, 197, 198, 199
    organic foods, 96–99
    processed foods, 96, 100, 102,
      155, 228
    and sleep, 138
    superfoods, 89, 90–92, 107–14
    travel food, 51, 52–56, 145
    trigger foods, 60, 61
food sensitivities, 5, 61
foot massage, as sleep ritual, 142
formaldehyde, 157, 162, 166, 177
formaldehyde releasers, 158–59
foundation, for everyday no-makeup
    makeup, 234
fragrance, in personal care products,
    159–60, 165
free radicals
    and antioxidants, 91, 188–89
    and foam rolling, 78
    minimizing damage from, 117–18
free thyroxin (FT4), 137
French-girl smoky eye, 240, *240, 241*
frizz, hair products for, 177
fruit enzymes, 187, 224

G

ghrelin, 137–38
ginger
    Ginger-Carrot Miso Dressing, 41
    Turmeric and Ginger Tonic, 114
gloss, in hair color, 175
gluten
    in beer, 103
    effect on intestinal wall, 59, 60
glycation, 100, 102, 183

glymphatic system, of brain, 73, 134

glyphosate, 96, 98

GMOs (genetically modified organisms), 96, 97, 228

Godfrey-June, Jean, 68

Good Hair (documentary), 177

GOOP Clean Beauty Shop, xi, 124, 142, 146, 157, 167

Grain Bowls, Two Ways, 26–28, *26, 29*

Green Goddess Dressing, 20

Green Grain Bowls, 27, *29*

green tea, antioxidants in, 91, 118, 189

greenwashing, 156, 168

Grilled Salmon and Avocado Salad, Two Ways, 108, *109,* 110

grocery store, salad bars at, 51

Grossman, Karyn, 211–14

grounding, 130

gut-associated lymphatic tissue (GALT), 58, 59, 61

gut system
    parts of, 58–59, 61
    promoting health of, 60–63
    and skin, 61–62, 94

H

hacks, food hacks, 48, 50–51

hair
    effect of adrenal fatigue on, 126
    effect of exercise on, 197
    effect of smoking on, 104–5
    foods for healthier hair, 180, 197
    Laura Lefkowitz on, 104–5
    supplements for, 94, 179, 180

hair color
    and breakage, 178
    color options, 174–75
    fading/brassiness/greenish tinge, 175
    hair dyes, 162

hair loss, Dendy Engelman on, 178–80

hair products
    for breakage, 178
    for frizz, 177
    ingredients in, 161–62
    product buildup, 177
    relaxers, straightening treatments, and perms, 177

styling products, 171–72
    for thinning hair, 177–78

hairspray, for top knot, 252

hairstyle tips
    for bangs, 257
    for beachy wave, 254, *254, 255*
    for blowout with body, 243–44, *244, 245*
    for high ponytail, 250, *250, 251*
    for perfect natural curl, 256
    for sexy Bardot-inspired tumble, 246, *246, 247*
    for short hair, 257
    for super-straight blowout, 248, *248, 249*
    for top knot, 252, *252, 253*

Hand Rolls, *18, 19*

hats, for sun exposure, 120, 121

Headspace app, 126

heat, for exercise, 68

heat-protecting product, for super-straight blowout, 248

heat styling, and hair breakage, 178

heat treatments, dermatological procedures, 192–93, 212

heavy metals, detoxification of, 66

herbicides, 96–97

highlighter
    for everyday no-makeup makeup, 233
    for red lip, 238

highlights, in hair color, 174–75

high ponytail, 250

Hirshberg, Gary, on herbicides, 96–97

homeopathy, 227

hormonal balance
    and acne and breakout-prone skin, 201, 210, 213, 214–15
    foods supporting, 197, 198, 199
    and personal care products, 154–55
    and skin care, 194–95, 197–99
    and sleep, 133, 134, 135, 137–38, 140, 146, 199

hormonal responses, and gut system, 59

hormone replacement therapy, 194–95

human growth hormone (HGH), and sleep, 134, 137, 139

hummus, Spinach and Lemon Hummus, *112,* 113

hunger
    gauging hunger with crudités, 48
    planning for snacks and easy dinners, 50, 51

hydration
    for detox organs, 66, 87, 104
    for dry and sensitive skin, 220, 222–25
    and jet lag, 145, 147
    for sugar cravings, 102

hydroquinone, 161

hypothalamic-pituitary axis, 135, 137–38

hypothyroidism, 137

I

Iced Matcha Latte, 111, *111*

immune system
    effect of adrenal fatigue on, 126
    effect of exercise on, 69
    effect of saunas on, 66
    effect of sleep on, 133, 134
    effect of smoking on, 105
    effect of sugar on, 100
    in gut system, 58, 61
    and jet lag, 145

immunoglobulins, 61

infections
    and antibiotic resistance, 62
    effect on intestinal wall, 59

inflammation
    and acne and breakout-prone skin, 201, 209, 213
    and dry and sensitive skin, 219
    and eczema, 228
    foam rolling for, 78
    foods causing, 5
    in gut system, 58, 59, 61
    and sleep, 133
    and visible aging, 183, 189

insecticide/Bt toxin, 96

insulin resistance, 137, 138, 198–99

insulin response, 134

intenSati, 68

International Agency for Research on Cancer (IARC), 102–3

International Fragrance Association, 159

intestinal flora
  avoiding threats to, 60
  compromising of, 59, 61, 62
  effect of antibiotics on, 62–63
  effect of colonics on, 86–87
  in gut system, 58
  probiotics for restoring, 63,
    86, 94
intestinal wall
  exposure to toxins, 59
  function of, 58–59, 61
  leaky gut, 59–60, 61
intrinsic aging, 194
Inverted Figure Four, 80, *80*
iPledge, 214
Italian Chopped Salad, *54*, 55
ivermectin, 211

J

jet lag
  Rafael Pelayo on crossing time
    zones, 146–48
  and sleep, 139, 145–48
Jivamukti yoga, 68
Juice Beauty skincare line, 156, 162,
  164–66, 186, 207
Junger, Alejandro
  on adrenal system, 126–27
  on colonics, 85, 86–87
  on gut health, 58, 59, 60–63
  on infrared saunas, 66
  on intestinal flora, 62–63
  meditation app of, 126
  12-hour fasting window, 141
  21-Day Clean Program, 5
Just Label It, 96

K

kale, Sautéed Cavolo Nero, 38
kidneys, capacity to detox, 3, 66, 104
Kimchi Turkey Burgers, 22
Kingsley, Philip, 177
kitchens, healthy food at eye
    level, 51
kohlrabi, Kohlrabi Slaw, 42

L

labels
  ingredients for dry and sensitive
    skin, 226
  of personal care products,
    156–58, 259
lactobacillus, 60
laser treatments
  dermatological procedures,
    192–93, 212
  for rosacea, 230, 231
lashes, curling, 234
lavendar oil, 204
Lawson, Blair, *234*, *235*
leaky gut, 59–60, 61, 133
leave-in conditioner, for perfect natural
    curl, 256
Lee, Kate, 233
Lefkowitz, Laura
  on acne and breakout-prone skin,
    214–15
  on skin and hair health, 104–5,
    194–95, 197–99
  on sleep, 135, 137–38
lemons
  benefits of, 92
  Canarino, *12*, 13
  Spinach and Lemon Hummus, *112*,
    113
Lenchewski, Shira, 48, 50–51
leptin, 137–38
L-glutamine, 60, 102
light exposure, skin products for, 190
light therapy, for acne and breakout-prone
    skin, 190, 209
lip balm
  for everyday no-makeup makeup,
    234
  for Sophia Loren cat-eye, 236
lip liner, for red lip, 238
Lipman, Frank
  on alcohol use, 103
  on sleep, 133, 134, 140
  on stress, 125
  on sugar habit, 100, 102
  on sun exposure, 120–21
  on supplements, 93–94
  on vitamin D, 118, 120

lipophilic toxins, 66, 160
lipstick, for red lip, 238
Little, Amanda, 97
Little Gem Salad with Vegan Green
    Goddess Dressing, 20
liver, capacity to detox, 3, 66, 73, 104
Loaded Miso Soup, 16, *17*
Loehnen, Elise, 126, *238*, *239*
lotions, as skin moisturerizers, 222
Lourie, Bruce, 65–66
low-level light treatment (LLLT), for hair
    loss, 179
lunches and dinners
  Asian Salmon and Avocado Salad,
    108, *109*
  Chicken Paillards with Fennel and
    Arugula Salad, 30, 32–33
  Chicken Paillards with Radicchio
    and Anchovy Salad, 31–32
  Citrus-Grilled Salmon and Avocado
    Salad, *109*, 110
  Clean Fish Tacos, 24–25
  Dashi, 15, *15*
  Grain Bowls, Two Ways, 26–28,
    26, *29*
  Green Grain Bowls, 27, *29*
  Hand Rolls, *18*, 19
  Kimchi Turkey Burgers, 22
  Little Gem Salad with Vegan Green
    Goddess Dressing, 20
  Loaded Miso Soup, 16, *17*
  Root Vegetable Soup, 23
  Steamed Fish with Dashi and Soba
    Noodles, 34, 35
  Sweet Potato and Avocado Grain
    Bowls, 28, *29*
lycopene, 95
lymphatic system
  dry brushing for, 84–85
  foam rolling for, 76, 78
  function of, 66–67, 68
  rebounding for, 68

M

McGonigal, Kelly, 125
magnesium, 100, 146
Maintenance of Wakefulness Test, 139

makeup products
>for acne and breakout-prone skin, 216
>blush, 234, 240
>chemicals in, 153–55
>concealer, 148, 216, 234
>eye liner, 236, 240
>foundation, 234
>highlighter, 233, 238
>lip balm, 234, 236
>lip liner, 238
>mascara, 234, 236
>organic ingredients in, 98
>powder, 234
>primer, 233, 234
>shadow, 240
makeup tips
>for everyday no-makeup makeup, 233–34, 234, 235
>for French-girl smoky eye, 240, 240, 241
>for red lip, 238, 238, 239
>for Sophia Loren cat-eye, 236, 236, 237
mango, Coconut Rice with Mango, 43, 44
mani-pedis, 166
maple syrup, 102
mascara
>for everyday no-makeup makeup, 234
>for Sophia Loren cat-eye, 236
masks, 206
Mason, Sherri, 164
matcha, Iced Matcha Latte, 111, 111
Mean Sleep Latency Test, 139
meditation
>for adrenal fatigue, 127
>apps for, 126
>environmental impact of, 127–29
>practice of, 71, 72, 74, 126
Mediterranean Chopped Salad, 56
melatonin, 141, 145, 146
memory, and sleep, 134
menopause, 138, 178, 179, 194, 198–99
menstruation, 215
mental health, effect of exercise on, 69
mercury, 59
metabolism, and sleep, 133, 134, 137, 138
methylisothiazolinone, 161
Metrogel, 229, 231
microbeads, 164, 187

microbiome, 86, 94, 134
>See also intestinal flora
microdermabrasion, 210, 230, 231
mindfulness practices, 72
mineral sunscreens, 123, 124
minoxidil, 178–79
miso
>Ginger-Carrot Miso Dressing, 41
>Loaded Miso Soup, 16, 17
moisturizers and creams, 184, 186, 220, 222
Moreno, Patricia, 68
muscle repair, and sleep, 134
myofascial release, 76

N

nail polish removers, 166
nails, supplements for, 94
nail salons, 166
nanoparticles, 124
napping, 140, 147
Naturopathica Alchemy oil concoctions, 166
Naturopathica sunblock, 124
nervous system, of gut system, 58, 59–60, 61
neuroplasticity, 72, 74
neurotransmitter production, 60
nightshades, 60
non-REM sleep, 139
NuGene Anti-Hair Loss Serum, 179

O

oil control, makeup products for, 216
oils
>and acne and breakout-prone skin, 202
>as skin moisturizers, 186, 222
olive oil, omega-3s in, 91
omega-3 fatty acids, 91, 94
oral contraceptives, for acne and breakout-prone skin, 214–15
organic foods, 96–99
organs, capacity to detox, 3–4, 66
oxybenzone, 123

P

pain, 127, 128, 129
palm nectar, 102
Paltrow, Gwyneth, viii, ix–xi
paper-towel-dry hair, for perfect natural curl, 256
parabens, 157, 158, 164
parasites, 60
parasympathetic nervous system, 125, 130, 134, 135
peels
>and aestheticians, 210
>skin products for, 189–90, 214
PEG, 160, 165
Pelayo, Rafael
>on crossing time zones, 146–48
>on sleep, 138–40
peptides, in skin products, 188
perimenopause, 138, 177, 199
perioral dermatitis, 213
peristalsis, 59, 60
permanent hair color, 174
perms, for hair care, 162, 177
personal care industry, standards of, xi, 153–55, 156, 168
personal care products
>Karen Behnke on, 162, 164–65, 166
>ingredients to avoid, 158–61
>labels of, 156–58
>petroleum in, 164–65, 227
>silicones in, 164, 172, 220
>toxins in, 153–55, 165
>See also hair products; skin products
Pestano, Paul, 167
pesticides, 59, 96–97
petroleum, in personal care products, 164–65, 227
phenoxyethanol, 157
phthalates, 159, 165, 166
physical body, in yoga, 71
phytonutrients, 97, 98
pillowcases, 142, 144
plastic containers, 50
plasticizers, 164
plated food, 48
platelet-rich plasma treatments, for hair loss, 180

polycystic ovarian syndrome (PCOS), 213, 215
pomade
 for high ponytail, 250
 for short hair, 257
 for super-straight blowout, 248
pomegranate seeds, antioxidants in, 91
porridge, Breakfast Porridge with Cinnamon and Blueberries, 10
powder, for everyday no-makeup makeup, 234
pre-dry hair
 for blowout with body, 243
 for super-straight blowout, 248
pregnancy, and acne and breakout-prone skin, 213–14
preservatives
 and eczema, 228
 food preservatives, 69, 96
 in personal care products, 157, 158, 162, 164
 in processed foods, 96, 100, 102, 155
primer, for everyday no-makeup makeup, 233, 234
probiotics
 multi-strain probiotics, 60
 restoring intestinal flora with, 63, 86, 94
 in skin products, 189
processed foods, 96, 100, 102, 155, 228
progesterone, 194, 197, 215
propylene glycol, 220
prostaglandins, 215
psychic sleep (yoga nidra), 144

Q

Q-tips, for Sophia Loren cat-eye, 236

R

radicchio, Chicken Paillards with Radicchio and Anchovy Salad, 31–32
radiofrequency treatments, dermatological procedures, 192–93

raw honey, 102
rebounding on mini trampoline, 68
recipes
 for detox life, 7–47
 for superfoods, 107–14
 for travel salads, 52–56
red lip, 238, *238, 239*
redness, resurfacing lasers for, 193
relaxers, for hair care, 177
REM sleep, 139, 141
restaurants, checking menu online, 48
resurfacing laser treatments, 192
resveratrol, 103, 189
retinoic acid, 209–10
retinoids, 184, 187, 189, 209, 211
retinols, 187, 189, 202, 230
retinyl palmitate, 123–24
rice, Coconut Rice with Mango, *43*, 44
Roasted Fennel, 40
Roasted Sweet Potatoes, 39
Rock, Chris, 177
Rolling Lunge, 81, *81*
Rolling Swan Dive, 83, *83*
roots, hair color for, 175
Root Vegetable Soup, 23
rosacea, 94, 105, 202, 213, 229–31
rose essential oil, 130
rose hips, 118
Roundup (glyphosate), 96, 98
Roxburgh, Lauren
 on foam rolling, 76, 78
 foam rolling sequence, 78–83

S

Safe Cosmetics Act, 168
sagging skin, radiofrequency treatments for, 193
salads
 Asian Chopped Salad, 52–53, *53*
 Asian Salmon and Avocado Salad, 108, *109*
 Chicken Paillards with Fennel and Arugula Salad, *30*, 32–33
 Chicken Paillards with Radicchio and Anchovy Salad, 31–32
 Citrus-Grilled Salmon and Avocado Salad, *109*, 110

 Italian Chopped Salad, *54*, 55
 Kohlrabi Slaw, 42
 Little Gem Salad with Vegan Green Goddess Dressing, 20
 Mediterranean Chopped Salad, 56
 travel salads, 52–56, 145
salicylic acid, 202, 225
salmon
 Asian Salmon and Avocado Salad, 108, *109*
 Citrus-Grilled Salmon and Avocado Salad, *109*, 110
 omega-3s in, 91
 vitamin D in, 120
sardines, 120
saunas, infrared saunas, 66, 67
Saunders, Heaven, *236, 237*
Sautéed Cavolo Nero, 38
scrunching, for beachy wave, 254
sea-salt spray, for beachy wave, 254
SELF (social interactions, exercise, light, food), 147
semi-permanent hair color, 174
Seneff, Stephanie, 96
serums
 for blowout with body, 244
 for high ponytail, 250
 as skin moisturizers, 186, 220, 222
 for super-straight blowout, 248
sexy Bardot-inspired tumble, 246, *246, 247*
shadow, for French-girl smokey eye, 240
shine spray, for perfect natural curl, 256
showers, water filters for, 167
side dishes. *See* snacks and side dishes
silicones, in personal care products, 164, 172, 220
Simply Being app, 126
skin
 dry brushing for, 84–85
 effect of adrenal fatigue on, 126
 effect of exercise on, 69, 197
 effect of smoking on, 104–5, 117, 118, 183
 effect of sugar on, 100, 102, 103, 104, 117
 elasticity of, 69, 102, 104, 144, 183
 environmental impact on, 117, 118, 120–21, 123–24, 225
 foam rolling for, 78

gut health reflected in, 61–62, 94
Laura Lefkowitz on, 104–5, 194–95, 197–99
minimizing free-radical damage, 117–18
personal care products absorbed by, 153
sun exposure on, 117, 118, 120–21, 123–24
supplements for, 94
See also acne and breakout-prone skin; dry and sensitive skin

skin cancer, 123–24

skin products
for aging, 183–84, 186–93
AHAs, BHAs, and fruit enzymes, 187
anti-inflammatories, 189
antioxidants, 188–89
cleansers, 186
collagen, 188
dermatological procedures, 190–93
light exposure, 190
moisturizers and creams, 184, 186
organic ingredients in, 98
peels, 189–90, 214
peptides, 188
retinoids, 184, 187
toners/waters, 186

sleep
and adrenal fatigue, 126, 127
and brain health, 72–73, 133, 134, 135, 137, 138, 139
effect of alcohol on, 104, 141
eye care, 148
and hormonal balance, 133, 134, 135, 137–38, 140, 146, 199
and jet lag, 139, 145–48
Laura Lefkowitz on, 135, 137–38
Frank Lipman on, 133, 134, 140
and napping, 140, 147
quality of, 138–40
restorative nature of, 126, 133–34
rituals for, 142, 144
sleep-enhancing tips, 140–41
stages of, 139
and sun exposure, 120

sleep debt, 139
sleeping pills/aids, 141, 148
SLES (sodium laureth sulfate), 160, 161

SLS (sodium lauryl sulfate), 161
Smith, Rick, 65–66
smoking
effect on hair, 104–5
effect on skin, 104–5, 117, 118, 183
smoothies, Chocolate Milkshake Smoothie, 9
snacks and side dishes
Acai Bowl with Bee Pollen, 106, 107
Bagna Cauda, 37
Kohlrabi Slaw, 42
Roasted Fennel, 40
Roasted Sweet Potatoes, 39
Sautéed Cavolo Nero, 38
Spinach and Lemon Hummus, 112, 113
soba noodles, Steamed Fish with Dashi and Soba Noodles, 34, 35
sodium benzoate, 157
Sophia Loren cat-eye, 236, 236, 237
soups
Loaded Miso Soup, 16, 17
Root Vegetable Soup, 23
SPF, in sunscreens, 123
spinach
benefits of, 92
Spinach and Lemon Hummus, 112, 113
spironolactone, 214–15
spot treatments, for acne, 206
spray sunscreen and sunblock, 124
stainless steel containers, 51
stem cells, for hair loss, 179
Stern, Eddie, on yoga, 71–74
steroidal creams, for eczema, 227, 228
stevia, 102
straightening treatments, for hair care, 162, 177
stress
and adrenal fatigue, 126
baseline response to, 72
breathing practices for, 71, 73
and dry and sensitive skin, 225
and earthing, 130
and eczema, 227, 228
effect on intestinal wall, 59
foam rolling for, 78
impact of, 125, 142
meditation for, 127–29
subtle body, in yoga, 71

sugar
in alcohol, 103, 104, 141
effect on intestinal wall, 59
effect on skin, 100, 102, 103, 104, 117
Frank Lipman on, 100, 102
nixing foods with added sugar, 50, 100, 102, 141
sulfur-based medication, 212
sunblock
for acne and breakout-prone skin, 206, 209
for anti-aging, 183
for dry and sensitive skin, 223
for minimizing free-radical damage, 118, 189
for sun exposure, 118, 120, 121, 123–24
sunscreen compared to, 123–24
sun exposure
environmental impact on skin, 117, 118, 120–21, 123–24
Frank Lipman on, 120–21
sunscreen ingredients, 123–24, 161
for vitamin D synthesis, 118, 120
wearing sunblock, 118, 120, 121, 123–24
SunFriend device, 120
sunscreen ingredients, 123–24, 161, 223
superfoods
antioxidants in, 91
definition of, 89, 90
examples of, 91–92
omega 3s in, 91
recipes for, 107–14
super-straight blowout, 248, 248, 249
supplements
for acne and breakout-prone skin, 94
beauty-specific supplements, 94
for dry and sensitive skin, 223
for hair, 94, 179, 180
Frank Lipman on, 93–94
vitamin and mineral supplements, 93
suprachiasmatic nucleus (SCN), 146
sweating
for detoxification, 66, 87
exercising in heat, 68
sweet potatoes
Roasted Sweet Potatoes, 39
Sweet Potato and Avocado Grain Bowls, 28, 29

sweet treats
Almond Butter and Sea Salt
Cookies, 45
Coconut Rice with Mango, *43*, 44
Detox Truffles, *46*, 47
sympathetic nervous system, 125, 135

T

tea tree oil, 202
teeth and gum care, 183
telomeres, 72
tequila, 103
testosterone, 194, 215
Text-Neck Massage, 82, *82*
texture spray
for short hair, 257
for top knot, 252
Thacker, Kirit, 144
thickening spray, for blowout with body,
243
thimerosal, 161
thinning hair
Dendy Engelman on hair loss, 178–80
products for, 177–78
threading, dermatological procedures
for, 192
thyroid gland, 137, 198
titanium dioxide, 123, 124
toluene, 161, 165, 166
toners/waters, 186, 206, 230, 231
tonics, Turmeric and Ginger Tonic, 114
Toomey, Taryn, The Class, 68, 75
top knot, 252, *252*, *253*
towel-dry hair, for beachy wave, 254
toxic triggers, 60, 61
toxins
alcohol as toxin, 104
avoidance of, 65
in cigarette smoke, 104
effect on intestinal wall, 59
exposure to chemicals, 3–4
in nail salons, 166

in personal care products, 153–55,
165
in processed foods, 96
and saunas, 66
See also detoxification; detox life
Tracy Anderson Method, 68
travel
flight bag, 121, 145–46
and jet lag, 139, 145–48
travel food
plastic containers, 51
salads, 52–56, 145
triclocarban, 161
triclosan, 161
trigger foods, 60, 61
trigger points, for pain relief, 129
truffles, Detox Truffles, *46*, 47
turkey, Kimchi Turkey Burgers, 22
turmeric
benefits of, 92, 94
Turmeric and Ginger Tonic, 114
21-Day Clean Program, 5

U

umbilical cords, toxic chemicals in, 4
urinary tract infections, 62
USDA-certified organic products, 156

V

vaginal mucosa, 194
vegetables
cruciferous vegetables, 91
dark, green vegetables, 91
raw vs. cooked debate, 95
Root Vegetable Soup, 23
vinyasa, 73
vitamin A, 93, 118, 187, 189
vitamin C, 118, 145, 186, 188–89, 204
vitamin D, 93, 118–21, 189
vitamin E, 118, 189

Vlachonis, Vicky
on dry brushing, 84–85
on meditation, 127–29
vodka, 103
volumizer
for beachy wave, 254
for top knot, 252

W

waiting 15 minutes, for cravings, 48
walnuts, omega-3s in, 91
water filtration, 167
Wechsler, Amy, 224–25
Weck jars, 51
weight gain, and sleep, 134
wellness and detox retreats, 144
Wendling, William, 167
Wi-Fi free zone, 141
Winfrey, Oprah, 126
World Health Organization (WHO), 62,
96, 102–3
wrinkles, resurfacing lasers for, 192

Y

yeast fungus, 60
ylang ylang, 130
yoga
benefits of, 71, 74
for detoxification, 71–74
effect on aging, 71–73
Jivamukti yoga, 68
restorative yoga, 127
yoga nidra (psychic sleep), 144

Z

zinc oxide, 123, 124
zonulin, 60

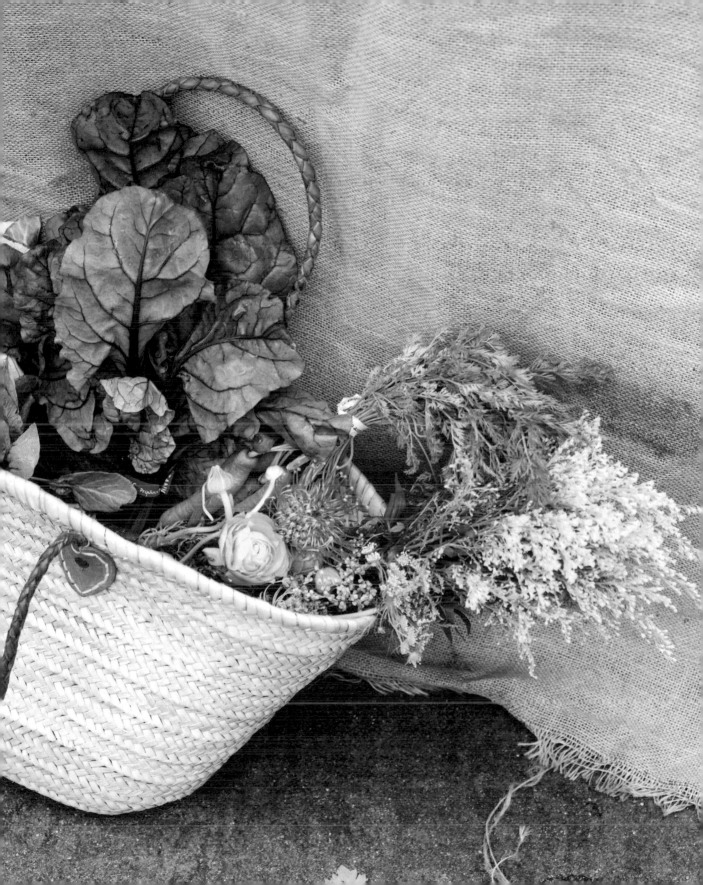

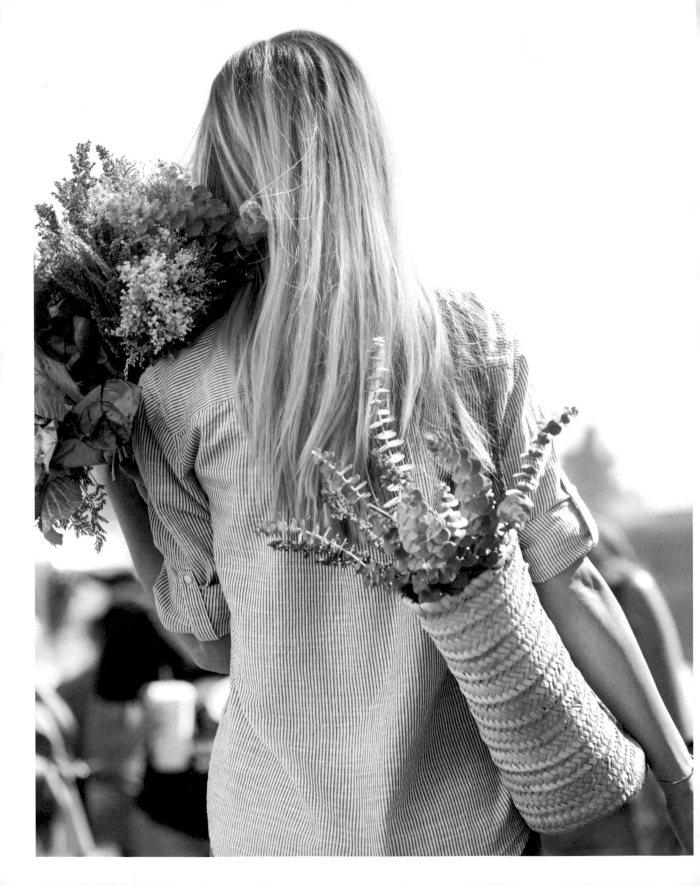